THE SOCIOLOGY
OF HEALTH CARE

THE SOCIOLOGY OF HEALTH CARE

Social, Economic, and Political Perspectives

Darryl D. Enos

Southern Illinois University

Paul Sultan

Southern Illinois University

Praeger Publishers
New York

362.1
E 59s

COPYRIGHT ACKNOWLEDGMENTS

From "The Struggle to Stay Healthy." Reprinted by permission from *Time*, The Weekly Newsmagazine. Copyright Time Inc., 1976.

From Margaret Clark, *Health in the Mexican-American Culture: A Community Study*. Copyright © 1959, 1970, by The Regents of the University of California; reprinted by permission of the University of California Press.

From Boyce Rensberger, "The Problem of the Incompetent Physician," © 1976 by The New York Times Company. Reprinted by permission.

Published in the United States of America in 1977
by Praeger Publishers
200 Park Avenue, New York, N.Y. 10017

© 1977 by Praeger Publishers,
A Division of Holt, Rinehart and Winston

Library of Congress Cataloging in Publication Data

Enos, Darryl D
  The sociology of health care.

  Bibliography.
  Includes index.
    1. Medical care—United States. 2. Social
medicine—United States. 3. Medical economics—
United States. I. Sultan, Paul, joint author.
II. Title.
RA395.A3E56   362.1'0973   76-17250
ISBN 0-275-56970-5

Printed in the United States of America

789   074   98765432

Acknowledgments

This book is an effort to integrate the perspectives of various disciplines on the important matter of health care. With the proliferation of information and activities in the health field, we witness the growth of specialization. Our effort has centered on the search for common themes, common interests, and issues that appear to transcend the superspecialized efforts so much in evidence today. Of necessity, we have been much dependent on the published views of leading scholars in the field. We have drawn shamelessly from the technical journals those views that appear to give a broad perspective to the behavior of this critical medical market. Our indebtedness to these authors and to the journals publishing their viewpoints will be evident to even the casual reader.

Preliminary drafts of much of the text material were circulated to our graduate seminars, attended largely by administrators in the health-care field, as well as by nurses and an occasional physician. We are much indebted to their spirited criticisms and constructive commentaries, particularly whenever the focus of text material seemed to do more to strengthen unwarranted popular prejudices than to represent a balanced portrait of reality. The angry chorus criticizing the malfunctioning of the medical market cannot obscure the reality that this sector is served by many remarkable individuals who know what they are doing and are proud of their service.

The text material also reflects, of course, discussion and debate with colleagues. Professors who have shared their views with us include Boulton Miller, Don Fogarty, Art Prell, and Ray LaGarce.

Development of the material required considerable library search of materials outside the health-administration field, and we are particularly indebted to the support of the staff of the Lovejoy Library of Southern Illinois University, Edwardsville. Staff members joined with us in the search for materials and always provided additional materials. They shared our enthusiasm and pleasure in uncovering materials to illuminate selected themes, and improvised arrangements for their review. We are particularly indebted to Bob Fortado of the documents section, Don Thompson of the Social Science section, and Joan Hewitt, head of the circulation department.

Two graduate assistants, Jacqueline Busby and Gerald Nicholson, labored

v

tirelessly in bibliographic search, article reviews, and the compilation of materials. Pam Horwitz also assisted us in these tasks. Jacqueline typed most of the manuscript through its several stages, and was assisted by Patti Agnuson and Vada Dillon.

Although our aim is to provide an integrated view of the health-care field, we realize that our prejudices have influenced the selection of themes for discussion. Our hope, of course, is that students, in reading this text, will share some of the pleasure and curiosity we have had in preparing it. We acknowledge full responsibility for any errors of judgment and fact, which our many friends, students, and colleagues have helped us to minimize.

D.E.
P.S.

CONTENTS

THE SOCIOLOGY
OF HEALTH CARE

PART ONE

Survey of
the Health System

1
HOW THE HEALTH-CARE SYSTEM OPERATES: AN OVERVIEW

During at least the next decade, our health-care system will become one of the foremost subjects of public concern in the United States. Although dramatic domestic problems of inflation, unemployment, and faltering confidence in government may appear today to be of substantially greater importance, the issues of the health-care system will soon receive an equal amount of public attention.

There are two sets of reasons for this prediction. The first concerns changing social attitudes about health care. Many of our leading citizens now believe that adequate health is a prerequisite to the good life, that access to good health care must now be made a right. But it is realized, too, that our health-care system is not the best in the world. As any casual review of the recent voluminous congressional testimony demonstrates, these changing attitudes mean that health policy is no longer a subject researched only by the medically or technically trained.

Second, various characteristics of the system, discussed later in this chapter, are resulting in enormous pressures for change in the way we organize, finance, and deliver medical care. Many of our society's problems, such as inflation, poverty, unemployment, and even foreign affairs, are associated with aspects of our health-care system. The growing economic and social importance of the system guarantees it will be of major importance to our political processes.

This book has five major goals. First, it seeks to describe the health-care system as a totality; that is, to describe all of its major components and the way they interrelate and affect one another.[1] It is common even

[1] When discussing the total range of attitudes, activities, and organizations affecting our health care, we use the phrase "health-care system." This includes, for example, planning functions and public-policy and legislative activities other than direct provision of medical care. When we discuss the part of our health-care system that is primarily concerned with the actual and direct provision of medical care to patients, we use the phrase "health-care delivery system." The latter is a very large and important part of the former.

for those working in the health field to be knowledgeable about only a few components of the total system. Numerous efforts at organizing doctors into large medical practices have demonstrated that physicians are often unfamiliar with parts of the health-care system, such as the public agencies affecting medical delivery or the academic programs training many of the health personnel that they employ. Overcoming this segmented understanding of the system is a contribution that the discipline of medical sociology can make. Our second goal, discussed more fully at the end of this chapter, is to give the reader some understanding of the concepts and conclusions of social science as they relate to our health-care system.

A third goal is to analyze in detail the major organizational, economic, and sociological trends that illuminate the inadequacies of our health-care delivery system and result in pressures for change. Fourth, we describe the occurrences by which society generally has come to be interested in the system and to discuss its merits. Here we analyze the political agencies, strategies and pressure groups, and public attitudes that influence health-care policy and will have significance for future directions. Fifth, we discuss the various major proposals for changing the system and their implications for consumers, providers, educators, and other organizations in society. We will give extensive attention to different ways of delivering care and to ideas for making services culturally relevant to various population groups.

The health-care system has numerous components, and there are many ways in which they influence one another. It has components that are primarily concerned with the actual delivery of medical care to patients. It has its recipient population (patients), and the recent involvement of laymen in forming plans and policy decisions for medical care has had consequences for physician behavior. The health-care system also has an elaborate network of agencies and activities revolving around the technology of medical care. The system has a set of values and rules about what is good and what is bad in health care. For example, one of the major barriers to group health delivery is the patient's fear that he will no longer have his own physician but rather will get whichever doctor happens to be available.

The health-care system also has an elaborate and changing manpower network. That is, we have developed patterns for selecting, training, and making use of the people who actually provide the medical care. The nature of the care the patient receives, and the cost of that care, are closely linked to this manpower network.[2] A brief example might best

---

[2] It is possible, for example, to predict with some accuracy what the manpower requirements would be for the various major proposals for national health insurance being considered by Congress. See, for example, Lien-fu Huang and Elwood W. Shomo, "The Impact of Archetypal National Health Insurance Plans on U.S. Health

clarify this point. The issue of task allocation between physicians and their nurses (what the doctor and nurse should be able to do in treating patients) is currently controversial. Should nurses, for example, be able to perform physical examinations in the absence of a physician? This question is related to other issues, such as providing medical care to those parts of our population and our country not adequately served by physicians. If we decide to provide more medical care to deprived citizens and underserved rural areas, we may well have to permit nurses to perform duties currently reserved for the physician. But that will require special advanced training for participating nurses, and educational programs will have to be developed. Thus the circle of relatedness between parts of the system continues.

The remainder of the chapter takes up three topics. We begin by briefly describing some of the major components of health-care delivery and the entire health-care system. This will provide the reader with a general understanding of the total system, as well as an introduction to our terms and definitions. The second topic is the major characteristic of the system, those features that make it what it is and that are often at the center of debate about it. The third topic introduces some of the historical occurrences that have made health care a controversial issue of increasing public concern.

SOME MAJOR ASPECTS OF OUR HEALTH-CARE DELIVERY SYSTEM

To understand the way we deliver medical care, it is important to recognize that the activities, attitudes, and techniques involved in its delivery are closely related to the activities and attitudes of those receiving that care. Health care involves both the styles of delivery and the styles of reception.[3] A physician can make a totally accurate diagnosis and prescribe brilliantly, but his patient can make that prescription ineffective through unwillingness to cooperate. A hospital can have very sophisticated programs for alcohol or drug abuse, but if the patient refuses treatment or leaves, these are useless. The overweight person can choose to suffer quietly with the recurring pains in his chest and arms, or he can decide to seek out medical attention and cooperate with the offered treatment. The nurse or the physician can decide that the call from the

Manpower Requirements," Prepared for Manpower Intelligence, Bureau of Health Manpower Education, National Institutes of Health, DHEW Publication No. (HRA) 75-1, February 1974.

[3] A dated but still intriguing book based on this concept is Benjamin D. Paul (ed.), *Health, Culture, and Community* (New York: Russell Sage Foundation, 1955).

frantic mother warrants an immediate appointment for the child, or they can decide the child can wait a few days for an appointment. Medical-care delivery occurs between human beings, even when it involves elaborate tests, machines, and computers.

In this light, our health-care delivery system makes certain assumptions about the population it serves and about the people (from physicians to bedpan specialists) who provide those services. Regarding the population served, it assumes that they have the capacity to pay for their medical care, either directly or through a third party, such as an insurance policy, a union health program, or the government. It also assumes that the patients will be inclined and able to initiate themselves into the delivery system, since in most cases the patient's choice to go to the doctor is the first step in his treatment. It assumes that patients will usually obtain care when needed and that they have some ability for self-care and self-diagnosis. It also assumes that patients will understand and follow treatment instructions and that they have the capacity and willingness to visit various independent medical providers. For example, the general practitioner who discovers that his patient is suffering from an unusual skin rash will provide that patient with the name of a good dermatologist but will normally not make the appointment, arrange for his patient to get to the specialist's office, or pay the new medical bill. After referral, the GP (general practitioner) may never see the patient again.

The common assumptions and attitudes about medical providers differ somewhat, according to who holds those attitudes and toward which providers. A very strong aspect of physicians' attitudes about themselves is that they are "professionals," members of an important scientific elite. This attitude often exists even before they begin practicing medicine, since most come from families of professionals and many have fathers or close relatives who are practicing physicians.[4] Relatedly, physicians learn, through their experiences in medical school, to be concerned about patients without becoming emotionally involved.[5] Many consumers respond to this by maintaining a blind faith in the doctor's wisdom and yet criticizing their aloofness.[6] Nurses, on the other hand, often regard their own status as inferior, while physicians see them as "obedient implementors of medical directives," and patients as the doctor's helper.[7] The status of other health professionals, from inhalation therapists to dietetic technicians, seems related to how closely they appear to approximate the characteristics of physicians.

We live in a time when the delivery of health care seems dominated

[4] Howard E. Freeman, et al., *Handbook of Medical Sociology* (Englewood Cliffs, N.J.: Prentice-Hall, 1972), p. 192.
[5] Ibid., p. 193.
[6] Ibid., pp. 269ff.
[7] Ibid., pp. 206ff.

by technology: large and frightening machines, computers containing our medical histories, extensive research, and the ever-present medical jargon. The pervasiveness of this technology often blinds us to a significant fact: medical care is delivered in the context of a social situation and is itself largely a social act. This social situation involves society's influence on medical providers and patients, relationships between various medical providers (doctors and nurses, nurses and laboratory technicians, etc.), and significant socioeconomic relationships between providers and patients. The physician is irritable because he had an argument with his wife, or he is pleasant because it has been a good morning; nurses working with the doctor may think the receptionist is dumb and poorly trained because she receives patients badly, or they may trust her efficiency; and the patient is comfortable because he knows the medical bills will be paid, or he is uncomfortable because the doctor is cold and uncaring. What probably matters most in the delivery of medical care is how the people involved think, act, and feel. Let us sketch some features of the major health-service providers.

PHYSICIANS

Physicians dominate the medical care provided to patients. They are usually the first and certainly the most important in deciding what the problem may be, how it should be treated, and what other health providers need to become involved. So called in-take physicians, usually GPs or internists, are very important, for they perform preliminary diagnosis, often prescribe treatment, and frequently refer patients to the other providers. Although some medical specialists are approached directly (e.g., pediatricians and obstetricians), in-take physicians remain important in referrals. (The discretion to decide which specialists get the bulk of referrals can serve as a powerful force to keep maverick physicians in line.)

Our rather uncritical faith in physicians is reinforced by the fact that they are an important elite in our society. As one author puts it:

> Since the turn of the century the American medical profession has enjoyed increasing affluence, the highest social status of any occupational group, and unchallenged control over not merely the social and economic conditions of its work, but . . . its definition as well.[8]

As an occupational group, physicians enjoy our nation's highest average income, over $50,000 per year.[9] The physician's personal and his occupational status cause and reinforce each other. Doctors are the primary

[8] Richard W. Wertz, *Readings on Ethical and Social Issues in Biomedicine* (Englewood Cliffs, N.J.: Prentice-Hall, 1973), p. 270.
[9] Paul S. Samuelson, *Economics,* 9th ed. (New York: McGraw-Hill, 1973), pp. 88–89.

source of healing, and we fear questioning their knowledge or opinions. As consumers, we usually have little knowledge of health care; yet few services are as important to us as these. If we do disagree with a physician's decision, our only real choices are not to receive care at all or to go to another physician. This monopoly, coupled with the small number of physicians available, helps explain their high income and unchallenged personal status.[10] To complete the circle, it is easy to believe that a doctor must be effective at practicing medicine since we can see that financially and socially he is "doing well."

NURSES

These preliminary comments on the nursing profession reflect two important and somewhat contradictory facts. First, even though two-thirds of all nurses work in hospitals or similar institutions, their professional functioning and the possibilities of limitations of their careers are largely controlled by the physicians with which they work. Second, the profession is experiencing constant pressures to change in ways contrary to many physicians' desires. We will discuss the network of professional relationships between physicians, nurses, allied health personnel, and administrative personnel more fully in a later chapter. It is sufficient here to note that many trends and proposed changes in health care involve expanded responsibility and status for nursing, which threatens some physicians and increases the nurse's independence from them. The use of nurses to give physical examinations to school children on public assistance and their central role in providing care in underserved areas of the county are two examples.

The nurse working in the doctor's office is the most directly influenced by physician control and supervision. As one author puts it:

> The office nurse . . . is likely to be continuously at the beck and call of the physician, who directs most of her activities. In this setting the nurse's opportunities for displaying her professional judgment are minimal.[11]

As Freeman notes, however, there is some flexibility in the accommodations within the work agreement between the nurse and doctor even in this situation of high nurse dependency on the physician. It is probably true that the greater administrative and recording duties occasioned by

[10] One of the great barriers to significant change in the health-care system is the threat that physicians may choose not to practice under certain kinds of programs or plans. "Health Maintenance Organizations," Hearings before the Subcommittee on Public Health and Environment, of the Committee on Interstate and Foreign Commerce, U.S. House of Representatives Serial No. 92-89. Testimony of the American Medical Association, 1972, pp. 333ff.

[11] Freeman, Handbook, p. 217.

Medicare and Medicaid have increased physician dependence on the nurse rather than the reverse.

Large numbers of nurses working in hospitals or similar medical institutions experience a somewhat different set of occupationally significant relationships. They function as the physician's deputy in carrying out his instructions, but the physician's orders are not as frequent nor quite as all-powerful in hospitals as they are in his own offices. Hospital nurses have a source of independence in performing their jobs that they do not have when working in the doctor's office. This source of influence is the hospital, its rules and regulations, and its administration. As hospital administration has become increasingly complex, with the growth in government financing and regulation and the emergence of consumer and "community" influence on hospitals, nurses are often in the position of performing middle-level administrative duties. Hospitals, like other large organizations in our society, seem to have more and more rules and procedures influencing the activities of the individuals associated with them. For nurses working in a hospital setting, this has been a source of some independence.

Nurses employed by colleges and universities, school districts, public-health agencies, industry, and community-service programs such as Head Start, are by far the freest in performing their duties. These nurses usually function rather independently, and in fact often decide when a physician's services are needed. Limiting this freedom, however, is the danger of physician disapproval of their actions. It is interesting to note that nurses are present where physicians are absent, and physicians are absent when there is little money to be made.

This relatively small percentage of the nursing profession, accustomed to a degree of professional independence, often forms the ranks of those on the front line seeking to expand the role of nursing in providing medical care. It is politically significant, however, that even in these careful efforts at increasing their professional responsibilities, nursing organizations and leaders often seek the support of a sympathetic physician, who can help make their case appear legitimate to the nursing school, governmental agency, or local medical society. The nursing profession is not in control of its own changes.

Other factors also influence the directions and uncertainty of changes in nursing. Educators and government officials, among others, frequently claim that there are too many nurses today. There is some scanty support for this, since the ratio of nurses to every one thousand in our population has increased by thirty percent during the past twenty years.[12] Training more and more nurses seems to be less important than earlier, and this has led to a declining interest in such programs as fed-

12 Ibid., p. 210.

erally funded nurse-training projects. Many nurses have a tendency to be uninvolved in both their profession and its organizations. About one-third of the registered nurses in this country are not employed in nursing, and the American Nurses Association has a membership of only one-third of those engaged in nursing. The irony is that while the nursing profession may be "Churning for Change," the number of nurses organized into potentially influential professional groups is significantly below full strength.

OTHER HEALTH-CARE PROVIDERS

From the viewpoint of the patient, the physicians and nurses are the most important, since the former determine the health need and the strategy for treatment and the latter are usually primary in carrying out the doctor's instructions. Other health-care personnel have traditionally been less visible to the patient though still important in health-care delivery.

The health industry has more than 4.5 million employees and is the nation's largest employer.[13] Significantly, our health-manpower "system" is characterized by a high degree of disorganization, chaos, and change. At the origin of this condition is the supply and training of health personnel. Until very recently, we have had no way to project the future employment demand for the various health occupations, and we are only now beginning to make use of projection techniques that permit educated guesses as to the number (for example) of inhalation therapists needed in Los Angeles during the next year or two. The number of people trained in the various professions has been largely determined by individual colleges or schools, with only vague statistical examination of community needs; by students who found a particular medical vocation attractive; or by teachers who like to teach nursing or physical therapy regardless of the need for personnel trained in these skills.

In addition, the number and variety of health-manpower positions, other than nurses and physicians, is bewildering and constantly changing. For example, one government study acknowledged that other allied health occupations that provide health-care services were too varied and the available statistics too few to permit detailed coverage in its report.[14] This California report identified some seventeen allied health positions, exclusive of nursing, for which the state's two-year community colleges provide instruction.

There is also a high level of instability in job retention among allied health professionals. One frequently finds evidence of employee turnover

13 Kenneth M. Endicott, "The Doctor Dilemma," *Manpower* (July 1972), p. 3.
14 California Department of Public Health, Office of Comprehensive Health Planning, *California State Plan for Health Statistical Supplement, California Health Manpower*, 1971, p. 28.

in hospitals in excess of thirty percent annually. Many of these employees are women and secondary wage earners, which permits them an occupational independence not enjoyed by the primary wage earners in the industry. In addition, a number of factors, including (but not restricted to) advances in medical technology, frequently create new jobs or replace old ones. Automatic chemical analyzers are performing more and more of all laboratory work, and nuclear medicine technicians or dialysis assistants are only two of the recent positions created by technology.

HEALTH-PERSONNEL EDUCATORS

There is a parochialism within health education and a relative absence of coordinated planning within and between educational institutions regarding society's needs for trained health personnel. It is important to note that this parochialism is not unique to educators in health care but rather related to characteristics common to our educational systems generally. Educators, particularly those in higher education, have a habit of developing secure personal "nests" through the creation of programs and curriculum constructed around their particular interests and talents. This, of course, provides them with some guarantee of being retained and with the happy situation of having created many of their own work conditions. This is not to say that academic faculty are always unconcerned with society's needs, or are immune from pressures to make their teaching "relevant." It is true, however, that tenure and the principles of academic freedom remove many faculty from the ultimate sanction of loss of employment and from the effectiveness of instructions or demands that they change their courses to meet the job market.

Nor are administrators of educational institutions unaware of this faculty lethargy. Even the most committed administrator, hoping to make his institution's curriculum more effective as a supplier of trained personnel, faces the reality that he must cajole and coax his teachers into course changes if there are to be any at all. And the administrator's efforts are further complicated by the fact that a community's educational institutions act independently, usually without any reliable information on employment demand for their area and almost always without any coordination of curriculum between themselves and other colleges or schools.

Despite this parochialism, divisiveness, and lack of communication, the forthcoming changes in our health-care system will require and produce changes in the education and training of health personnel. It is our sad, though tentative conclusion that comprehensive change in the institutions educating health personnel will be seriously delayed. Many educators perform a major service in describing the problems and alternative solutions and policies for our health-care system. Unfortunately, because of the nature of the academic industry, many of these innovative programs will take effect long after the need for them is apparent.

GOVERNMENTAL AND OTHER REGULATORY, RESEARCH, AND PLANNING AGENCIES

Like the catalog of health-manpower positions, the governmental and quasi-public agencies regulating or affecting (though not providing) our medical care are numerous and changing. They are best understood with reference to the functions they perform. Some control the quantity and quality of the health personnel and facilities providing care. An example is the National Board of Medical Examiners. Others perform largely planning, and evaluation and information-collection activities, such as Health Systems Agencies (HSAs) and Professional Standards Review Organizations (PSROs). Others (particularly the various public foundations and some agencies of the U.S. Department of Health, Education, and Welfare) encourage medical research and programmatic experimentation.

The influence of governmental agencies is growing along with public expenditures, which totaled $28 billion in the 1970–71 fiscal year. Most observers believe that some form of national health insurance (NHI) is inevitable. Regardless of the form it takes, the influence that NHI will have on health care will be enormous as the system adjusts to new government regulations and resources. As we discuss later in this chapter, the passage of Medicare and Medicaid in 1965 resulted in the momentous growth of public pressures for changes in the health-care delivery system. But unlike NHI those programs cover only a portion of our citizens.

MISCELLANEOUS ASPECTS OF HEALTH CARE

No discussion of our health-care delivery system is adequate without attention to hospitals, the drug industry, and the growth in consumer influence, to mention only three major subjects. Our effort in the preceding pages has been to introduce the reader to a few basic concepts about the health-care delivery system, generally, and about some of its major components, specifically. More-detailed analysis of these components is provided in later chapters.

CHARACTERISTICS OF THE HEALTH-CARE SYSTEM

The American health-care system has certain major characteristics that critically influence the way it delivers medical care, selects and trains its personnel for that delivery, and influences the health of our citizens. Not surprisingly, these characteristics are frequently under attack by critics of the system. The following characteristics are the most important for our consideration.

1. Most observers agree that the health-care system is a nonsystem: it operates largely on the basis of an infinite number of daily individual decisions by providers and consumers of medical care; it is influenced by the politics of give and take and by the inadequate communication between the numerous medical groups, consumer groups, and governmental agencies. As yet, it is not a planned system. There is no agency in control.

2. Most medical care is provided by physicians operating in an office setting. Here physicians function as relatively independent solo practitioners or as members of a very small group of doctors. Although there is a continuing decline in the ratio of generalists (GPs, internists, family physicians, pediatricians) to specialists, the major organizational connection between physicians in most communities remain the referral to specialists by generalists. Coordination between physicians or between physicians and hospitals in this setting is often inadequate.

3. Almost all medical care in this country is provided on a fee-for-service basis.[15] As economists put it, the pricing mechanism dominates. The physician provides medical care and then charges a fee for each unit of service he has given. The fee is usually somewhat similar to fees charged for similar services by other local medical providers, but physicians (as well as hospitals) feel free to increase their fees without much fear of losing business. The majority of patients do not deny themselves needed medical care because the prices have increased. But high fees can be a barrier to care, particularly for the low-income. For the middle-income, these fees are often paid by a third party, such as an insurance company. The control of fees by medical providers, rather than by the principles of supply, demand, and competition, is exemplified by two classic situations. Beginning in the 1970s, physicians all over the nation were confronted with rapidly accelerating premiums for malpractice insurance. In most cases, these costs have been passed on to either the consumer or payer of medical services. In a second case, it is frequently alleged that too many hospital beds have been constructed and that hospitals are experiencing unusually high vacancy rates. The irony is that hospitals often appear unconcerned about the situation. Their strategy has been to increase fees for the services provided, thus covering the "overhead" of excess capacity. The patients have not publicly complained, probably because most of their bills for hospitalization were paid by their insurance companies or union plans. Here again, it is

[15] Harry Schwartz, *The Case for American Medicine: A Realistic Look at Our Health Care System* (New York: McKay, 1972), p. 29. Although Schwartz presents a perspective contrary to our own, his book is a good example of the arguments of those supporting the existing system.

reasonable to assume that consumers ultimately pay through increased insurance premiums.

4. Although physicians do not control the system as a giant elite in close communication, they do dominate and influence it and have much to say about any changes that occur. Thus, as we have already noted, physicians determine the strategy of any personnel involved in treating a patient—excepting, of course, those situations, such as underserved areas or populations, in which nurses conduct these activities. In addition to dominating the care provided to individual patients, it has been frequently shown that doctors as a group have a very powerful voice in decisions about general public-policy changes in medical care, such as those that occurred during congressional considerations of Medicare and Medicaid in the 1960s. Consideration of this power and its limits are included in later chapters.

5. Our medical system is largely curative in nature. Medical care is usually sought and provided when there is reason to believe that an illness exists. There is some preventive medical care, such as physical examinations and inoculations, but care most often occurs after problems develop, rather than as an effort to keep people healthy.

Many observers believe that these characteristics produce a grossly inadequate health-care system. The "nonsystem" characteristic means that there is little coordinated planning; hence, the quality of care is adversely affected by lack of communication between physicians, and waste occurs in duplication of unneeded medical facilities and programs. In one view, the predominance of solo and small-group forms of physician practice results in less than full use of health personnel, facilities, and equipment. Inflation in the costs of medical care is the consequence.

The fee-for-service characteristic leads physicians to concentrate in the higher-income areas of the country. Depressed urban areas and poor rural areas are seriously underrepresented in physician services. Fee-for-service also encourages inflation of medical costs because physicians have a hand in setting their own fees; and as fees rise, an increasing percentage of our population find adequate health care inaccessible. Physician dominance retards the experimental use of other health personnel, for physicians usually resist innovative programs. The curative nature of our health care means that treatment often comes too late to be effective. Our mortality and illness rates compare unfavorably with those of other industrialized nations.

These and other charges have become ever more frequent as the pressures for change have expanded during the past decade. We turn now to the historical occurrences producing these pressures.

PRESSURES FOR CHANGE

The criticism of the health-care system, particularly of physicians and hospitals, is not strictly a recent phenomenon. Around the turn of the century, George Bernard Shaw spent a good deal of time poking pins into the "scientific arrogance" of physicians. The contemporary public discussions and debates, however, really have their roots in the 1960s, and it is there that we begin our description of the growth in the pressures for change.

Among the many pressures to change the health-care system, some are attitudinal, some institutional, and some economic. In the first place, the costs of medical care for any American citizen have risen enormously in the last few years. These data are fully reviewed in chapter 3, but we can note here that medical costs have been increasing at an annual rate of more than ten percent for the past decade. Everyone, except the very wealthy, finds it increasingly difficult to pay his medical bills. In most cases, economy cannot be realized by cutting back on the amount of medical attention we receive. We cannot limit our consumption of emergency care or medical attention to catastrophic or long-term afflictions. In many situations, we cannot defer or ignore our needs for attention, even if the costs are high.

Although the amount of money individuals must pay for care has increased dramatically, the total amount of money spent for medical care, both privately and by government, has also increased tremendously. Health care is this nation's largest single industry and is one of its most rapidly growing industries. We spent a little more than $11 billion for health care in the 1949–50 fiscal year, $75 billion in 1970–71, and over $130 billion in 1976. In addition, the publicly funded portion of that expenditure has increased significantly. Thus, the growth in the total health-care bill has made it of major economic significance, while the increased dollars and the higher percentage paid from public monies have made it a concern for citizens as well as for politicians and students concerned with the behavior of the medical sector.

As the economics of the health-care system have become critical, changes have also been occurring in public attitudes about who should receive medical care, how much they should receive, and under what conditions. Beginning in the middle and late 1950s, academic authors, civil-rights leaders, and some political leaders began to draw our attention to poverty and the living conditions of minority groups. Although the civil-rights confrontations in places like Alabama and North Carolina tended to focus on educational needs and the right to be served at a lunch counter, they ultimately raised questions about other rights, such as the right to an income and to medical care. In 1959, Oscar Lewis argued that many people live in an all-encompassing and self-reinforcing condition known as the "culture of poverty."[16] Three years later, Michael Harrington told us that the poor in our society live in "The Other America." We had begun to pay attention to poverty in our midst and to the fact that it affected all aspects of life, including health.

During his campaign for President in 1960, John F. Kennedy chose to make the poverty of many of our citizens a political issue. The fact that much of that year's presidential campaign was televised meant that the issue could rapidly become of major social importance. Kennedy's concern for poverty did not result in much legislative action, but his assassination seemed to. His successor, Lyndon Johnson, achieved passage of the Economic Opportunity Act in 1964, which established programs that included health services for some low-income program recipients. In 1965 almost as an afterthought, Congress passed and Johnson signed into law a bill that provided medical assistance to the aged (Medicare) and to many of the indigent of all ages as well (Medicaid). The health-care system in this country would never be the same.

There are two basic ways that Medicare and Medicaid resulted in pressure for changing the health-care system. First, it was a partial institutionalization of the idea that accessibility to medical care was a right and that fixed or very low incomes should not stop citizens from receiving services. In that sense it was a major step toward national health insurance.

But there were also more pragmatic and political ways in which it influenced the health-care system. Federal contributions to personal health care now exceed $30 billion annually, compared with $3 billion before these programs were launched, and millions of people now receive care who had very little before. This massive influx of government dollars and millions of low-income patients severely tested the system and found it deficient in many ways.

We will later discuss in depth the programmatic and administrative features of Medicare and Medicaid, but the following are their basic characteristics. A person who is on Public Assistance (Medicaid) or is aged (Medicare) receives some form of identification (usually a card) that says he is entitled to receive any of a list of medical services for which the provider will be paid a fee by the government. This "recipient" takes his card to the medical provider when he needs services, and if the provider is willing to participate in the program, the physician or hospital bills the state for the services rendered.

One of the problems has been that numerous providers, particularly physicians, are unwilling to give services to Medicaid and Medicare re-

16 Oscar Lewis, *Five Families* (New York: Basic Books, 1959).

cipients. Their reasons vary from philosophical opposition to the programs, to frustration over fees they regard as too low, to the delay in compensation from the government agencies. One also suspects that a few physicians may find it distasteful to treat low-income citizens.

The fee-for-service and solo-practitioner aspects of the system have also worked against the rational administration of Medicare and Medicaid. Government agencies paying for these services must budget funds well in advance of the time when patients will seek care. But with thousands of independent providers, and their millions of patients, making decisions that result in fees of over $30 billion, predicting costs in any exact way is almost impossible. In the 1970s many state Medicaid agencies, confronted with the bankruptcy of their program, began seeking alternatives to the independent practitioners' fee-for-service system or tightening eligibility standards for those seeking care.[17]

There is some evidence that Medicaid and Medicare have contributed to the inflation of medical costs that has been with us for many years.[18] The problems of increased costs, the difficulties with cost predictability, and the unwillingness of many physicians to participate have been pronounced in both these programs since their inception. The enormity of government's expenditure in these programs have caused many public officials to feel the necessity of finding solutions to the problems, frequently by making basic changes in the health-care system.

Medicare and Medicaid have committed us programmatically to massive public support for health services for those who cannot afford it. But institutional and economic trends in the industry make it clear that the entire system is changing, not just that part of it pertaining to care for the low-income and elderly.

SUGGESTED READINGS

ALTMAN, STUART H., "Present and Future Supply of Registered Nurses" (Washington, D.C.: GPO, DHEW Publication No. (NIH) 72-134, Division of Nursing, National Institute of Health, Public Health Service, November 1971. An analysis of the adequacy of the supply of nurses and the determinants of their labor-force participation rate.

[17] See Darryl D. Enos, "Health Maintenance Organizations Attract Federal, State Attention as Health Care Alternatives," California Journal (September 1971).
[18] For a physician's perspective on inflation, see Spyros Andreopoulos (ed.), Primary Care: Where Medicine Fails (New York: Wiley, 1974), p. 140. See also "Health Maintenance Organizations," Hearings before the Subcommittee on Public Health and Environment of the Committee on Interstate and Foreign Commerce, U.S. House of Representatives, Serial No. 92-89, 1972, p. 386.

CAMPBELL, RITA RICARDO, *Economics of Health and Public Policy* (Washington, D.C.: American Enterprise Institute, June 1971). An attempt to explain the disappointing boxscore for the United States in health and morbidity data.

COHEN, HARRIS S. and WINSTON J. DEAN, "To Practice or Not to Practice: Developing State Law and Policy on Physician Assistants," *Milbank Memorial Fund Quarterly*, Vol. 52, no. 4 (Fall 1974), pp. 349–75. An examination of the legal status of paramedics, physician assistants, and nurse practitioners.

GOLDSTEIN, HAROLD M. and MORRIS A. HOROWITZ, "Restructuring Paramedical Jobs," *Manpower*, March 1973, pp. 2–7. A field study providing evidence of the variance between formal job descriptions and actual job duties.

JONES, D. C., P. C. COOLEY, A. MIEDEMA, and T. D. HARTWELL, *Trends in Registered Nurse Supply* (Washington, D.C.: GPO, DHEW Publication No. (HRA) 76-15, Public Health Service, Health Resources Administration, Bureau of Health Manpower, Division of Nursing, Bethesda, Maryland, March 1976). A comprehensive review of nurse-supply studies for their policy implications.

KENNEDY, EDWARD M., "Health Care in the Seventies," *Journal of Medical Education*, Vol. 47 (January 1972), pp. 15–22. A critical commentary on the health-care delivery system.

MCNERNEY, WALTER J., "Why Does Medical Care Cost So Much?," *The New England Journal of Medicine*, Vol. 282, no. 26 (June 25, 1970), pp. 1458–65. A critical survey of the health-care system that focuses on cost considerations.

MCTERNAN, EDMUND J., *Educating Personnel for the Allied Health Professions and Services* (St. Louis: Mosby, 1972), pp. 1–10. A treatment of the origin, education, and training of allied personnel.

New Health Practitioners, Robert L. Kane, ed. (A conference sponsored by the John E. Fogarty International Center for Advanced Study in the Health Sciences and the Association of Teachers of Preventive Medicine, National Institute of Health, Bethesda, Maryland, May 14–15, 1974. Washington, D.C.: GPO, DHEW Publication No. (NIH) 75-875). Each chapter provides a position paper by a manpower specialist concerning the redesigning of job activities in the health-care delivery system.

RECORD, JANE CASSELS and MERWYN R. GREENLICK, "New Health Professionals and the Physician Role: An Hypothesis from Kaiser Experience," *Public Health Reports*, Vol. 90, no. 3 (May/June 1975). A discussion of the changing status and responsibility of the physician in delivery of patient care.

SCHEFFLER, RICHARD M., "Physician Assistants: Is There a Return to Training?," *Industrial Relations*, Vol. 14, no. 1 (February 1975). An analysis of the advantages of the physician assistant.

SCHWARTZ, HARRY, *The Case for American Medicine: A Realistic Look at Our Health Care System* (New York: McKay, 1973). A defense for the current medical system.

YETT, D. E., "An Economic Analysis of the Market for Nurses," *The U.S. Medical Care Industry: The Economist's Point of View* (Ann Arbor: Michigan

Business Papers No. 60, Division of Research, Graduate School of Business Administration, University of Michigan, 1974. A statistical study of the supply of nurses.

YETT, D. E. and F. A. SLOAN, "Analysis of Migration Patterns of Recent Medical School Graduates," *Inquiry*, Vol. 11, no. 2 (June 1974), pp. 125–42. Discusses why many trained nurses and other medical personnel choose not to practice in the health-care system.

2

SYSTEM TRENDS:
PROFESSIONALISM AND
SPECIALIZATION

In chapter 1, we provided an overview of the health-care system. We emphasized the essential personal aspect of health-care services, even though the system is characterized by increasing technology and size. We noted that much of the delivery of services reflects the judgment of the solo practitioner, supported when necessary by hospital care. We briefly identified the major providers within the system, acknowledging the strategic role of the physician and the reluctance of those concerned about the status quo to admit change in the delivery system. Resistance to change is found, not only in those providing services, but also in the educational facilities training such personnel. Finally, we noted an increasing popular awareness of the need for improved health-care service. Public pressure for government assistance has taken the form of Medicare and Medicaid programs, identified as precursors of a fully nationalized health-insurance program.

In this chapter, we will review the role of professionalism in the medical field in order to identify the value structure that is unique in many ways. In this and the following chapters, our purpose will be to identify major trends of the medical market, along with the concerns frequently expressed about the need to improve access to medical care. In this chapter, we will also discuss professionalism, specialization, and licensing arrangements as they affect our search for quality care. In the following chapter, we will view the major economic dimensions of the medical market, involving levels of expenditure, price and cost adjustments, and changes in funding sources.

PROFESSIONALISM VERSUS COMMERCIALISM

Professional integrity represents the historic stamp upon the medical sector. We begin by outlining the evolution of this concept and of its vital service, simply because it is now challenged from several quarters. As we will see, allegations are made that professional principles sometimes disguise the more pervasive economic interests of health-care providers. Furthermore, professional autonomy is now challenged by government intrusions into the medical market and, more recently, by public insistence on the determination of standards for appropriate medical service. It has also been challenged by consumerism and by economists who contend that a restricted access to any profession (ostensibly designed to improve the quality of service through restrictions of supply) has the effect of raising professional income. In effect, a restriction of services intensifies the scramble for attention while improving the economic status of providers.

The case has been made that professionalism has emerged in response to change, particularly change that tended to be destructive of traditional value systems. For example, Stephen Kunitz contends that medical professionalism reflected the economic and social turmoil of rapid industrialization during the turn of the century.[1]

The urbanization and industrialization of the Progressive era led to overcrowding, poor diets, unsanitary conditions, and increased insecurity. There was a concurrent erosion of family structures, long the source of discipline and morality. Old problems emerged with what appeared to be unprecedented severity, including unemployment, alcoholism, juvenile deliquency, prostitution, political racketeering, epidemics, crime, and mental illness. Two forces emerged to deal with these severe issues: the government proposed social legislation, and clusters of private citizens responded with intensive study and personal commitment. The "expert" emerged, with expertise identified by his research and understanding of the issue and by his personal decision to dedicate inordinate amounts of his energy in a problem-solving capacity to serve society.

Thus, professionalism in medical services became a reality. Not only was society seeking authority and professional expertise, but it felt more comfortable or assured when men of stature were handling issues of sensitivity to society, whether these included brain surgery or the rehabilitation of women of the streets. The notion that guilds could preserve the integrity of job standards and pride in craft skills was fused with yet another ideology: service to humanity through years of intensive study, adherence to strict standards for individual performance, and an overriding concern for public rather than personal welfare. In exchange for such altruism, such groups had a modest request: a license or exclusive charter that would recognize the exclusive responsibility (and privilege) of their activity.

The logic for this evolution can be better understood if one appre-

[1] Stephen J. Kunitz, "Professionalism and Social Control in the Progressive Era: The Case of the Flexner Report," *Social Problems*, Vol. 6, no. 22 (October 1974).

ciates the rampant commercialism of medical practice during much of the nineteenth century. Licensing laws to control the practice of medicine collapsed in the 1830s and 1840s, and until 1880 there was no control over the licensing of physicians, their training, or their standards of practice. Throughout the nineteenth century, proprietary medical schools were open virtually to anyone who could pay the required fees. The M.D. degree alone was a license to practice. An enterprising spirit abounded. The poor who could afford the fees of proprietary education were assured both an income and social status. For the wealthy, securing the M.D. degree might involve modest costs and offer enhanced prestige. We have no statistical series to confirm how such arrangements benefited the ill.

One index of the state of the art was the suspicion and hostility displayed by many in the medical profession to advances being made in the new science of microbiology. As Kunitz explains, "It is an entertaining irony that the germ theory was actively resisted in this country because many physicians regarded it as a threat to free trade." He further observed:

> Quarantine was regarded by most physicians before 1880 as an unwarranted infringement on personal liberty and commerce, and the germ theory, of course, would have rationalized quarantine. The resistance to this theory may well have been the result of the lower educational attainments of Americans as opposed to European physicians. Isolated from the laboratory, generally unfamiliar with microbiological research, and politically opposed to the implications of the theory, many physicians resisted it until well into the 1880s.[2]

A further clue to the prevailing attitude of American medicine involves a comparison with the much-respected reputation of the German medical practice. William Welch, first dean of the medical school at Johns Hopkins, wrote in 1880:

> I was often asked in Germany how it is that no scientific work in medicine is done in this country. . . . The answer is that there is no opportunity for, no appreciation of, no demand for that kind of work here. In Germany, on the other hand, every encouragement is being held out to the young men with taste for science.[3]

The Carnegie Foundation undertook an analysis of the entire educational structure, with a study of medical education by Abraham Flexner as part of that larger project. In his study, Flexner urged the consolidation of medical schools into major centers of excellence, and the organization of specialty boards to define education standards. Those standards would involve control over entrance to medical schools, the policing of

[2] Kunitz, "Professionalism and Social Control," p. 20.
[3] Quoted by S. Flexner and J. T. Flexner, *William Henry Welch and the Heroic Age of American Medicine* (New York: Viking, 1941), p. 113.

the educational sequence of the schools, and the licensure of graduates. Licensure would not be provided for graduates of "schools scandalously defective in teaching facilities."

Flexner acknowledged that examination for licensure was the power to destroy. But it was also, in his view, a lever with which the entire medical field would be lifted. In essence, the issue of restriction and control was motivated not by economic gain but by the quality of service citizens have a right to expect. His expressions are both eloquent and incisive:

> Medicine, curative and preventive, has indeed no analogy with business. Like the Army, the police, or the social worker, the medical profession is supported for a benign, not a selfish, for a protective, not an exploiting, purpose. The knell of the exploiting doctor has been sounded, just as the day of the freebooter and the soldier of fortune has passed away.[4]

But did not such licensure privileges create the opportunities for abuse, and even deny access to care desperately required? Did it not, in fact, empower a small group of professionals to determine the terms and conditions under which medical service might be provided? Again, Flexner explained:

> Such control in the social interest inevitably encounters the objection that individualism is thereby impaired. So it is, at that level; so it is intended. The community through such regulation undertakes to abridge the freedom of particular individuals to exploit certain conditions for their personal benefit. But its aim is thereby to secure for all others more freedom at a higher level. Society forbids a company of physicians to pour out upon the community a horde of ill-trained physicians. Their liberty is indeed clipped. As a result, however, more competent physicians are being trained under the auspices of the state itself, the public health is improved; the physical well-being of the wage-worker is heightened; and a restriction put upon the liberty, so-called, of a dozen doctors increases the effectual liberty of all other citizens. Has democracy, then, really suffered a set-back? Reorganization along national lines involves the strengthening, not the weakening, of democratic principles, because it tends to provide the conditions upon which well-being and effectual liberty depend.[5]

The licensing of professionals required the establishment of internal rather than external definitions of professional integrity. Thus, medical schools and examining boards were given new roles: they had the task of improving physicians' skills to protect the public from charlatans.

In historical perspective, this program has involved the restriction

---

[4] *Medical Education in the United States and Canada* (New York: Carnegie Foundation for the Advancement of Teaching, Bulletin 4, 1910), p. 173.
[5] Ibid., p. 155.

of the physician flow, a process that assured the rising productivity of those who served and enlarged rewards for the profession as well. By maintaining a policy of exclusion (or restriction of numbers), it was able to control one blade of the demand-and-supply scissors that cut the pattern of medical care. And as the rewards to physicians increased because of such scarcity, it was not surprising that physicians should conclude (as does much of society) that a person tends to be paid what he is worth and be worth what he is paid. The proof of the rising integrity (value) of physician services is reflected in the increased amounts of money consumers paid for such services.

BIOCHEMISTRY VERSUS THE SOCIOLOGY OF MEDICAL CARE

The move to professionalism encouraged, in turn, a view of medical science that has major ramifications for the character of the health industry. Clearly, the Flexner report sets the standard for this century: medical education must focus on the basic science of medicine—on pure research, the biochemistry of body function, and physiology.

Medicine can, as an alternative, be viewed as the preservation of health, with contributions toward an understanding· to be secured from a study of the culture and its stresses. Disciplines that contribute to understanding the individual in that environmental setting include sociology, economics, demography, and psychology. Medical science opted for a micro rather than macro view of health, for individual medicine rather than population medicine, for laboratory research rather than community research, and for biomedical research rather than the sociology of health. It was, of course, quite logical to identify, through biomedical research, the sources and causes of infection, for the major triumphs of medicine involve the discipline and tenacity of those committed to pure research. This preoccupation with research has given a unique character to contemporary medicine in the United States. Kerr L. White makes the point with characteristic force:

> Full-time medical school faculties selected medical students in their own image. They looked for those well grounded in physics, chemistry, and biology, who were motivated by curiosity about disease processes rather than for students grounded in the humanities and the social sciences, motivated by desires to meet needs of people. Both motives are laudable and medicine needs both groups of disciplines; however, emphasis on the former excluded the latter. Because faculties were increasingly concerned with molecular events, because they selected students with the same interests and discouraged patients with chronic,

emotional, minor or terminal problems from applying for help from teaching hospitals, the earlier mechanisms for training general practitioners seemed obsolete and the apparatus for doing so was dismantled. Primary care was no longer regarded as the responsibility of medical schools, and perhaps not even of physicians.[6]

In effect, the research focus of medical schools has set a tone within the entire structure of this service sector: the most respected in the prestige hierarchy are those with demonstrated research capabilities. The most valued member of the medical department is the individual receiving generous government or foundation grants. Distinguished colleagues are those participating in elaborate laboratory research, making regular contributions to the medical journals, giving papers at national professional meetings.

The research orientation has naturally spawned respect for field specialties and has led to what in turn has been called the era of superspecialties. It can be reasoned that specialization in the medical field is but one variant on the general specialization found in all occupational groups. With the explosion of knowledge, individuals are attracted to unusual (but confined) segments of the field. The paradox of the medical field is that the press for specialization has proceeded, not because of, but in spite of market demand. Most physicians serve in general practice and most people seek the services of a general practitioner. But fewer than ten percent of the medical-school graduates "major" in general practice. This undoubtedly reflects the value structure within the medical school: as the number of specialists increases, the generalist comes to be considered as a nonexpert, as a person who is soft or even sentimental in his view of society, rather than rigorous and scientific. Research enjoys enhanced status, while the individual interested in the sociology of medicine or in general practice is further denigrated. Rashi Fein confirms the view that medical schools have nurtured such specialization:

> The culture of the medical school, the nature of its faculty, the heavy emphasis on clinical teaching in the hospital (the world of the specialist), all tend to reinforce the pressures that already exist. Trained in the hospital where one sees the sickest patients, where things are happening, where time is compressed . . . it is no small wonder that specialists become the role model. These pressures in themselves might be sufficient, yet the nature of modern medical practice adds to them. There are significant disadvantages to being a primary care physician, particularly in individual solo practice, a type of practice that places heavy demands upon the physician.[7]

[6] Kerr L. White, "Health Care Arrangements in the United States, AD 1972," *Milbank Memorial Fund Quarterly*, Vol. 50, no. 4 (October 1972), pp. 19–20.

[7] Rashi Fein, "On Achieving Access and Equity in Health Care," *Milbank Memorial Fund Quarterly*, Vol. 50, no. 4 (October 1972), p. 180.

THE GENERALIST VERSUS THE SPECIALIST

Superspecialization has constricted our access to medical services. The specialist expects—and requires—hospital-based facilities and colleagues. Thus, physicians cluster around major metropolitan areas where there are concentrations of both facilities and other specialists. Although the United States has 132 physicians per 100,000 population delivering patient care, the ratio of such service is 320 nonfederal physicians per 100,000 population in Washington, D.C., while only 69 in Mississippi and 75 in Alabama.

Such specialization has also caused the fragmentation of services. As David Mechanic has observed:

> Specialization in the absence of aggregation of personnel and integration of services has resulted in growing fragmentation of care and poor medical care from a community point of view. Such functions as preventive care, follow-up care, health education and wise management of patients' difficulties in the context of family and community conditions have been difficult to maintain in systems of fragmented services where no person or agency has responsibility for the whole person.[8]

Specialization has also encouraged the decline of solo practice. In horse-and-buggy days, the physician made house calls without hesitancy because he carried in his black bag most of the technology for treatment. Today, in contrast, he typically has access to a vast array of testing and treatment procedures, but these require ready access to laboratory facilities, collaboration with medical colleagues, or a hospital:

> He requires an emergency admission unit, an outpatient facility and a modern hospital and laboratory if he is to deliver his . . . [modern] brand of care. He is almost helpless alone. No wonder he hesitates to make a house call, for by his standards, alone at the home, there is little he can do. Is it worth the patient's money to have him come?[9]

Charles Code contends that about eighty percent of all medical information applied in medical practice today has been acquired over the last sixty years, with an accumulation that no one person could possibly absorb. There is no contemporary form of the renaissance man in the medical field. Given that reality, the only way to handle the amassed information is through specialization. Although the obligations for group practice flow naturally from this situation, and although the prospect of abandon-

[8] "Ideology, Medical Technology and Health Care Organizations in Modern Nations," *The American Journal of Public Health*, Vol. 65, no. 3 (March 1975), p. 243.
[9] Charles F. Code, "Determinants of Medical Care: A Plan for the Future," *The New England Journal of Medicine*, Vol. 283, no. 13 (September 24, 1970), p. 681.

ing solo practice is disagreeable or even frightening to many rugged individualists, medical technology offers no simple alternative. And although solo practice remains a dominant form of providing care, it is being steadily abandoned. In Minnesota, for example, those providing general practice accounted for ninety-five percent of the physician stock in 1910, with combined specialists representing the other five percent. In 1965, only fifty-two percent were in general practice, with forty-eight percent in combined specialty practice.

> Nationally, the trend is clear; increasing numbers of physicians are seeking the personal security and satisfaction of specialization. They look for a body of knowledge they can contain and be highly skilled in applying. To be able to deliver what he knows is the best, the doctor today is forced to limit the breadth of his practice—to specialize. The trend has been fired by the demand of the American public for the ultimate in medical care.[10]

Code draws the analogy between the solo practitioner and the one-room schoolhouse. He anticipates that the 1970 stock of sixty thousand GPs will decline by about twenty thousand per decade, to reach a zero level by the year 2010.

> The general practitioners, particularly the soloist, is not replenishing his ranks. He is overworked and overtaxed beyond his mental and physical capabilities; his plight has become recognized, and his numbers diminished. This appears to me a natural physiologic—or psychologic—or sociologic consequence of advance in medicine. I see no reason to fight this natural trend toward specialization.[11]

The supply of primary doctors, including family practitioners, internists, and pediatricians, fell from 94 per 100,000 population in 1931 to 53.2 per 100,000 in 1967.[12] Of the 278,500 physicians involved with patient care, only 20 percent (57,000) are now in the practice of general medicine. The bulk, then, are absorbed in no fewer than 61 specialties, with the AMA officially recognizing 43 of these by issuing specialty certificates.[13] From the decade 1955–65, physician-directed services rose by 81 percent, hospital-directed services 65 percent, the growth in the number of physicians 22 percent. But the increase in the number of physicians involved in patient care was only 12 percent, or less than the 17-percent population growth. It remains true that about 60 percent of the present physician

[10] Ibid., p. 681.
[11] Ibid. For further analysis, see I. J. Fahs and O. L. Peterson, "The Decline of General Practice," *Public Health Report*, Vol. 83 (1968), pp. 267–70.
[12] Mary Overpeck, "Physicians in Family Practice, 1931–1967," *Public Health Reports*, no. 85 (June 1970), pp. 485–94.
[13] J. N. Haug, G. A. Roback, and B. C. Martin, *Distribution of Physicians in the United States, 1970* (Chicago: American Medical Association, 1971).

stock is involved in the direct care of patients and are solo practitioners.[14] Most solo practitioners are specialists. These data suggest a decline in the number of physicians who define themselves as GPs, family practitioners, or those concerned with primary patient care. With the decline of that specialty, we can anticipate the decline of the solo practitioner as well. We can expect these declining trends to be sustained in the future, despite belated efforts of some medical schools to revitalize general practice, and the advance of the Family Practice Specialty Board.

EMOTIONAL NEED VERSUS TECHNICAL VIRTUOSITY

It is now recognized that the emotional aspects of disease and sickness are substantial. As White has explained, the way people feel and the way they behave in response to environmental and cultural influences has a great deal to do with the form, duration, and intensity of their symptoms and disability.[15] Persons trained in primary practice have to cultivate skills in listening, counseling, sympathizing, and in understanding what others might regard as trivial, nonmedical aspects of the health field. These skills may be acquired, of necessity, by specialists forced into general practice. But it remains true that major attention in medical education is given to the superspecialists' skills in dealing with the relatively rare or uncommon afflictions. Again, as White makes the point:

> Medical care, medical education and medical research were focused increasingly on the acutely ill and on patients who responded promptly to treatment. The chronically ill, the terminally ill and the emotionally disturbed were whisked away from the teaching hospitals as "uninteresting" for study and "unsuitable" to the clinicians and investigators of the day, and "unsuitable" for teaching about acute problems. Presumably these problems were of considerable "interest" to those who suffered from them.[16]

There are certain major afflictions that are of particular interest to health specialists. Significantly, the afflictions the patient often regards as serious may be diagnosed by the specialist as trivial, commonplace, or (at the other extreme) terminal. If the patient persists in seeking treatment or cure, he may be put down as a "crock." Physicians are not attuned to the problems of helping people live in lifestyles that could reduce the risk of affliction, or even of assisting people to die more comfortably. The dominant trait of the physician is one of "curing," not "caring."

[14] Fred Anderson, "The Growing Pains of Medical Care," *The New Republic,* January 17, 1970, p. 16.
[15] White, "Health Care Arrangements in the United States," p. 20.
[16] Ibid., p. 18.

There are substantial gaps between hospital-centered training of the physician and the flow of treatment actually provided to the public. For a typical population of 1,000 in one year, some 720 people visit a physician in an ambulatory setting. From the 720 physician visits, only 100 are admitted to a hospital at least once. But only 10 of these, in turn, were admitted to a university hospital. Because of this filtering process, the medical students' exposure to the full range of procedures is limited. It is important, therefore, that there be an increased effort for the physician to relate to his patients in an ambulatory setting, and that he appreciate the impact of external environmental influences as well as internal psychic elements in the diagnosis and treatment of his patients. The enormous qualitative and quantitative gaps between what a patient expects from his physician and what he in fact receives may well reflect the hurried pace of the specialist practitioner. Again, as White makes the point, general practitioners may be disappearing, but the general problems patients bring to them are not.[17]

The structure of the existing educational process is demanding, with pressures that require attention to detail, long hours of exhausting study, and masochistic rigors. The experience may tend to squeeze from the individual those idealistic traits that were person-centered. In one view, the physician emerges with an obsessive, compulsive personality. He may have deferred marriage and the privilege of having a family or purchasing a home.

Let us recapitulate: the Flexner report identified the unhappy consequences of commercialized medicine, and contended that access limited only by the costs of education would flood the medical market with pragmatic and opportunistic medical practitioners, with a kind of Gresham's Law at work: bad service would drive out good service. With the sponsorship of the prestigious Carnegie Foundation, governments cooperated with the AMA to restrict the number of medical schools, raise entry and graduation standards, and dampen the flow of persons serving the medical market. The result was less total medical service to the American public and improved income for the physician. Between World War I and World War II, the focus of medicine shifted from family practice to research, exalting the breakthroughs in biochemistry that led to remarkable triumphs of disease control. But the preoccupation with pure research led to a depreciation of the importance of patient contact.

With the research orientation came splintering of functions and the emergence of the superspecialist. It is an axiom of economics that the division of labor permits dramatic improvements in total productivity.

[17] Kerr L. White, "Organization and Delivery of Personal Health Services: Public Policy Issues." In John B. McKinley (ed.), *Politics and Law in Health Care Policy* (New York: Prodist, 1973), p. 346. See also Kerr L. White, "Life and Death and Medicine," *Scientific American*, Vol. 229, no. 3 (September 1973), pp. 23–33.

Division of labor characterizes the structure of our present physician service but sometimes, from the patient's viewpoint, with disappointing consequences. In the medical industry, specialization and superspecialization abounds. This reflects the increasing of medical knowledge and the fact that advances in our understanding have involved sophisticated technology, research teams, and dependence on hospital facilities with their diagnostic and laboratory aids. This superstructure has, in turn, been supported by an increasing number of paraprofessional workers.

Within this structure, medical-school students quickly absorb the value structure: the "important" services to health are achieved in the laboratory, not through general practice in Small Town, USA. He wants to absorb as much as possible and contribute to advances through his own research. Since he cannot master the entire field, he can establish his credentials through specialized attention to a selective field.

Research and specialization have produced a fascination with "exotic" or "interesting" forms of illness. The common criticism emerges: "America is the best country in the world for serious illness." While the present system provides adequate care for episodic, specific illnesses, it is short on personalized lifelong programs of prevention and rehabilitation. The system provides for "sporadic bursts" to meet individual health needs:

> Today, we must wait until we are ill (preferably very ill) before modern medicine can bring its sophisticated techniques into play. Hospitals, medical researchers, and, to a surprising extent, private practitioners prefer it this way: Illness is impersonal, isolatable, scientific. . . . People, thought of in terms of what's needed to prevent illness, are not nearly as tractable.[18]

The point is clear that a satisfactory health system must give added attention to the consumer and to the peculiarities of his emotional as well as physiological needs during a time of illness and accidents. It will have to integrate preventive and curative systems; also, it must assume responsibility for "health maintenance," especially where such attention does not center on repair but on lifestyles that sustain good health. As we have noted, our educational process has little that prepares specialists to be generalists or that gives the health-care specialists an awareness of or concern for the vast range of external influences that have a major influence on health.

Americans take pride (and properly so) in leading the world in technological development. We have fallen in love with "pure" as opposed to "applied" research, confident that the spillover benefits of pure research will inevitably (and rapidly) be passed on to consumers. It is not

[18] Fred Anderson, "We Can Do It Better, Cheaper," *The New Republic*, January 24, 1970, p. 14.

illogical to conclude that conceptual ignorance inhibits our capacity to control disease. With the appropriate medical knowledge in hand (reflecting the germination of successful research), there is no medical problem that will remain insoluble. As Andreano and Weisbrod point out, after World War II the United States alone seemed to acquire a posture of believing that knowledge per se was the key to adequate medical care. Meanwhile, much of the rest of the world deployed resources to apply known remedies to known afflictions. The former strategy involved the development of new information; the latter, the delivery of traditional information to remedy existing health problems.

These historic interests in scientific explorations that characterize the United States health industry have generated remarkable breakthroughs. But often these remedies were expensive:

> The achievement of dazzling technology became a goal itself. Heart transplants became possible, but at a cost of $40,000 or more, and 80 percent of the patients died within four months. People with previously fatal kidney defects could be saved by the use of new kidney dialysis equipment, but at costs of thousands of dollars per year, continuing indefinitely. The lives of persons who suffered from severe infections caused by a lack of oxygen could be saved by hyperbaric chambers, but these cost three quarters of a million dollars each to install and $600,000 per year to operate. It is understandable that the federal government and the consumer have become increasingly impatient with the growing gap between knowledge and its delivery and, at the same time, increasingly troubled by the high cost of closing the gap.[19]

LICENSING AND JOB CONTENT

Licensing provisions specify work functions for professional specialties. Probably no profession, including the construction trades, is characterized by such exclusionary entrance or admission policies as the medical profession. The analogy of the industrial worker and craftsman are appropriate. The former is intended to perform a single function well. The production process is designed to minimize dependence on individual specialties. In contrast, craft workers possess a bundle of skills, some held in reserve for relatively rare occasions. The purchasers of such services are obligated to pay for the large inventory of capabilities, even though few of these may be used for a specified job or function. The pressure of consumers to secure production and services at reasonable prices has compelled the substantial reorganization of American industry. Today the

19 Abraham Ribicoff, "The 'Healthiest Nation' Myth," *Saturday Review*, 22 (August 1970), pp. 18, 19.

bulk of labor services assumes an industrial rather than a craft form. The medical sector, however, has tenaciously resisted any tendency for the "belt-line" production of services. The entire industry has been physician- and craft-centered. Physician dominance and control of the industry was very much extended through the implementation of the Flexner report. The study's impact reduced the number of medical schools from more than two hundred in 1900 to only seventy-six in 1930, and the physician emerged at the very center of the health-care system:

> Physicians became preeminent in this system, the ultimate arbiters of what constituted "good" medical care, who received it, and how much it cost. The predominant form of practice was fee-for-service. Access to the system was achieved through the sponsorship of a privately practicing physician. The enforcement of quality standards on individual physicians and on medical schools was accomplished through physician-dominated accreditation groups at the state and national level, which to a large extent determined the number and level of training of physicians. . . .[20]

The physician determines his own job functions. He is in charge. However, he appears to be caught in an administrative trap, for he has assigned to himself the full range of duties, many of which could be performed by persons with much less elaborate training. Individually and collectively, physicians are apprehensive about sharing job functions with others. Perhaps such anxiety reflects a concern that such scattering of responsibility might involve an erosion of control, influence, economic status, and an increased risk of malpractice suits.

A federal government's white paper reports on the misallocation of human resources related to obsolete job structures:

> The Joint Council of National Pediatric Societies . . . has stated that 75 percent of the pediatric tasks performed by a physician could be done by a properly trained child-health assistant. A significant proportion of the tasks performed by obstetricians, similarly, can be performed by nurse-midwives without any loss in the quality of care. And experience with several physicians'-assistants programs has demonstrated that ex-medical corpsmen, or comparably trained individuals, with some additional training can assume a large number of tasks performed now by general practitioners.

> With regard to dental services, it has been amply demonstrated that one chairside assistant, efficiently used, increases a dentist's productivity by 50 percent; a second assistant adds another 25 percent; and by properly utilizing all the skills of the dental team, a dentist can more than double his productivity.

[20] Ralph L. Andreano and Burton A. Weisbrod, *American Health Policy* (Chicago: Rand McNally, 1974), p. 26.

. . . Nurses in hospitals are still spending only 35 percent of their time in caring for patients, the remainder being utilized for administrative tasks. Nurses in physicians' offices spend even less time on the care of patients.[21]

We appear to be caught, then, in arrangements in which the subspecialties in medical care each guard those prerogatives that have been identified as properly belonging to them. When any formal motion is made to redesign jobs, to reallocate function, or to reassign duties, there is a reflex action to preserve the status quo. Critical functions are not fully separated from the casual or supportive function. Creative and productive energies are dissipated in administrative, reporting, and other support activities that could readily be performed by specialized aides.

Such difficulties are compounded by licensing and certification arrangements that are largely controlled by the professional subspecialty itself. Admission standards for medical schools, the delineation of function for nurses, the cultural difference in status between registered nurses and practical nurses, all serve to complicate the task of rationalizing function.

Significantly, the attitudes of the physician, just as they have been socialized by the values of medical colleges, in turn permeate the value structure of hospitals and other care facilities. The struggle to establish integrity through licensing and through well-defined job responsibilities has affected almost every other specialty within the structure. Glenn Wilson of the University of North Carolina Medical School explained to a congressional committee just how pervasive the guild system is within the field. Such numerical growth of allied and supporting personnel is of particular significance, as attempts are made to lighten physicians' burdens and responsibilities:

> The decade of the sixties witnessed an explosive public demand for health services which was vastly beyond the capacity of the providers. The initial lethargic response of both the educational institutions and the providers only increased the frustration. One consequence of this frustration has been the creation of a wide variety of new health-professional roles to fill the void. There are currently 422 different job descriptions in the health field. Although increasing emphasis is being placed upon the health-care team, the nation runs the risk of further fractioning the delivery of service at a time when the public is clamouring to be treated as a whole person. As new professional groups have emerged, they have inevitably formed national organizations, have taken on all the trappings of a guild, each asserting, under the banner of good patient care, that they hold an important answer to the national health-care

[21] "Towards a Comprehensive Health Policy for the 1970's," A White Paper, HEW (Washington, D.C.: GPO, 1971), p. 11.

problem. One needs only to re-read the history of the feudal era in Europe to see how a tight guild structure immobilized that society.[22]

SUMMARY AND RECAPITULATION

In this chapter, we juxtaposed the professionalism of medical services with commercialism. During the nineteenth century, proprietary medical schools provided a broad range of educational experiences, but there was little uniformity in graduation standards. Physicians advertised freely, often providing their own patent medicines. Through the implementation of the Flexner report, there was a restriction on the number of medical schools and a decline in the flow of graduates. As standards were raised, the quality of medical services increased while the volume of low-cost care declined. The physician emerged as the individual "in charge," enjoying government approval for licensing boards and internal regulation of quality standards in the medical field.

Flowing from this reach for excellence was a redirection of energies from simple practice to research. The focus of medical-school training became biochemistry and physiology, to the neglect of the sociology of population medicine.

The triumphs of research that led to the control of major epidemics and "killer" diseases had other consequences. With increased knowledge of disease control came specialization. And with specialization came a fragmentation of services, so commonly viewed as a major flaw in today's delivery system. In brief, most physicians do not have either the skills for or the interest in treating the whole person, rather than the specialized areas of affliction. Expertise in the treatment of the parts has been secured at some loss in the continuity of care and in the physician's understanding of the whole range of environmental and other external elements that could effect the patient's recovery prospects.

Specialization creates other problems as well. Those with single-purpose skills must locate in densely populated areas and, as a consequence, we notice the urbanization of medical services. Related to the problem of distribution is the issue of income. With a fee-for-service standard determining levels of income, it is important to secure a practice in affluent areas. The redistribution of medical service is thus away from rural America, and more particularly the thinly populated areas with low to moderate incomes, to urban and particularly high-income areas. Core-city areas of major metropolitan areas, increasingly dominated

[22] Statement submitted, *Medical Policies and Costs,* Hearings before the Subcommittee on Consumer Economics of the Joint Economic Committee, Congress of the U.S., 93rd Congress, 1st Session, May 16, 1973, p. 138.

by minorities and problems of crime and unemployment, have become high-risk service areas for the physician and have been avoided.

Specialization has even further consequences. It encourages a clinical view of medical services, with an appearance of impersonality and the dominance of technology. Most service is hospital-based, adding to both the cost of care and the apprehension of patients caught up in a seemingly impersonal and authoritarian system.

The research orientation of medical training has further adverse consequences. In the screening process determining who will secure hospital attention in university-based medical centers, there is a natural curiosity for the unusual afflictions. These patients become the students' first exposure to the afflicted population, and tend to reinforce this medical interest in uncommon problems. Interest in the rare afflictions discourages an interest in caring for the ordinary afflictions.

We have touched on only a few of the problems that have prevented the rational attention to health-care needs. First, the attention of the health-care system is local rather than national. Clearly most physicians have responded to market realities and potential earnings, not to existing needs unsupported by income. Physicians have resisted any "dilution" of job status that might come with the restructuring of job content; such resistance involves substantial extravagances in the use of medical talent for report-writing, and administrative services. The occupational structure within the industry is characterized by hierarchies of occupational pockets, each with its own certifying process, each jealously protecting prerogatives and traditional job structures. There is tragically little occupational mobility within the industry, for a posture of exclusion is often the unfortunate by-product of professional enclaves. Physicians have been attracted to specialty services rather than general practice, accounting for a redundancy of talent in the former and a serious scarcity of service in the latter. Further, the industry has grown enchanted with "pure" research intended to identify the root cause of many illnesses, rather than with the broad dispensation of knowledge reflecting existing wisdom and traditional technologies. There is little doubt that the tradeoff decision favoring the future over the present will benefit future generations. But the unattended sick in our present society are bearing the cost of decisions they had no part in making.

SUGGESTED READINGS

"The American Medical Association: Power, Purpose and Politics in Organized Medicine," *Yale Law Journal*, Vol. 63, no. 7 (May 1954), pp. 938–1022. A treatise on the subject of AMA control of the health-care system. It sets the stage for the contemporary thrust of the AMA in preserving professional integrity.

BOWMAN, ELIZABETH, "Senate Alters Health Manpower Programs," *Congressional Quarterly Weekly Report*, July 10, 1976, p. 1833. Examines the theory that the National Health Service Corps program is designed not only to subsidize students in their education, but also to ensure that we can overcome the geographic maldistribution of health professionals.

CASSEDY, JAMES H., "An Early American Hangover: The Medical Profession and Intemperance, 1880–1860," *Bulletin of the History of Medicine*, Vol. 50 (1976), pp. 405–13. A discussion of the evolution of professional standards for medical care.

CHAPMAN, CARLETON B. and JOHN M. TALMADGE, "Historical and Political Background of Federal Health Care Legislation," *Law and Contemporary Problems*, Duke University Law School, Health Care, Part I, Vol. 35, no. 2 (Spring 1970), pp. 334–47. The political history of early efforts to involve the federal government in health care.

COHEN, HARRIS S., "Professional Licensure, Organizational Behavior and the Public Interest," *Milbank Memorial Fund Quarterly*, Vol. 51, no. 1 (Winter 1973), pp. 73–88. An account of the restrictive policies of the AMA concerning the licensing of physicians.

CULLISON, SAM, CHRISTOPHER REID, and JACK M. COLWILL, "Medical School Admissions, Specialty Selection, and Distribution of Physicians," *Journal of the American Medical Association*, Vol. 235, no. 5 (February 2, 1976), pp. 502–5. A critique of the specialization of physicians.

CULLISON, SAM, CHRISTOPHER REID, and JACK M. COLWILL, "The Rural–Urban Distribution of Medical School Applicants," *Journal of Medical Education*, Vol. 51 (January 1976), pp. 47–49. A timely discussion of the distribution of physicians and the efforts to attract students of rural medical schools in hopes that they will return to their home communities.

DEVER, G. E. ALLEN, "Locational Characteristics of Selected Medical Manpower in the United States: 1970," *Atlanta Economic Review* (November/December 1974), pp. 41–46. Portrays the ratio of service to population for key medical specialties.

FAHS, I. J. and O. L. PETERSON, "Towns Without Physicians and Towns With Only One: A Study of Four States in the Upper Midwest, 1965," *American Journal of Public Health*, Vol. 58, no. 7 (July 1968), pp. 1200–1211. A study conducted to identify the degree of neglect of physician services to rural America.

GOLDMAN, MARTIN E., "Something There is That Doesn't Love a Wall: The Need for a Conceptual Approach to Professional Responsibility," *George Washington Law Review*, Vol. 43, no. 3 (March 1975), pp. 713–28. A general review of the issue of professional responsibility, including definitions of responsible behavior for lawyers and accountants.

MORROW, JOHN H. and ARCH B. EDWARDS, "U.S. Health Manpower Policy: Will the Benefits Justify the Costs?," *Journal of Medical Education*, Vol. 51 (October 1976). An essay on the anticipated increase of active physicians, which is expected to produce an increase of four percent in the proportions of national product expended for medical care.

SENIOR, BORIS and BEVERLY A. SMITH, "The Number of Physicians as a Constraint on Delivery of Health Care: How Many Physicians Are Enough?," *Journal of the American Medical Association*, Vol. 222, no. 2 (October 9, 1972), pp. 178–83. Raises the questions of the adequacy of physician supply and their distribution.

STEVENS, ROSEMARY, *American Medicine and the Public Interest* (New Haven: Yale University Press, 1971). A detailed account of the physicians' trends to specialization.

TANCREDI, LAURENCE R. and JOHN WOODS, "The Social Control of Medical Practice," *Milbank Memorial Fund Quarterly*, Vol. 1, no. 1 (January 1972), pp. 99–125. A critical examination of the licensure procedures for establishing competency for medical service.

WAITZKIN, HOWARD B. and BARBARA WATERMAN, *The Exploitation of Illness in Capitalist Society* (Indianapolis: Bobbs-Merrill, 1974). A radical critique of professionalism providing summaries of social theories of medicine, including the contributions of Parsons, Mechanic, and Freidson.

3

SYSTEM TRENDS: EXPENDITURES, COSTS, AND FUNDING SOURCES

The health market represents one of the most important, yet most neglected sectors of the American economy. We now spend more than the equivalent of one month's earnings per year for health care. In terms of total dollars, we spend more for health services than we do for food, or for national defense, or for all levels of education. Expenditure levels are now soaring well above $130 billion annually. All of this represents an effort to provide adequate health services as a "right" rather than as a privilege. Given the option of subsidizing the demand or socializing the delivery system itself, we have opted for demand subsidies. The rapid increase of public reimbursements has not, however, been matched by a proportionate increase of health services. What are the reasons for this?

DEMAND PRESSURES AND THE PRICE RESPONSE

In the 12 months ending June 1975, each person in the United States had spent $547 for health care. For this same time period, personal income per capita was $5,633. For an average family of 4, then, health-care expenditures were $2,188. In affect, each individual was spending a startling 9.7 percent of his personal income for health services.

The massive outpouring of funds has undoubtedly served to raise costs and prices in the medical market. Indeed, for the first 3 months of 1976, medical-care services rose at an annual rate of 14 percent, physician fees at 14.2 percent, and hospital-services charges at 20.1 percent. This contrasts sharply with the annual index rate for all consumer purchases of only 3.9 percent for the same period. If the medical-care index were removed from the consumer price index, actual costs during the first quarter would have increased at an annual rate of only 2.4 percent. Thus, medical-care inflation in that quarter accounted for close to 40 percent of the inflationary problem.

In reviewing these data Michael H. Moskow, director of the administration's wage-price watchdog agency, noted that the medical market was "different," lacking any conspicuous economic rewards for either efficiency or cost reduction. He further noted that the government pays for more than 42 percent of total health-care costs. When we add to this the reality of other third-party payments (involving private insurance) and consider, too, that the physician is largely in control of the nature and extent of services to patients, we may well conclude that the consumer is a "passive participant" in the spending spree. In 1975, third-party payments covered 67.4 percent of all personal health-care expenditures, including 92 percent of all hospital bills, and 65.5 percent of all doctor bills.[1] Clearly, demand "pull" must be a major force accounting for these remarkable upward price adjustments.

The magnitude of the expenditure increase may be cast in even more vivid terms if we broaden the time span of historic comparison. In fiscal 1929, we spent about $3.2 billion for health services. For a population of 123 million, this amounted to only $26 for each individual. Some 88 percent of the total bill was paid directly by consumers themselves. This compares, as noted above, with the less than one-third of out-of-pocket payments made today. In fiscal 1975, private insurance paid approximately one-quarter of the health bill. As noted above, governments paid about 40 percent of the tab, with the federal government picking up a 28-percent portion, state and local governments a 12-percent portion. Interestingly, the 1929 per capita expenditure level of $25.72 had actually decreased to $25.47 in 1940. The spiral of both expenditures and prices appears to be a post–World War II phenomena. Analytically, the challenge is to identify the extent to which the expenditure flow has induced the price increase in contrast to the possibility that autonomous price increases necessitated an enlarged expenditure flow.

In fiscal 1975, hospital care accounted for 45 percent of all medical expenses. But as noted above, only 8 percent of such hospital bills were paid by out-of-pocket expenditures by patients. Private insurance paid over 36 percent of the hospital bills, and public funds over 55 percent. The next largest category of expenditure involved payments for physician services, absorbing 21 percent of medical-care spending in fiscal 1975. For this vital aspect of care, private insurance paid 39 percent of the bill, public funds 26 percent, and patient out-of-pocket expenditures 34 percent. We see why patients are much more likely to be concerned about the bill for physician services than for hospital care.

[1] These data are provided in the Council on Wage and Price Stability Report in a thirty-page study, with highlights reproduced in The St. Louis Globe Democrat, "Medical Care Costs Spiral," April 26, 1976.

Of most concern to the patient are his out-of-pocket expenditures. These averaged $155 per capita in fiscal 1975. Twenty-three percent of direct payments went for physician services, 11 percent for hospital-care costs, and a substantial 66 percent for "other" health-care costs, such as dentistry and drugs. Philanthropy and industry provided $6 per capita for health services, with 41 percent of that modest total serving hospital care.[2]

What might account for the ten-fold increase of spending levels from 1950 to 1975? It has been estimated that population growth accounts for only about 15 percent of the expenditure increase. An expanded use of health resources, including technological improvements, may account for another 37 percent of the enlarged flow. This leaves a considerable "unexplained residual," which is mostly attributed to the increase in the cost of services.

Between 1950 and 1965 the annual increase of the medical-care component of the Consumer Price Index (CPI) was 3.5 percent. This compares with the overall 1.8-percent annual change of the CPI. From 1965 to 1975, however, the annual rate of change of health-care prices almost doubled to 6.5 percent. The CPI showed an accelerated annual rate of change, too, increasing at an average rate of 5.5 percent.

Undoubtedly the unequal price increases among the various medical-care components help explain the shift in the distribution of resources for spending. For example in fiscal 1950, hospital care absorbed 35.5 percent of expenditures. By fiscal 1975, that proportion had increased sharply to 45.2 percent. During this same period, hospital-care prices increased more sharply than other health-care service costs. If hospitals were getting proportionately more, who was getting proportionately less? The fiscal 1950 share for physicians services, 25.9 percent, was reduced by 1975 to 21.4 percent. Dentists experienced a similar decline in their share, from 9 percent in fiscal 1950 to 7.3 percent in fiscal 1975. Prescriptions and drugs declined even more sharply, from 15.8 percent in 1950 to 10.3 percent in 1975. Note that the costs of prescriptions and drugs were much more stable than other components in the health-care price index.

There are divergent geographic patterns in health-care costs. A National Industrial Conference Board report indicates that in 1974 a typical four-person family in Los Angeles spent $901 in medical care, compared to only $650 for a similar family in Buffalo, St. Louis, Cincinnati, or Pittsburgh. There are unexplained variations in costs that run as high as ten percent between cities that are in close proximity, such as Chicago and Milwaukee. The Intermediate-budget families faced the highest costs in Los Angeles, San Diego, Dallas, San Francisco, Baltimore, and New York

2 Ken Goldstein, "Health Care Expenditures," The National Industrial Conference Board, Road Maps of Industry, No. 1780, March 1976.

City. Low-cost cities include Minneapolis, Buffalo, Cincinnati, Pittsburgh, and St. Louis. Levels of existing costs do not fully correlate, however, with the geographic patterns of cost increases. The leading cities for average annual increases include Detroit, Baltimore, Atlanta, Philadelphia, and New York City. Those with the lowest cost increases include Minneapolis, Buffalo, Dallas, Boston, and St. Louis.

Tracing the patterns of medical-care costs over time must take account of the economic-stabilization program. Beginning in August 1971, the health sector was covered by mandatory economic controls, with that stabilization effort sustained until April 30, 1974. Even though controls were in effect for ten months of fiscal 1974, medical-care prices began to accelerate several months before the end of the program.[3] Part of this increase in the price of hospital services (as with other industrial prices) has been attributed to "catch-up" efforts on the part of the industry, as well as a precaution against the reimposition of price controls. It is paradoxical that concern about "uncontrolled" inflation in this sector may have the perverse effect of exacerbating the problem.

We have noted that hospital care continues to command an increasing share of the medical-expenditure flow. The cost and price pressures in this sector will be given detailed attention later. But we should note parenthetically that admissions in community hospitals increased from 26,831,000 in 1966 to 32,752,000 in 1974. The average length of stay, however, diminished slightly, from 7.6 days in 1966 to 7.4 days in 1974. If we multiply admissions times the average length of stay, we get total patient days. These increased from 203,741,000 in 1966 to 242,393,000 in 1974. Clearly, the greater demand on facilities helps explain price increases. But note, too, that hospitals were not operating at full capacity during this period. The occupancy rate was only 76.4 percent in 1966, and this dropped to 75.4 percent in 1974. Throughout the period it ranged from a low of 75 percent to a high of 78.5 percent. For the period, admissions increased 22 percent, hospital days 19 percent. But total expenses increased much more sharply, from $9.7 billion to $30.1 billion, or an increase of 310 percent. Expenses per patient day increased from $43.58 to $110.77, for a 252-percent adjustment. In related terms, therefore, cost pressures seemed much more intensive than could be reasonably attributed to demand pressure. To recapitulate: an increase in the level of use of 19 percent was concurrently associated with a 25 percent unused capacity and cost increases per patient of 252 percent.[4]

Spending for nursing-home care reached an estimated level of $7.5 billion in 1974 and was then increasing by twelve percent annually. This is the fastest-growing expenditure category for government funding, re-

[3] Nancy L. Worthington, "National Health Expenditures, 1929–74," *Social Security Bulletin,* February 1975, p. 3.
[4] Ibid., p. 4.

flecting reclassification of expenditures previously made by the Office of Economic Opportunity (OEO) as well as the impact of Medicare payments.

Government expenditures for health services continue to expand at a rate about double that of the private sector. At the federal level, Medicare and Medicaid programs account for eighty percent of the overall rise in public spending. Each program involved $11 billion for benefits and administration in 1974. In effect, the two programs account for seventy-five percent of total government expenditures and eighty-eight percent of federal government expenditures.[5] In July 1973, Medicare coverage was extended to pay cash benefits for individuals suffering disability for a two-year period and for persons with chronic kidney disease. It was estimated that 1.7 million disabled persons and 9,300 persons with chronic renal disease were eligible for Medicare coverage, adding to the expenditure flow.

Other cost pressures within the medical sector reflect the fact that it is labor- rather than capital-intensive. Many medical personnel have been seeking "catch-up" wage and salary adjustments, reflected in part by militant unionization procedures. Hospitals have concurrently increased the ratio of supporting personnel to each patient in a bid to improve the quality of care. The change in the patient/supporting-personnel ratio has been statistically much more significant than wage and salary adjustments in raising labor costs. Medical technology has not, for the most part, been labor-saving, but tends to set in motion a fresh demand for additional personnel with high levels of skills. Technological breakthroughs, in effect, involve large capital-intensive investments, which require additional technically proficient and well-trained personnel. Another circumstance is that specialization of services, long considered a key to economies of scale in most economic sectors, appears to have had a perverse effect on medical-care costs. Ken Goldstein notes how the penchant for medical specialization has added to costs: "One method of achieving greater productivity is by increasing the specialization of tasks, where possible. But the increased specialization of physicians has exacerbated the shortage of general practitioners."[6] The "scarce" general or family practitioner has been able to raise fees for services. When he is not available, an increasing number of patients have rushed to the emergency facilities of community hospitals.

A further obvious factor accounting for greater expenditures is our insistence on improving the quality and quantity of services at the same time. There have, however, been some improvements in productivity over time. For example, the AMA reports that the typical physician in the late

[5] Ibid., p. 7.
[6] Ken Goldstein, "The Rising Cost of Medical Care," National Industrial Conference Board, Road Maps of Industry, No. 1779, March 1976, p. 2.

1930s saw an average of fifty patients per week. By the late 1960s, his average weekly load had increased to about 130. This has the effect of improving physician productivity; but with the primary reliance on a fee-for-service structure, the heavier case load is more likely to be reflected in improved physician income than lower patient costs.

Medical-care expenditures continue to increase because of the popular illusion that by spending more money, we can in fact purchase more substantial amounts of quality care. But as a nation we are reluctant to acknowledge the problems of drug abuse, venereal disease, obesity, sedentary lifestyles, and other consquences of self-indulgence that fall outside the influence of most medical-care providers. As health providers emphasize, we continue the spree of self-indulgence, confident that a concurrent spending spree for health services can "cover" any threatened risk to health.

ANOTHER VIEW OF THIRD-PARTY PAYMENTS

Probably the most important force encouraging increased spending is the rapid growth of third-party payments. These induce the illusion that the costs of securing immediate services are minimal or nonexistent. This is equally true for private insurance as for public reimbursements. In the former case, such costs must be met by premium payments. Here, an individual may rightly conclude that his personal costs are minimal if the employer meets the entire premium cost. He does not typically consider that such fringe benefits are provided as a substitute for wage benefits otherwise available. In the latter case, the taxpayer pays the bill. Several of the taxes providing revenues for the public sector are regressive, meaning that those with only modest resources pay a disproportionate amount. Even so, an individual may logically conclude that he gains much more as a patient-consumer than he loses as a taxpayer. Indeed, the only certain way of coming out ahead is to make certain your individual medical-care services are more substantial than all applicable taxes and premium payments. But what is true for the individual cannot, of course, be true for the collective.

Let us reconstruct the data showing the steep trend toward third-party payments. The American health system is distinguished by its heavy reliance on private insurance schemes. In 1974, benefit payments for all forms of private insurance involved some $23 billion, a level that had doubled in the few years since 1968. As noted earlier, about sixty percent of benefits from this source pays for hospital care, and one-third pays for physician services. There has been very little shift to third-party payments when we move from hospital and physician categories to "other" health services. For example, only sixty-eight cents of every ten dollars spent for dental care is reimbursed by private insurance plans.

Nineteen sixty-seven was a threshold year in the American health sector. For the first time, out-of-pocket payments for health services were less than half of total health-care expenditures. Since that year, out-of-pocket payments have declined steadily so that now they involve no more than one-third of total expenditures. Paradoxically, however, because the costs of such services have increased so sharply, the fact that the out-of-pocket *share* has declined has not prevented the absolute dollars of personal expenditure from increasing. Indeed, per capita direct expenditures by consumers is now double what it was in 1950.[7]

Let us compare the role of third-party payments for the three major categories of health-care consumption. In 1950, direct payments by the consumer for hospital care were 34.2 percent (16 percent of the bill was paid by private insurance, 45.7 percent by the government). By 1974, out-of-pocket contributions were only 10.4 percent (private insurance more than doubled to 35.4 percent, and public support increased to 52.9 percent). This was truly the golden age for the expansion of private insurance in hospital care.

For physicians' services, private direct payments in 1950 were 84.8 percent (insurance benefits paid 10 percent of the bill and the government 5 percent). By 1974 private direct payments declined to 38.8 percent. Private insurance benefits were then about equivalent to out-of-pocket costs: 37.3 percent. The most dramatic increase has been the government's share: 27.8 percent. Although the government still ranks third as a contributor to physician fees, the rapid increase may well account for physician anxieties about his future autonomy in the medical market. In round numbers, the government's share of support in this market has increased by some 20 percentage points in 25 years; thus it is not difficult to understand why some physicians have anticipated the time when government becomes the major purchaser of their services.

When we turn to the third largest category of health-care purchases, a catch-all category that includes dentists' services, other professional services, drugs and drug sundries, eyeglasses, nursing-home care, and the like, we find less conspicuous increases of third-party payments. Direct payments by private parties in 1950 represented 88.8 percent of the total, with insignificant support by private insurance companies. Government support provided 7 percent of these benefits. By 1974, the out-of-pocket share declined to 67 percent, private insurance benefits increased to 5.2 percent, and public support rose to 25.7 percent.[8]

[7] Data are provided by Nancy L. Worthington, "National Health Expenditures, 1929–74," *Social Security Bulletin*, February 1974, pp. 13–20.
[8] Ibid., p. 14.

A CLOSER LOOK AT HOSPITAL COSTS

Because hospital costs have moved up so sharply and because hospital services account for some $41 billion of spending (compared with expenditures for physicians of $19 billion), let us take a closer look at the sources of cost pressures within hospitals.

First, and most conspicuous, has been the rush to advanced forms of technology in all hospitals. In 1960, only 18 percent of nonprofit private hospitals had an electroencephalograph, and this ratio increased to 45.1 percent in 1972. Only 11 percent had an intensive-care unit in 1960, and this increased to 68 percent in 1972. Few hospitals provided cobalt therapy in 1960, but 18 percent provided this service in 1972. There is a spreading interest in intensive-care units for victims of heart attacks, severe burns, and traumatic shock. There is, in addition, pressure for hospitals to provide more community services, including home-care programs, family planning, and outpatient psychiatric care.[9]

Another cost consideration is the rapid increase of plant investment, requiring $22.5 billion in 1972. The stock of capital has increased by a factor of 8 in only 22 years. It is surprising that the profitmaking hospitals have one-half the capital investments of their nonprofit counterparts. This suggests that investments in medical technology and plant facilities in profitmaking hospitals are constrained by considerations of returns. By inference, one possible cost-push factor is the absence of constraints on capital and technological investments for those units that are not obligated to yield a surplus. Much of this capital growth has undoubtedly been encouraged by the Hill Burton program. Beginning in July 1947, this act provided over $2.6 billion for construction and modernization of about 350,000 beds in general hospitals. From 1950 to 1972, the number of beds per 1,000 civilian residents increased from 3.35 to 4.28.

There has been a gradual decline in the average length of hospital stays, from 8.3 days in 1969 to 7.9 in 1972; therefore, one would expect that this would provide for some reduction of visit costs. But with the compression of hospital visit time, there is a need to pack a greater intensity of service into the shorter time frame. This has served to increase costs. It is also possible that the decline in the length of stay accounts particularly for the 25-percent vacancy rate. As a consequence, daily costs per case have been increased, as hospitals make a bid to cover their overhead costs of idle capacity.

[9] *Medical Care: Expenditures, Prices and Costs.* HEW, Social Security Administration, Office of Research and Statistics, DHEW Publication No. SSA 74-11909, GPO, 1973, p. 31.

One remarkable phenomenon is the rapid increase in the volume of outpatient care provided by hospitals. There are six individuals treated on an outpatient or ambulatory basis for every one treated in the hospital. This, however, is a somewhat misleading index of service. The number of patient *days* provided for inpatients is double the number of persons seen on an ambulatory basis. The growth of outpatient services is of much interest to government and others concerned about cost reduction. Outpatient visits per capita have risen sharply—some sixty-seven percent from 1965 to 1972. From 1969 to 1972, they were increasing at an annual rate of ten percent.[10]

One problem in attempting to identify the "real" increases of medical services lies in the medical-care component of the consumer price index. That index does not take account of the full range of medical services provided, nor indeed of the changing market basket of services from year to year since the base period. Nursing-home care and private-duty nursing are not priced in the index. There are problems of weighting as well. For example, hospital charges are assigned a weight of about twenty-seven percent, but we have noted above that hospital-care expenditures account for close to fifty percent of medical expenditures.

The measurement of hospital costs has always posed problems simply because we lack any historic index of those costs. The Bureau of Labor Statistics (BLS) does measure the charges for semiprivate rooms, but this is hardly a representative index. First, that charge excludes consideration of drugs, tests, and blood costs, as well as the use of operating rooms or intensive-care units. With the "depackaging" of hospital costs, these supplemental items assume an increasing proportion of total costs. Second, changes in the mix of services can involve substantial adjustments of patient-day costs not reflected in the room cost alone.

The American Hospital Association provides an estimate of patient-day costs by dividing the aggregate of all expenses (including expenses for the treatment of outpatients) by the number of inpatient days. This expense index has obvious limits. It is overstated to the extent that outpatient services are substantial; it is understated because it omits any charge to the patient that is not billed by the hospital, such as physician fees.

A third cost index is the "adjusted" patient day. This estimates the cost of services to ambulatory patients and compares it to the cost of inpatient care. Thus, if treatment costs for outpatients were twenty percent of the average treatment costs for inpatients, five episodes of outpatient are equivalent to inpatient care. Total expenses are then divided by the equivalent of full-time patients. A final measure divides total hospital expenses by the number of admissions to get an index of costs per case. Adjustments are sometimes made to take account of the outpatient visits.

[10] Ibid., pp. 34–35.

From 1950 to 1972, the BLS index shows that semiprivate room charges increased from an index level of 57.3 to 173.9. Total expense per patient day increased from $32.23 to $105.21. Expense per admission increased from $244.54 to $830.13. Most categories of hospital costs increased at an annual rate of about 13 percent from 1965 to 1972.[11]

In spite of these cost pressures—some would say because of them—the hospital sector has been able to realize profits. From 1950 to 1971, net income per patient day for nongovernmental community hospitals increased from 29 cents to $3.00. Indeed, the average annual increase of net income for this period was 13.9 percent for nonprofit hospitals. Annual increases in net income per patient days were 7.7 percent for profitmaking hospitals. These surpluses reflect the more extensive use of hospitals, the growth of third-party payments ensuring reimbursements, retrospective payments by the government, and the flow of Medicare and Medicaid reimbursements to hospitals. Net income per patient day for nonprofit hospitals in 1971 was $2.63; for the profitmaking hospitals it was $6.43. Together, both enjoyed a $547 million surplus.[12]

Studies of the cost pressures in hospitals indicate the increase in costs that hospitals must absorb in their purchases of supplies, along with more extended levels of purchases for each patient treated. One is a price effect, the other the quantity effect involving an effort to improve services. From 1971 to 1972, as a case in point, the wage-and-price effect raised hospital costs by 6.2 percent, and the quantity effects required a 7.8 percent increase. The labeling of additional expenditures as "improvements of service" may be somewhat misleading, for it reflects the intent rather than the measured consequence of additional purchases. For most years since 1950, the distribution of these two alternative explanations for higher costs is about equally divided.

Because hospitals are labor-intensive enterprises, it is tempting to identify wage increases as a prime cause of the cost pressures. There has been considerable union activity in this field, along with the application of minimum-wage laws, to confirm this view. Indeed, in 1950 the average annual earnings of the hospital employee was only $1,817. By 1972, this had increased to $7,062, for an annual percentage increase for the period of 6.4 percent.

But there were additions of staff too. In 1950, there were 1.78 employees per daily census. By 1972, this had increased to 3.10 persons, for an annual percentage increase of 2.6 for the period.

Interestingly, there is discernible pattern for patient-day costs that can be related to hospital size (as measured by bed capacity). Put simply, expenses per patient increases with the size of the hospital. For most cost categories, there is a dip in hospital costs from the smallest size (6 to 24

11 Ibid., p. 37.
12 Ibid., p. 39.

beds) when we shift to a hospital capacity of from 25 to 49 beds. Beyond this size, however, payroll and nonpayroll expenses increase steadily per adjusted patient day. For example, total costs per adjusted patient day in 1972 were $94.61. For the 25–49-bed category, these costs were $69.36, but they increased steadily to $115.34 for hospitals with 500 beds and more. Undoubtedly the larger hospitals often provide more elaborate care, with more specialized (and expensive) services. They house cardiac-care units, cobalt-therapy units, EKG, EEG, and organ banks. They are likely to be located in urban areas, where they must bid for skills at higher wage rates. We do know that the average length of patient stay increases with hospital size, as do the occupancy rate, the average earnings of hospital employees, the number of supporting personnel per average daily census, and the average value of plant assets per daily census.[13]

The many sources of cost pressure on the hospital industry are well summarized by an HEW study:

> Factors contributing to the overall rise in hospital expenses include technical changes, increased demand, and rising costs of labor and supplies. Most other industries increased their output by combining organizational improvements in productive activity with the substitution of capital equipment for labor. In the hospital industry, organizational change has been slow. Improvements in medical technology have led to changes not only in the types of cases treated by hospitals but also in the methods of treatment, which now require more expensive equipment as well as more highly skilled labor.
>
> Because of rising income, increasing insurance coverage, and changing demographic characteristics of the population, the public also demands more—a larger number of more costly services—from hospitals now than it did two decades ago.[14]

It is probable, as we shall later discuss, that the dominance of the nonprofit hospital has had a costly influence on the resource mix. At first, one might intuitively conclude that not-for-profit institutions would provide services at cost or with minimal (if any) price markups. But although markups may be minimal, the expense of providing quality services certainly is not.

INCREASES IN PHYSICIAN COSTS AND INCOME

In recent years there has been a substantial increase in payments for physician services. The increment or net addition to physician income was $13.5 billion from 1950 to 1972, with about half of the increase taking

---

[13] Hospital Statistics, 1972, American Hospital Association, 1973.
[14] Medical Care: Expenditures, Prices and Costs, p. 38.

place in the 6 years following the enactment of Medicare and Medicaid. Attempts to assign causes for the increase in expenditure reveal that from 1965 to 1972, price or rate increases for physician services account for 65 percent of the gain. Population increases account for 11.4 percent, and "all other" considerations, including improvements in the quality of care, represent 24 percent of the total.[15]

From 1960 to 1971, the net income of self-employed physicians increased at about 5.2 percent annually. But in 1967, there was a 14 percent jump in physician income, reflecting an increase in the fee structure for services, a greater use of physician services, and the improved opportunities for physicians to collect for services because of Medicare. In 1971, the IRS placed the median net income of physicians at $32,371. But this is thought to underestimate the total, for it does not include income from dividends, salary, interest, rent, or other sources. In addition, the data include returns from partially retired physicians or from those working for less than a full year. The IRS estimate contrasts with a *Medical Economics* survey for the same year, which places the median net income from the practice of self-employed physicians at $42,700. By this account, the IRS data may underestimate income from practice by about 25 percent. There is, of course, considerable range of salaries obtained by field specialty, with the obstetrician-gynecologist making one-third more than general practitioners. Business deductions account for about 42 percent of gross receipts obtained by physicians, with the operating costs slightly higher for partnerships than for those engaged in solo practice. But partnerships proved to be much more profitable than solo practice. For example, in 1971 those in partnerships had a median net income of $39,163, compared with $30,447 for those in solo practice.[16]

Many elements account for increases in the costs for physician services. As noted previously, the physician is in a unique position to influence the level of demand for his personal services, for his prime responsibility is to define a regimen of needed care, typically involving his active participation. Since this has always been the case, it is less obvious why this reality should account for the sharp increases in the demand for physician services, unless one makes the strained assumption that physicians are now more often captives of economic incentives than previously.

A second reality is the sharp trend to specialization. Economists since Adam Smith have emphasized how specialization makes possible rapid advances of labor productivity and hence cost reduction. But as suggested in chapter 2, quite the opposite appears to be the case in the medical field. First, patients pay more for specialized rather than generalized medical attention. Second, the specialization process has produced conspicuous geographic distortions in labor supply, obligating specialists

15 Cooper and Worthington, *Social Security Bulletin,* January 1973.
16 Ibid., p. 58.

to serve densely populated areas. The scarcity of medical services in rural America has led, in turn, to a larger income for physicians serving those areas. The income differential relative to income provided by service has not served as an inducement to additional supply. The emphasis on specialization may be more a consequence of professional pride than of a desire to increase one's income. If physicians do not respond to market signals in the allocation of service, the cost problem can be further aggravated. One study notes the sharp change in the mode of physician practice:

> Physicians have become increasingly specialized. In 1949, 54 percent of all physicians were in general practice. By 1973, this proportion had dropped to 15 percent, with the remaining 85 percent made up of medical, surgical, and other specialists and subspecialists. Although much primary care formerly performed by general practitioners is now being performed by internists and pediatricians, there is little doubt that this increased specialization has had an impact on the quality of physicians' services as well as the amount spent for them.[17]

Related to the cost factor is the rapid growth of the incorporation process for medical practice. In 1969 only five percent of all private practice physicians were incorporated, whereas by 1974 the figure had reached forty percent. The trend continues. It is possible that in a corporate structure, economic incentives acquire additional attention. Corporate physicians care for twenty to forty percent more patients per week on the average than their self-employed counterparts. There is no evidence that the increase in volume has diminished the unit cost of such service to the patient.[18]

Until recently, the formal report of physician costs included the "customary" fee. This fee was set at a level sufficiently high to allow gratuitous or low-cost services to the poor. Through this form of price discrimination, the rich paid for services rendered to the poor. Economists have reasoned that the revenue-maximizing behavior of the physician requires that he alter his price for certain segments of the market, that he behave as a discriminating monopolist. In contrast, the AMA views the physician as serving as a collection agency for medical charities. As Reuben Kessel explains, "The income of these charities is derived from a loading charge imposed upon well-to-do patients. This income is used to finance the cost of hiring doctors to provide medical care for the poor who are sick." Kessel quotes one physician:

> I don't feel that I am robbing the rich because I charge them more when I know they can well afford it; the sliding scale is just as demo-

[17] Nancy Worthington, "Expenditures for Hospital Care and Physicians' Services: Factors Affecting Annual Changes," *Social Security Bulletin*, November 1975, p. 9.
[18] R. Craigin Lewis, "What Future for Incorporated Physicians?" *Medical Economics*, November 26, 1973.

cratic as the income tax. I operated today upon two people for the same surgical condition—one a widow, whom I charged $50, the other a banker, whom I charged $250. I let the widow set her own fee. I charged the banker an amount which he probably carries around in his wallet to entertain his business friends.[19]

Kessel, in his widely reprinted discussion of monopolistic influences exerted by the physician, contends that the physician is primarily interested in maximizing income through a differentiated price structure. He charges each segment of his market a price that reflects the limit of its ability to pay. Technically, he is a discriminating monopolist. The truth of the matter—in Kessel's view—is that the differentiated cost structure for services is simply rationalized as a program to support attention to the poor. As he further charges, why should physicians alone assume such "charitable" activities? Many private corporations give generously to charities, but do not justify such charity by charging various customers different prices for a similar product.[20]

Some evidence to support Kessel's view emerged when the government became the major agent for reimbursing physicians for their services to the poor. With "reasonable" payments from this source assured, it was no longer necessary for physicians to charge high rates to their more affluent patients to "cover" charitable services to the poor. One would expect, therefore, that the rate structure for physician services would then decline. But this did not, in fact, happen. Simply stated, since the government was presumably taxing the rich to pay for medical services for the poor, there was less reason for the physician to do the same thing. But because physician rates did not decline (but rather increased) we are left with the conclusion that physicians charge what their markets will bear. Elliot Richardson, when secretary of HEW, offered a singularly unconvincing "explanation" for this cost increase:

Incentives that have led to inflationary medical costs are not too difficult to discern. When Medicare was introduced, it provided that physicians would be paid their customary fees. Some had been giving care free of charge or at prices below what they considered to be their value, and hardly customary. Hence, there was a rather rapid jump in the cost of physicians' services after the birth of Medicare.[21]

Another variable that influences the demand for physician services is the availability and accessibility of such services. This suggests that demand-and-supply elements interact with each other to produce the pat-

[19] "Who Pays the Doctor?" *The New Republic*, Vol. 135 (July 9, 1956), pp. 10–11.
[20] For a full elaboration of Kessel's argument, see "Price Discrimination in Medicine," *Journal of Law and Economics*, Vol. 1 (October 1958), pp. 20–25.
[21] U.S. Senate Committee on Labor and Public Welfare: Hearings before the Subcommittee on Health, Part I. Health Crisis in America, 1971, 92nd Cong., February 22–23, 1971, pp. 11, 12.

tern of expenditure, with the possibility that the supply variable is the more active aspect. For example, Fuchs and Kramer challenge the widely held view that services and expenditures are largely explained by the pa-tient—by his income, his insurance coverage, or his sensitivity to the cost of services. In their empirical analysis, they found the supply factors more important: technology and the number of physicians appeared to be the decisive determinants of physician use and the expenditures for physician services. "Indeed we find that the elasticities of demand with respect to income, price and insurance are small relative to the direct effect of the number of physicians on demand."[22] Rashi Fein has observed that total expenditures for physician services are, to some extent, "administered"; that is, prices are not set by market forces, but by providers, who largely control the market. Further, use is also largely administered: it is deter-mined by the physician.[23]

Fein follows the logic of physician "presence" as the determinant of spending for physician services to several policy issues. First, if physician supply creates its own demand, the proposition that we can reduce the risk of inundation of the system by constraining demand through deduct-ibles and coinsurance loses much of its force. The levels of deductibles may have to be large indeed to offset the lure of physician presence. He also notes:

> Increasing the number of physicians may be justified on various grounds, but the argument that such increases will reduce prices and redistribute physicians is not one of them.[24]

AGE DIFFERENCES IN MEDICAL-CARE SPENDING

A key to health-care planning involves analysis of the age structure of the population, for obviously both morbidity and mortality patterns are a function of age. Because one can construct population pyramids dis-playing the frequency distribution of the population by both age and sex categories, and because these data reflect known values, we have in hand a remarkably effective predictive instrument. It is possible to anticipate how each age category will have changing numbers with year-by-year progressions of time. In more refined analysis, each age category can be

[22] V. R. Fuchs and M. J. Kramer, "Determinants of Expenditures for Physicians' Serv-ices in the United States, 1948–1968," DHEW Publication No. (HSM) 73-3013. GPO, December 1972, p. 2.
[23] Rashi Fein, "Some Health Policy Issues: One Economist's View," *Public Health Reports*, Vol. 90, no. 5 (October 1975), p. 390.
[24] Ibid., p. 391.

"adjusted" for anticipated mortality values by age. The only major uncertainty is the birth rate, or numbers entering the base of the population pyramid. We then identify the morbidity patterns by age group and can project with reasonable assurances future patterns of health-care needs.

What are the patterns of care for the major age groups, the young (under nineteen), the intermediate group (aged nineteen to sixty-four) and the aged (sixty-five and over)? In fiscal 1973, the under-nineteen group represented thirty-five percent of the population, but absorbed only fifteen percent of health expenditures. In contrast, the intermediate group represented fifty-five percent of the population and absorbed fifty-five percent of the expenditure flow. Those sixty-five years and over represented ten percent of the population, but absorbed twenty-eight percent of health-care expenditures. In effect, the economies (or skimping) of medical attention for the young permitted the generosity of expenditures for the aged. On the average, the aged person is twice as likely to have one or more chronic conditions and be limited to certain activities. He is incapacitated more frequently and is confronted with more costly treatment. Indeed, for the senior group the expenditure for health services was almost three times the national average, more than six times that for the young-age category, and nearly triple that for persons in the intermediate-age category.[25]

We have noted that private funds contribute about sixty percent of total physician expenses, with the government making up the remainder. But the proportions of the sources of funding do not hold up when we consider age. For the young- and intermediate-age groups, private sources of funding (including insurance) account for over seventy percent of the total spending, whereas for the senior group, private sources account for about one-third of expenses. With the introduction of Medicare and Medicaid, the government has emerged as the major "buyer" of medical care for the aged. The two programs account for eighty-five percent of public funds spent for the aged. Those sixty-five and over receive all of the Medicare funds, and about forty percent of Medicaid funds.[26] In fiscal 1973, public funds financed only about twenty percent of total physician services. For the young- and intermediate-age groups, public expenditures paid about ten percent of physician services; but for the aged, government contributed about sixty percent.

There are sharp variations in hospital use by age category as well. As one would expect, while nursing-home care involved 5 percent of aggregate expenditures, this involved about 1 percent of the outlay for persons in the two younger age groups. Hospital care absorbed over 48 per-

[25] Barbara S. Cooper and Paula A. Piro, "Age Differences in Medical Care Spending, Fiscal Year 1973," *Social Security Bulletin*, May 1974, p. 3.
[26] Ibid., p. 6.

cent of expenditures for those 65 and older. Nursing-home care absorbed 14 percent of the total health-care budget for those in this age category. Per capita expenditures for hospitalization for those under 19 was only $51; for those 65 and over, such costs were $509, greater by a factor of almost 10. Clearly, as our population becomes increasingly aged, we can anticipate sharp increases in the costs necessary to support the senior population.

Great Britain, facing similar prospects of an aging institutional population, has made major efforts to secure home-care and intermediate-care facilities for its elderly. Such a shift in the resource mix is clearly necessary to avoid inordinate pressures on the delivery system. Further, home care is often more humane than institutionalized care.[27]

THE INTERACTION BETWEEN HEALTH AND EDUCATION

One of the major puzzles of medical economics is that income and good health are not strong correlates. However, there is a strong relationship between good health and higher education. The mystery of these relationships deepens when we realize that education and income are highly correlated. We are left with the puzzle of isolating the root cause of good health. These interrelationships are complex, and identifying both the *directions* and multiple causes of health are indeed challenging. For example, some would contend that an individual may have little education because of his poor health. Or he may be in poor health because his education is meager. Whatever the direction of causation, there is a strong measure of association between the two.

In his econometric model, Michael Grossman found a positive and statistically significant relationship between education and health. He identified "health time" as the complement of the number of restricted-activity days due to illness and injury or the complement of the number of work-loss days. He found a lower measure of disability among the

[27] Though not focusing only on the problems of the aged, Brian Abel-Smith, senior advisor to the British secretary of state for social services, cautions on the risks of excessive hospitalization: "We showed not simply . . . the number who *could* be treated or cared for in hospital, but the number who *should* be in hospital. It is believed that the hospital should not be overused, not only because it is so costly but because it is dangerous: Unnecessary admission to a hospital may make the patient sicker and also make him think that he is sicker than he is. Moreover, the artificial community contacts of hospital visiting are no substitutes for living in the community. The patient's involvement with the community is seen as part of the quality of patient care." The search for alternatives to hospital care requires an inventory of community resources and of personnel capable of giving care. As Abel-Smith explains, "Some people clearly need health services, others only need social services, but many need both." "Value for Money in Health Services," *Social Security Bulletin*, July 1974, p. 24.

better educated.[28] Myron J. Lefcowitz also found evidence to indicate that levels of education were causal elements in determining an individual's health status.[29] In his analysis, levels of education determine both income and standard of health.

Mordechai E. Lando analyzed 1970 census data to secure information on work-related health conditions. He uncovered clear evidence that the proportion of the work population suffering disability declined as the years of schooling increased. He also found that for each educational level, the overall proportion of disability is lower for women than for men. This is true for all age categories except for cases of complete work disability: here the proportion is about equal for men and women at each educational level.[30]

However, there are other elements comingling with education that might explain the relationship. For example, we know that age and education are negatively related. That is, the more youthful segments of the labor force are likely to have more education than older workers. And we know, too, that younger workers are less likely to be disabled because of illness or accidents. Could not age, then, be a factor that explains the apparent causality in the education/income relationship? Lando attempted to track this possibility by classifying the data by both age and education and then viewing the disability status of each segment. Even after the data were standardized for age, increased schooling was still associated with better health.

There were substantial differences in disability by race. For example, those with complete disability totaled 4.1 percent for the whites in the sample and 7.4 percent of the blacks. For the category "No years of completed education," about one-quarter of the sample for both races suffered complete disability, indicating the harmful effects of illiteracy on good health. The incidence of complete disability drops sharply for both racial segments as education increases, with only 1.1 percent among whites and 1.7 percent among blacks completing 4 or more years or more of college.[31]

The decline of disability with years of schooling is so precipitous that one is tempted to conclude that future relief from morbidity must be achieved through improved education rather than by investments in health-care provisions themselves. This contention gains considerable support from the widespread conviction that the major causes of affliction

[28] Michael Grossman, *Demand for Health,* National Bureau of Economic Research, Occasional Paper, 119, 1972.
[29] Myron J. Lefcowitz, "Poverty and Health: A Re-examination," *Inquiry,* March 1973, pp. 3–13.
[30] Mordechai E. Lando, "The Interaction Between Health and Education," *Social Security Bulletin,* December 1975, p. 17.
[31] Ibid., p. 18.

involve individual recklessness and neglect. Again, however, we must be cautious about directions and elements of causation. The better-educated may work at less physically taxing jobs and be less vulnerable to industrial accidents that interfere with the regularity of work. An individual with an attractive occupational status may find his job more challenging and attend work more regularly, in spite of the headache, hangover, or minor afflictions. The less-educated worker confronted with arduous tasks may decide to stay at home.

SOME POLICY IMPLICATIONS

The disquieting statistics on cost and price movements in the medical market help explain the rising levels of concern about the market's behavior. Since 1965, approximately fifty percent of the anticipated increase in the flow of medical services has been dissipated by price increases imposed by medical-care providers. The comfortable assumption that the enhanced revenue flow will eventually overcome short-term hindrances to supply seems to be less persuasive today than in the past. The steady increase in the supply of hospital capacity has not had any discernible effect on dampening the remarkable cost increases for hospital services. Nor has the substantial influx of foreign medical-school graduates appeared to constrain upward pressures on the fee structure for medical services. With soaring costs and prices, the medical market is displaying a unique form of economic weightlessness.

Two additional considerations have compounded public anxieties about the behavior of this aberrant market. First, we experience the steady drumbeat of newspaper and television accounts of the "rip-off" within the medical reimbursement systems. We are confronted with weekly exposés of fraudulant testing laboratories, evidences of kickbacks, billing for services not performed, and, even more disconcerting, the performing of unnecessary surgery. The distinguished New York Times series on the medical crisis estimates that some 12,000 individuals succumb annually because of unnecessary surgery. The resulting skepticism about the integrity of health-care providers has led, in turn, to a further source of cost pressures. Suits for maloccurrences are increasingly common. It is estimated that excessive testing and other forms of "defensive medicine" (to avoid later law suits) now cost $10 billion annually. Malpractice insurance premiums have soared to $4 billion annually, and the public has been exposed to periodic accounts of $1-million settlements in "celebrated" cases of patient abuse. It is unfortunate that an industry so dependent on a sense of altruism and service has now been stigmatized by portraits of "fast-buck artists" exploiting and sometimes thwarting well-intentioned programs to broaden our access to medical services.

Equally chilling is the realization that expenditures for Medicare and Medicaid have tended to follow the physician rather than the eligible patients. We witness a renaissance of Say's Law of Markets, with evidence that hospital beds beget patients and that surgeons beget surgery. The distressing inference is that the flow of services is carefully calibrated to reflect the providers' interest in using his facilities rather than in meeting patient needs.

It is not surprising, therefore, that the government is seeking alternative solutions to the cost problems. It is proposing to replace retrospective budgeting with prospective budgeting; it is seeking out standards of care through the peer-review activities within Professional Standards Review Organizations (PSROs); it is encouraging local and regional planning through the establishment of Health Systems Agencies (HSAs); it is encouraging consideration of alternative delivery forms, or more specifically, health-maintenance organizations. Whether these small efforts—only $100 million is expended annually on planning functions—can alter the direction of $100 billion or more of total spending remains to be seen.

Concurrent with the knowledge that the demand pressures have not set in motion the full measure of supply responses is the unfavorable ratio of providers to population. The ratio of active nonfederal physicians to population varies on a scale of three to one from state to state. For nurses, the ratio nationwide is four to one. There is serious concern, on the one hand, about the lack of access to physicians (particularly for rural Americans) and, on the other hand, about the consequences of unnecessary services where the ratio of physicians to population is large. One study identified a curious variation of from three to four times in the rates of common surgical procedures by region. Some of the variation could be attributed to variations in the incidence of disease, but the more significant contributing factors appeared to be the number of available hospital beds, the number of board-certified surgeons, and the number of other doctors who performed surgery.[32]

The geographic disparities of service exacerbate our health-service problems, for these are, in turn, related to income level and race. Looking at whites versus blacks for 1965, for example, the ratio for life expectancy was 70.2 to 63.6 years; for maternal mortality, 22.4 to 90.2 per 1000 live births; for infant mortality, 21.5 to 40.3 per 1000 live births; for tuberculosis mortality in all forms, 3.4 to 12.8 per 100,000 population; and for mortality from influenza and pneumonia, 24.4 to 55.4 per 100,000 population. As Walter J. McNerney has observed,

[32] C. E. Lewis, "Variations in the Incidence of Surgery," *The New England Journal of Medicine,* no. 281 (1969), pp. 880–84.

. . . these differences are not genetically determined, as indicated by the fact that they were more economically than racially related. Similarly, there was wide variation in the prevalence of chronic conditions that limited activity (29 percent versus 4.2 percent) between families with income under $2,000 and those over $7,000.[33]

With this preview of issues confronting the medical sector, we can now turn to the specifics of the medical-supply system.

SUGGESTED READINGS

COOPER, BARBARA S. and PAULA A. PIRO, "Age Differences in Medical Care Spending, FY 1973," *Social Security Bulletin,* May 1974. An analysis of the increased spending on medical care by senior citizens.

DEPAMPHILIS, DONALD M., "Forecasting Medical Care Expenses," *Business Economics,* September 1976, pp. 21–32. A technical discussion of cost estimation and projections.

FEIN, RASHI, "Health Care Cost: A Distorted Issue," *AFL-CIO American Federationist,* Vol. 82, no. 6 (June 1975), pp. 13–17. Discusses the rising costs of health care.

FELDSTEIN, MARTIN S., The Medical Economy," *Scientific American,* Vol. 229 (September 1973), pp. 151–56. A discussion of the cost problems of the health-care sector containing several graphs portraying industry trends.

GILEHART, JOHN K., "What Goes up, Isn't Coming Down," *National Journal,* April 17, 1976, p. 522. Estimates the expenditure increase for Medicare and Medicaid, as well as the anticipated growth of overall expenditures.

Health in the United States: A Chartbook (Washington, D.C.: GPO, DHEW, Public Health Service, Health Resources Administration, National Center for Health Statistics, DHEW Publication No. (HRA) 76-1233). A graphic display of features of the health-care industry.

LANDO, MORDECHAI E., "The Interaction Between Health and Education," *Social Security Bulletin,* December 1975, pp. 16–22. A commentary on the phenomenom that increased education leads to a greater expenditure on health care and, in turn, a lower rate of illness.

LESPARRE, MICHAEL, "An Interview with Michael H. Moskow, Ph.D., Director of the Council on Wage and Price Stability," *Hospitals, Journal of the American Hospital Association,* Vol. 50, no. 11 (June 1, 1976), pp. 31–38. An interview dealing with sources of cost pressure.

National Health Insurance Resource Book, rev. ed. Prepared by the staff of the committee on Ways and Means for use by its subcommittee on Health. (Washington, D.C.: GPO, U.S. House of Representatives, August 30, 1976.) A profile of the expenditure and cost trends of the health-care industry, including funding sources for health care.

[33] Walter J. McNerney, "Why Does Medical Care Cost So Much?" *The New England Journal of Medicine,* Vol. 282, no. 26 (June 25, 1970), p. 1460.

NEWHOUSE, JOSEPH P., CHARLES E. PHELPS, and WILLIAM B. SCHWARTZ, *Policy Options and the Impact of National Health Insurance* (Santa Monica: Rand Corporation, R-1528-HEW/OEO, June 1974). An examination of National Health Insurance's influence on the price and income elasticity of consumer demand.

PHELPS, CHARLES E. and JOSEPH P. NEWHOUSE, *The Effects of Coinsurance on the Demand for Physician Services* (Santa Monica: Rand Corporation, R-976-OEO, June 1972). A discussion of third-party funding and its role in consumer-cost reduction.

REYNOLDS, ALAN, "The High Cost of Health," *National Review*, July 20, 1973, pp. 780–84. Critical survey of the cost problems surrounding the health-care industry.

SCITOVSKY, ANNE M., "The Higher Costs of Better Medical Care." In Anselm L. Strauss, ed., *Where Medicine Fails* (Chicago: Aldine, 1970), pp. 43–51. Speculates that the proliferation of services for patients is a major source of cost pressure.

TUCKER, JAMES F., "Medical Care: Rising Costs in a Peculiar Marketplace," *Economic Review*, March/April 1975, pp. 6–18. A statistical study that points up the aberrant behavior of the health-care market sector.

WORTHINGTON, NANCY L., "Expenditures for Hospital Care and Physicians' Services: Factors Affecting Annual Changes," *Social Security Bulletin*, November 1975. A statistical study of expenditure and cost trends for the medical sector.

PART TWO

Delivery and Reception of Health Services

4
THE PHYSICIAN-PATIENT RELATIONSHIP

Medical service is an interaction between people. The quality of that personal relationship is a major determinant of the effectiveness of its delivery. The individual's perception of the care he receives involves much more than impressions of sophisticated medical hardware or even the technical virtuosity of the practitioner. More than anything else, it reflects his perception of whether his physician—and the supporting staff—*care*. In his classic statement a generation ago, F. W. Peabody emphasized the significance of this emotional component.

> The good physician knows his patient through and through, and his knowledge is dearly bought. Time, sympathy, and understanding must be lavishly dispensed, but the rewards to be found in that personal bond forms the greatest satisfaction of the practice of medicine. One of the essential qualities of the clinician is interest in humanity, *for the secret of the care of the patient is in caring for the patient.*[1]

The purpose of this chapter is to examine some dimensions of the "medical transactions." Our focus will be less on the physiological effectiveness of the transaction and more on its psychological and sociological aspects. The case can be made that many patients do not expect, nor do they require, the kind of emotional support advocated by Peabody. Stated simply, the patient is looking for a cure, not TLC. But our position is that the subtleties and complexities of the medical transaction have enormous implications for the perceived adequacy of health care. For example, at a national conference of physicians dealing with the malpractice crisis, Senator Edward Kennedy explained:

> The family doctor has been replaced by an amazing array of specialists, each interested in a specific illness rather than in a whole human being.

[1] F. W. Peabody, "The Care of the Patient," *Journal of the American Medical Association*, Vol. 88 (March 19, 1927), pp. 877–82. Italics added.

And every patient is reminded of this each time he or she receives a bill from a physician. Jack Jones, M.D., who a generation ago was a friend, personal counselor, and family doctor, has become Jack Jones, M.D., a professional corporation. A generation ago, when I was a child, no family would ever have given consideration to suing their doctor. But who would be reluctant to sue a professional corporation, which has charged a high fee and spent a minimum amount of time in examining a left eye or a right elbow? It would be interesting to know how often those doctors who still spend time getting to know their patients and offering their reassurance and advice in addition to medical treatment are sued for malpractice.[2]

Dr. Sidney Wolfe, director of the Public Citizens Health Research Committee (a Ralph Nader organization), confirmed the Kennedy viewpoint, describing the doctor–patient relationship as "beleaguered."

Aside from the more apparent attributes of modern medicine, such as increased specialization, the use of penning a prescription to avoid having to talk any more to the patient, and more machines, all of which are very understandably depersonalizing to the patient, there is an increased patient perception of the low regard many doctors have for their [the patients'] human rights.[3]

A *Newsweek* report on the effectiveness of medical services offered the following commentary:

In the last decade, the number of primary-care physicians has declined from 59 for every 100,000 persons to 40. As more and more young doctors succumb to the lure of the specialist's higher income and prestige, the population of GPs has become not only smaller but older and less well qualified. "We've had no significant planning for the numbers and kinds of physicians we need," says former U.S. Surgeon General Dr. Jesse Steinfeld. "The thing has grown up willy-nilly."

The educational process of the specialist has tended also to steer the young physician away from the role of comforter of the sick and toward the job of technologist. "Ninety percent of patients only need a guy who'll take an interest in them," says Dr. Joel Posner, a University of Pennsylvania Hospital fellow training in pulmonary disease. "We're being trained to handle the other ten percent, and very well, but we're not keyed up to deal with the grandmother who has aches and pains."[4]

Our concern in this chapter, of course, goes far beyond the neglect of grandmother's aches and pains. We are concerned with the attitudes of both patient and provider in medical transactions. We will view, at the outset, some statistical aspects of these interactions. Second, we will re-

---

[2] *National Conference on Medical Malpractice*, Arlington, Virginia, March 20, 1975 (Washington, D.C.: GPO, 1975), p. 7.
[3] Ibid., p. 63.
[4] "How Good Is Your Doctor?" *Newsweek*, December 23, 1974, p. 48.

view the socializing, or "acculturating" influence on the postures of both patient and physician. And finally, we will view some of the major policy issues that reflect the public viewpoint of the effectiveness of contact with the medical industry.

THE VOLUME AND FORM OF MEDICAL TRANSACTIONS

The relationship of individuals with the medical-industry provider takes place constantly and in heavy volume. Robert W. Jamplis, president of the American Group Practice Association, estimated that there are about 300,000 doctors involved in patient care, and that each physician sees about 138 patients per week. He concluded that this involves, then, some 2 billion doctor–patient encounters each year, or to be conservative, 5 million such encounters every day.[5] If the incidence of malpractice suits is an index of patient dissatisfaction with those encounters, the results are encouraging. There are some 20,000 malpractice claims filed each year, which means only 1 claim for every 100,000 patient–doctor encounters. Clearly, the negative aspect of a single unhappy episode (involving litigation) secures much more publicity than the 100,000 that presumably provide satisfactory service.

The average person living to seventy will have approximately four hundred contacts, as a patient, with both doctors and dentists during his lifetime; and, as we emphasized earlier, because many of those contacts may involve emergencies, pain, and stress, the reception afforded the individual seeking relief or cure assumes obvious psychological significance.

There was, in 1973, 1 physician for every 562 persons in the United States. That ratio has declined steadily since 1950, when the population–physician ratio was 672. By international standards, the American population is generously endowed with a large physician stock. For example, in 1971 the population–physician ratio in Nigeria was 1 to 43,500, in India 1 to 4,820, and for the Philippines 1 to 9,100. The last ratio is of interest because of the large numbers of Philippine-trained physicians serving in the United States.

Within the United States, there is no clear relationship between physician services and health. For example, the Western and North Central states have relatively few physicians, but have the highest life expectancies found in the United States. But in the South, where there is an equally thin physician supply, life expectancy is lower.[6]

[5] *National Conference on Medical Malpractice,* p. 3.
[6] *Health: United States, 1975,* DHEW Publication No. (HRA) 76-1232, Health Resources Administration, National Center for Health Statistics, Rockville, Maryland (Washington, D.C.: GPO, 1976), p. 105.

The geographic distribution of physicians is heavily biased toward metropolitan areas. In 1973, there was 1 nonfederal physician providing patient care for approximately every 500 individuals living in the largest metropolitan areas, contrasted with 1 for every 2,000 to 2,500 patients in small, nonmetropolitan counties. The bias in the distribution of medical specialists is even more pronounced. But apparently population densities alone do not fully explain the location of physicians. In Vermont, which has the same population density as Iowa, there is 1 physician for every 565 persons. In Iowa, there is 1 physician for every 999 persons. The amenities of life that determine physician location are not apparently a function of population density alone.

Only five percent of the population accounts for more than one-third of all outpatient physician visits. And some twenty-two percent of the population accounts for about seventy-five percent of all physician visits. This is not to imply that these twenty-five percent have trivial needs. Clearly, the individual's view of his own symptoms of illness can trigger interest in diagnosis. But there are substantial sociological and cultural elements that encourage (or discourage) an individual's impulse to play the "sick role."

Outside of a hospital setting it is estimated that, from 1971 to 1974, there have been about 1 billion physician contacts each year. The fact that the physician stock serving the public had increased about 10 percent during the same interval suggests some decline in the volume of patient contacts per physician. In 1971, practicing physicians reported working an average of 53.6 hours per week, with an average of 46.3 hours devoted to direct patient care.[7]

Government programs to reimburse the aged and indigent for medical services have increased the proportion of the population making physician visits. In 1964, about twenty-eight percent of those classified as "poor" had not seen a physician in the past two years. By 1973, that percentage had dropped to seventeen percent. For the more well-to-do, the proportions dropped from eighteen to thirteen percent. There has been an even sharper increase in physician visits by the minority poor. The percentage that had not seen a physician for two years dropped from thirty-three to nineteen percent from 1964 to 1973. And when one looks at annual physician contacts, the contrast is even more striking. In 1964 the poor had fewer physician visits per year than the nonpoor, but by 1973, these findings had been reversed.[8] There were more physician contacts for women than for men, with 5.6 for the former and 4.3 for the latter. There were 5.7 visits per year for persons with a family income under $5,000, compared with 5.1 visits for those with a family income over $15,000.

[7] Ibid., p. 286.
[8] Ibid., pp. 287, 288.

Over two-thirds of outpatient physician contacts occurred at the physician's office. Home visits accounted for only one percent of all physician visits, compared with over five percent a decade ago. The reluctance of physicians to make home visits undoubtedly has symbolic and emotional significance to the public. As the president of Stanford University explained:

> It is always easier to contemplate the simple verities of a bygone era than to disentagle the complex realities of today. Thus, we yearn for the time when good old Jean Hersholt, Hollywood's favorite MD, went around with his battered old black bag curing the sick and comforting the worried. No amount of legislation is going to restore Jean Hersholt, or Dr. Christian, MD, to life. But one suspects that some such subconscious yearning, fueled by populist dislike for professionalism and for the mysteries of arcane specialties, plays a part in the motivation behind congressional efforts to solve the problems of medical manpower distribution in the United States of the 1970s.[9]

In a *U.S. News and World Report* interview with AMA head, Malcolm C. Todd, Todd acknowledged that physicians had been preoccupied with scientific, economic, and political affairs and had not given enough attention to human needs. He also acknowledged that physicians must teach their nurses and receptionists to respond to telephone calls in a manner that would have the patient feel someone is paying attention to him. And on the question of housecalls, he explained:

> Surprisingly enough, there are still about fourteen million physician housecalls being made in this country every year. That's down from what it used to be, but we must realize that probably the most inefficient procedure a doctor goes through is making a housecall.
>
> Q: Why is that?
>
> A: Well, say I'm called at two o'clock in the morning by someone who has a pain in his chest. It sounds to me like he's probably had a coronary. By the time I can go out to his house, give him a hypodermic, and call an ambulance, we could lose a lot of lives. The best procedure is to send an ambulance with oxygen and all the other supportive equipment that can be used while the patient is en route to the hospital. I can be at the hospital when the ambulance arrives.
>
> The same thing applies to a pediatrician who gets a call from a mother who says her child is sick. It's in the middle of office hours, and the most inefficient thing for that doctor to do is leave fifteen other kids—some of whom may be sicker than the child at home—and go rushing out there. He should advise the mother of what to do, send out any

9 Richard W. Lyman, "Public Rights and Private Responsibilities: A University Viewpoint," *Journal of Medical Education*, Vol. 51 (January 1976), p. 9.

> prescription needed, and then go see the child after office hours if necessary.[10]

Todd acknowledged that part of the problem of inadequate relationships was the patient contact reflected within medical training itself. There has been an increasing reliance on testing for diagnosis and prescription. In many cases, the doctor makes a private analysis of test results, simply hands the patient the results, "and—boom!—he's out of the office carrying a prescription. He's really had only a few minutes of the doctor's time." He also acknowledged the increased difficulty of establishing close personal relationships with physicians who are specialists:

> We have specialists, of course, because medicine today is so complex and it's impossible for one doctor to master all fields. But now it's almost getting to the point where a man is going to be a left-leg amputator or a right-leg amputator. We recognize we need more family practitioners.[11]

One of the central issues of patient–physician interaction is the patient's concern that he may not, in fact, have symptoms that justify the physician contact and is thus exposed to the risk of ridicule. Another concern is that the physician may not appreciate the harmless nature of the symptoms and involve the patient in an elaborate treatment regimen that is both costly and painful. From the physician's viewpoint, there is some risk that the examination process may involve such patient anxiety that medical problems might develop where none, in fact, exist. Paradoxically, in this case, the transaction between the physician and patient contributes to the patient's illness. In the first contact, the doctor seeks to determine what pathological symptoms exist. However, "no consultation can be purely diagnostic, because any interview involves interaction between doctor and patient which begins to modify the situation being presented."[12] Patients may develop symptoms that the physician seems to suspect, or they may organize undefined feelings of illness into terms suggested by the doctor. As one observer notes:

> Many doctors hesitate sometimes to order barium-meal examination lest an anxious person become converted into an "ulcer sufferer" and an acute peptic inflammation thereby organizes into a chronic ulcer. Perhaps the doctor, by demanding physical symptoms from the patient as the passport of entry to the consultation, and by selecting certain symptoms for investigation and observation, may actually condition a patient into developing a definite illness much less amenable to treat-

---

[10] "Are Doctors Doing Their Job? An Interview with Dr. Malcolm C. Todd, President of the AMA," *U.S. News and World Report*, July 1, 1974, p. 30.
[11] Ibid.
[12] Kevin Browne and Paul Freeling, "The Doctor–Patient Relationship" (Edinburgh and London: E. and S. Livingstone Ltd.), chapter 1.

ment or to healing by the passage of time than the original anxiety state.[13]

Some patients are so dominated by physicians that their illness adjusts to the doctor's expectations, real or perceived.

Overall, about one-half of all visits to a physician's office are for conditions that the doctor judges not serious. There is an inclination toward such nonserious visits among children and young adults; about six of ten visits fall into this category. The occasions for serious episodes increase with age, with only three out of ten visits for those over sixty-five involving nonserious problems. We have noted that males have less impulse to visit a physician than females, but when they do, there is a slight tendency for their visits to involve more serious problems.[14]

As we will elaborate more fully in the chapter following, these visits are much colored by cultural, social, and economic considerations. A person may not want a moderate impairment to prevent his regular attendance at his job, particularly if there is no provision for sick pay. In playing the sick role, he suffers an interruption or loss of income. There are, of course, acute episodes of illness in which an obviously severe impairment precludes work. But most episodes are less clearcut than this, and we must acknowledge the cultural reflex in which individuals "permit themselves" to be disabled. We have, on one hand, the concern that many individuals do not have the intelligence, energy, or interest in undertaking preventive examinations. And we have opposite anxieties that when health services become a right or appear costless, the system is confronted with the "moral hazard" of overuse. The system will be inundated by the worried well.

THE PHYSICIAN'S VALUE STRUCTURE

In almost all studies of occupational prestige in the United States, physicians receive top ratings. The current public disenchantment with all forms of institutional organization, including government, the church, institutions of learning, the military, and the corporate structure, has encompassed the health establishment as well. Although all institutions are exposed to the crisis of public confidence, the decline of faith in medical institutions is less pronounced than for other institutions. In *relative* terms, medical professions have still maintained their favored position.

Clearly, society bestows honor, respect, and prestige on this elite group. Such social and economic status is warranted, because physicians

[13] Ibid., p. 2.
[14] *Health: United States 1975*, pp. 298–99.

receive unusually challenging assignments involving a remarkable measure of responsibility. The more difficult, extended, and rigorous the training period, the more rewarding must be the offsetting incomes during the
"practicing years" of the physician. Medical education can require up to
twelve years of training for some specialties. The costs to the student involve not only tuition, books, and direct-support costs while studying, but
also the opportunity cost represented by income forgone during the extended years of study. The loss of such opportunity—involving deferred
gratifications and other creature comforts—is sharply revealed to the medical student as he compares his work week, lifestyle, and modest resources
with those of his peers enjoying "fast-track" advances in corporate enterprise following completion of an MBA program. As one study explains,

> If, after having selected this type of personality (obsessive-compulsive,
> with acquisitive propensities) into American medical schools, we sub-
> ject students to a lengthy education experience that frequently requires
> deferment of marriage, postponement of a family, and delay in acquir-
> ing a home and the material accoutrements of contemporary American
> life, we should not be surprised that many doctors are preoccupied with
> money. This becomes all the more pressing when they have to repay
> loans for their medical education and take out mortgages for equipping
> their offices.[15]

We find confirming evidence in the filtering process that determines
who may secure medical education.

> As standards rose and as the costs and length of education expanded,
> medicine became staunchly middle-class. The unmarried student could
> expect expenses of $10,000 or $11,000 for the four-year degree, fol-
> lowed by an ill-paid internship and a two- or three-year residency. A
> 1963 study noted that over 80 percent of the average medical student's
> expenses came from his own earnings and savings and from those of
> his family. The relatively arduous economic process of gaining a medi-
> cal education, coupled with a delay in professional and economic grati-
> fication through internship, residency, and perhaps the lean years of
> practice, brought to medicine a new spirit of mercantilism. The physi-
> cian was tempted to feel that, for demanding a spartan youth, society
> owed him a rich return. And indeed, to become a practicing physician
> was to enter the most highly paid of all occupations.[16]

A second conditioning influence is the experience of the medical
school itself and of the acculturation process. The elevated status of the

15 Kerr L. White, "Health Care Arrangements in the United States, AD 1972," *Mil-
bank Memorial Fund Quarterly*, Vol. 50, no. 5 (October 1972).
16 Rosemary Stevens, *American Medicine and the Public Interest* (New Haven: Yale
University Press, 1971), pp. 355–56. See also Marian E. Altenderfer and Margaret D.
West, *How Medical Students Finance Their Education*, USDHEW, Public Health
Service, 1965, pp. 70–71.

doctor is emphasized throughout medical school, internship, and residency. The symbols reinforcing physician status are numerous, ranging from white clothing (symbolic of the doctor) to freedom in treating patients. If an attending physician tells an intern that he is incapable of treating a patient in the hospital, the trainee cannot successfully challenge the physician's judgment. This kind of unquestioned power is something the medical student looks forward to exercising when he reaches the full status of "doctor."

Physician status is in part based on beliefs about his superior knowledge and skills.

> It is characteristic of a profession that its members believe that their work is special and worthy of note and esteem, and that laymen also accord it prestige. Professionals share a collective identity with those who have gone through similar training, as well as attachment to the work itself. The extended training that professions typically demand develops the sense of identity that is indispensable if members are to care about what happens to their profession. With this, the profession can fulfill some of its social functions. It can control its members through pressures and sanctions not available to the layman, who is hardly able to judge performance.

Confidence in the physician's superior knowledge and skill has numerous dimensions. Other health providers, such as nurses or allied health personnel, do not enjoy the status or income of the doctor, which can be given as proof of professional superiority. It is clear that physicians view their medical capability as substantially superior to that of other health providers. One study, for example, found that medical students trained in the use of a health team considered the team useful, but made use of it only in unimportant functions.

The "rite of passage" from medical school to internship, residency, and certification is long and arduous, encouraging cynicism, some loss of humanitarianism, and attention to the status and worthiness of the physician.[17] Medical students are taught that becoming too close to their patients can be dangerous. Courses emphasize the physical rather than psychological aspects of the doctor–patient relationship. And, of course, young doctors feel the need to succeed as practicing physicians in order to prove that the masochistic and expensive training they have been through has been worth it.

There is considerable ambivalence about what the public might rea-

[17] In the words of a classical study of physician education, a "rite of passage" is that series of instructions, ceremonies, and ordeals by which those already in a special status initiate neophytes into their charmed circle, by which men turn boys into fellow men, fit to be their own companions and successors." Becker, Geer, Hughes, and Strauss, *Boys in White* (Chicago: The University of Chicago Press, 1961), pp. 352–53.

sonably expect as a consequence of this extensive educational experience. In one view:

> Other than affirmations made by their professional organizations, I know of no evidence to suggest that physicians are more or less altruistic than other groups of our society. I also know of no reason why they should donate their services during their working hours; other groups in society are not called upon to do this, and it is difficult to enforce standards and monitor performance when physicians are not clearly paid for their services.[18]

From a different point of view:

> I have always believed that the department of medicine and its faculty set the tone and the values of the ends of medical education—ends which must relate directly to society's needs and are, therefore, inevitably utilitarian. . . . And all too frequently we have had to settle for the technologist with the big research team, who seems to have left his humanity and social conscience in the trash can of Grover's Corners.

> Whatever the reason, professors of medicine have, by their contemporary model, downplayed the art and science of clinical medicine and the importance of community public health measures while stressing the role of super-specialized technocrat.[19]

There has been little research on the attitudes of physicians after they leave their medical training. We do know, however, that physician services are concentrated in middle- and upper-income urban areas where the most money can be made. Only a few are willing to practice in impoverished or rural areas. The values of physician status and cohesion seem to have resulted in the profession's reluctance to publicly criticize its own ranks.

CONSUMER PERCEPTIONS OF THE PHYSICIAN

Of essence in the physician–patient transaction is the patient's feelings of "sociological ambivalence."

> Sociological ambivalence, a socially induced tendency to be both attracted to and repelled by, to need and at the same time to fear the services of a group, characterize attitudes toward the medical profession.

At least under our current system of health-care delivery, consumers know they need physicians to receive medical attention and often to maintain

---

18 White, "Health Care Arrangements," p. 25.
19 John Knowles, "The World of Health and the American Physician," *Journal of Medical Education*, Vol. 49 (January 1974), pp. 52–53.

life itself. Although the doctor may experience admiration and loyalty from patients and the public, stories about the insensitive, incompetent, or even cruel doctor also are quite common. We often trust rather blindly and yet are suspicious of "money-hungry, fee-splitting, arrogant" doctors.

Sociological ambivalence has numerous sources. The personalities and elevated status of doctors can produce both admiration and jealousy. Doctors are seldom meek and almost never poor. Their position in the structure of health-care delivery is also a source of ambivalence. As we have noted, the physician controls the care we receive and thus has an awesome influence over our lives. The physician is really our only choice for receiving health care, at least within the realm of "traditional" medicine. Whatever we feel about physicians, most of us must eventually face the necessity of asking for their help.

As we approach the physician for help in maintaining what is so vital to us, life and health, we encounter another essential in the doctor–patient transaction, the imbalance of knowledge about the subject of that transaction. Most laymen know very little about their own bodies, physiology, and biologic processes, and even less about diagnosis or treatment. The esoteric and complex nature of medicine, its language and techniques, reinforce our own ignorance. Except for an occasional "personal health" course in high school or college, few laymen receive formal instruction in health and medicine.

In addition to having less knowledge, patients enter the relationship to be helped by the physician. Patient dependency on the doctor is largely psychological, while his dependency on the patient is largely economic. Patients can sometimes escape the dependency on physicians, but "shopping around" for doctors is infrequent, particularly in times and locations where there are too few of them available. The cost to a physician of having a patient leave him is seldom dramatic.

Sociological ambivalence, patient ignorance, and patient dependency are not always appreciated by the health provider. The physician may receive excessive praise from one patient and excessive blame for failures from the next. Because of malpractice problems, the physician is increasingly sensitive to the need for involving his patients in basic medical decisions. And yet he recognizes the psychic pain he can cause by such candor about the uncertainty of outcomes or even the impossibility of a cure. He may even have a major commitment to treating the poverty stricken or ethnic minorities and yet be constantly frustrated by their "different" perceptions of pain, by other medical symptoms, or by the oppressive consequence of inadequate nutrition and housing.

The ideal doctor–patient relationship in our culture assumes the patient will work with the physician in achieving and maintaining his health. Here the patient is considered responsible for and interested in his own health; he is helpful in assisting the doctor with identification of symptoms and is compliant and obedient in following doctor's orders.[20] The physician assumes the right to evaluate the patient's conformity to these rules, and he is quick to chastise the uncooperative individual. But an essential of the doctor–patient transaction is that the latter has little ability (and only infrequently assumes the right) to evaluate the performance of the former. This reality is usually based on one or more of the following patient attitudes: "Only doctors can evaluate doctors." "Physicians are well-educated and regulated by government or professional societies." "I know there are incompetent doctors, but mine is excellent." "I don't want to take the chance of attempting to find another doctor."

Another reality elevating the stature of the physician is the clear dependence of allied health personnel on his judgment. Allied health personnel, nurses, and medical psychologists usually enter a case only as support for and under the supervision of the responsible doctor. Usually only physicians have authority to admit patients to hospitals except in cases of extreme emergency. Thus, doctors must identify the "best" mix of medical services for the patient but also control patient access to other services.

Although our rather blind faith in physician wisdom and skill, and their power over hospital and other services contribute to physician dominance in health-care delivery, the major bulwark for that dominance is that they are a self-controlling profession. Put another way, we have long practiced the rule that only doctors can regulate doctors and what they do.

Patient–doctor transactions may be classified as "doctor dominated" in one extreme or as a "partnership" in the other. In the former, the physician is seen as the skilled, educated professional to whom one comes for help. Since his knowledge is precise and medicine is a science, he controls and dominates the occurrences. He decides what the patient should or needs to know, and what other medical providers need be involved. Decisions about treatment are "medical" rather than value or attitude judgments, and patients have little or no involvement in them. It is assumed that the patient will carry out the doctor's instructions, and failure to do so is treated as errant behavior to be punished by physician anger. The doctor is God. The patient is ill and compliant.

The "partnership" model involves a very different set of attitudes. Here the belief is that both doctor and patient are whole human beings, rather than scientific diety and biologic processes.[21] The personal attitudes and characteristics of the patient and his socioeconomic condition are known to affect his symptom-illness perceptions, his attitudes and behavior regarding healthfulness, and his compliance with medical technol-

[20] Howard E. Freeman, Sol Levin, Leo G. Reeder (eds.), *Handbook of Medical Sociology*, 2nd ed. (Englewood Cliffs, N.J.: Prentice-Hall, 1972), p. 322.
[21] Kong-Kyun Ro, "Patient Characteristics and Hospital Use." In Victor R. Fuchs (ed.), *Essays in the Economics of Health and Medical Care*, National Bureau of Economic Research (New York: Columbia University Press, 1972), pp. 70–71.

ogy and treatment. The doctor gets to be human too. He has his limits, his frustrations, and his needs. He cannot treat all patients with equal effectiveness, for his own perceptions of patient attractiveness have some influence on the treatment offered.[22] Medicine involves facts and precision, but it also involves guesswork.

SOME STATISTICAL FEATURES OF MEDICAL EDUCATION

The elitism—some would say aristocracy—involved in medical education can be further understood by review of the admission criteria, and the socioeconomic status of families of medical-school students. Most physicians come from professional, upper-middle-class families. They are predominantly males and predominantly white. Over forty percent of the students entering medical school have fathers who are professionals, a third of them physicians. About one-third of all medical students come from families with earnings in the top three percent of incomes nationally.[23]

Efforts to improve minority representation within the upper reaches of the occupational structure have a long way to go. If we represent the blacks as 12 to 13 percent of the total population, we find that only 2.2 percent have M.D. and D.O. degrees, 2.3 percent are dentists, 0.6 percent are optometrists, 2.3 percent are pharmacists, 4.1 percent are podiatrists. Only in the registered-nursing category does the black representation of 7.5 percent indicate more than a trivial proportion of the total. For those of Spanish heritage, the figures are even more dismal. Some 3.7 percent of those practicing with M.D. and D.O. degrees are of Spanish origin, probably reflecting the substantial influence of foreign medical graduates. For all other categories of professional service listed above, the figure is less than 2 percent, with the exception of registered nurses, where the Spanish-heritage representation is 2.1 percent.[24]

When we look at the "allied" medical services, however, we find a

[22] Freeman, et al., *Handbook*, p. 17.

[23] Alan Reynolds, "The High Cost of Health," *National Review*, July 20, 1973. In 1963–64, 14 percent of medical students belonged to the 1 percent of the country's families with incomes in excess of $25,000 a year. While some 36 percent of U.S. families had incomes of less than $5,000, these accounted for only 14 percent of medical students. "The attainment of medical education has not only been a traditional object of prestige in this country, but also one of privilege." Cecil G. Sheps and Conrad Seipp, "The Medical School, Its Products and Its Problems," *The Annals of the American Academy of Political and Social Science*, Vol. 399 (January 1972), p. 44.

[24] *Minorities and Women in the Health Fields: Applicants, Students, Workers*, Bureau of Health Resources Development, DHEW Publication No. (HRA) 75-22, May 1974.

much more conspicuous presence of blacks, particularly females. Some 40.4 percent of all lay midwives are black, as are 25.2 percent of nursing aides, orderlies, and attendants, 21.9 percent of practical nurses, 21 percent of dieticians, and 18.9 percent of health aides. Significantly, only 4.7 percent of health administrators are black. The highest penetration within these occupations for those of Spanish heritage is for dental laboratory technicians (6.3 percent), opticians, lens grinders and polishers (6.5 percent), and health aides (4.2 percent).

During the 1970s there have been attempts by governmental agencies and medical schools to increase the numbers of women and minorities in medical schools, and, therefore, eventually their presence in the physician supply. Government currently accounts for slightly more than 50 percent of the total operating costs of medical schools as compared with only 30 percent 10 years ago, and this increased financial support has been accompanied by growth in government influence over who is admitted to medical schools. Recent figures indicate some success in reducing the dominance of white male medical students. The year 1972 saw the largest increase ever recorded in women applicants, as they comprised 16.8 percent of all medical-school entrants (an increase of some 35 percent from the previous year). Minority admissions increased by 10.7 percent, with black Americans having the highest numeric increase and American Indians the highest percentage increase. A total of 19 more Mexican-Americans enrolled in first-year classes in 1972 than in 1971.[25] The lengthy period of physician education means that it will be a number of years before these moderate increases in minorities and women change the physician supply.

Many of the reasons for the disproportionately high percentage of white upper-middle-class physicians are found in the realities of medical school. As has always been true of other institutions of higher education, a very small percentage of medical-school applicants are women or minorities. Premedical education stresses biology, physiology, and other "hard sciences," which have never attracted large numbers of women or minority students. Medical schools place heavy emphasis on prior grade-point averages and effective performance on the Medical College Admission Test (MCAT), which again discourage women and minorities. But the major deterents to women and minorities are undoubtedly financial and attitudinal. Often the families of medical-school students must contribute substantially to payment of educational expenses, an obligation difficult for low-income minority families to meet. The important contribution of the incomes of "working wives" to the support of medical students probably discourages women. Few husbands seem willing to put their wives through medical school. It is particularly difficult for students

25 W. F. Dube and Davis G. Johnson, "Study of U.S. Medical School Applicants, 1972–73," *Journal of Medical Education*, Vol. 49, no. 9 (September 1974), pp. 857ff.

in poor families to forgo all opportunities to earn an income during the long years of medical study.

One attitude favoring white middle-income males is that medical schools prefer applicants from prestigious colleges and universities, places where minorities and women are usually less evident and successful. In addition, it has been claimed that "No other occupational choice . . . has as strong a father–son determination as medicine."[26] This means, of course, that one predominant generation of upper-middle-class white male doctors tends to produce the next generation in its own likeness. Individuals considering medicine as a profession probably believe that medical schools judge them on factors other than past academic success, such as race, ethnic origin, and economic background. It is reasonable to believe that this may sometimes be true, and therefore applicants other than white middle-income males probably suffer from both imagined and actual bias. In the 1970s a higher percentage of women applicants to medical schools have been admitted than male applicants. This may not reflect reverse discrimination but simply the fact that the self-selection process is very much more severe for women than men.

The importance of the socioeconomic background of physicians stems from the simple reality that background helps shape attitudes and attitudes are important in health-care delivery transactions. As long as physicians are primarily middle-income white males (often from a "professional" family), we will have a physician pool that does not fully understand the medical and related problems and attitudes of minorities, women, and consumers who suffer discomfort with and alienation from physicians. Mexican-American women, for example, are very modest and often become highly anxious and seek to avoid treatment having any implications of sexuality if the physician is a male.[27] Many argue that male surgeons are insensitive to the trauma of women undergoing hysterectomies and mastectomies and that they are too quick to operate.

THE "SPECIAL CASE" OF THE FOREIGN MEDICAL GRADUATE

The largest "minority" in the pool of practicing physicians are foreign medical graduates. Almost half the physicians licensed in 1972 were FMGs.[28]

[26] Rashi Fein and Gerald I. Weber, *Financing a Medical Education* (New York: McGraw-Hill, 1971), p. 77.

[27] Margaret Clark, "Health in the Mexican-American Culture" (University of California Press), 1970, pp. 229ff.

[28] Charles C. Sprague, "National Health Policy: Objectives and Strategy," *Journal of Medical Education*, Vol. 49, no. 1 (January 1974), p. 9.

The debate over the appropriate flow of physician services has taken an international perspective, for the influx of foreign medical-school graduates reflects the attractions of the domestic market. The 1965 amendments to the Immigration and Naturalization Act terminated the traditional national-origins quota system and encouraged entry of individuals with professional and occupational skills thought to be in short supply nationwide. Physicians soon began to appreciate that they had an opportunity to immigrate to the United States, leaving the question of their ability to meet American licensing requirements for later resolution. In a little over a decade from 1962 to 1973, the number of FMGs increased four times more rapidly than that of the total physician supply. FMGs now approach twenty percent of all physicians, and fill one-third of all internships and residency training posts. In 1972, more graduates of foreign medical schools entered the United States than physicians graduated by our own schools, and forty-six percent of all newly licensed physicians in that year were FMGs.[29] As of 1972, for the total physician stock in the United States of 356,534, 288,525 were graduates of U.S. schools, and 68,009 graduates of foreign schools. In 1973, 12,285 foreign medical school graduates entered this country. In that same year, U.S. schools graduated 10,391 students. There is an emerging group of American-born FMGs who have secured their medical training abroad, undoubtedly because of their failure to gain admission to American schools. In 1974, an estimated 6,000 Americans were enrolled in medical schools abroad, a figure that can be compared with the 50,716 students in American medical schools. In 1972, Latin American universities had 2,045 American students enrolled, with 91 percent of these attending the Universidad Autonoma de Guadalajara in Mexico.

The interest of students in securing admission to medical schools has increased at astonishing rates. Some admissions officers joke that about three out of every two college freshmen now aspire to become a doctor. AMA president, Malcolm C. Todd, pointed out that the 114 medical schools in this country accepted 14,000 freshmen for the academic year 1973–74. "I was on the Yale campus last autumn and 52 percent of the freshmen wanted to be doctors. Another 37 percent wanted to be lawyers. That doesn't leave many for anything else."[30] The increase in the number of applicants explains the higher proportion of applicants rejected and the impulse for American students to find alternative sources for education. From 1969 to 1974, the number of applicants to medical schools increased by 72 percent. During the spring of 1974, 42,000 seniors sent transcripts and test scores to our 114 medical schools. More than 27,000

29 "Graduates of Foreign Medical Schools in the United States: A Challenge to Medical Education," *Journal of Medical Education*, Vol. 49, no. 8 (August 1974), p. 813.
30 *U.S. News and World Report*, July 1, 1974, p. 32.

of the 1974 applicants were turned down, even though admissions directors agreed that at least half of the rejected students were qualified.[31]

Because of the press of American students in European medical schools, many European countries have abandoned open-admission policies and established quotas. In France, for example, foreign quotas have been cut from fifteen to five percent, and now admission to French medical schools is allowed only if the student can prove he has been accepted by a medical school in his own country! With access to the European schools limited, the flow to the Mexican university has increased even more sharply. More than three thousand students are now registered there, paying $5,000 tuition fees for the first year and $4,000 for each subsequent year. Although the program is rigorous, it does not compare with American demands. As a consequence, when students from the UAG take the National Board of Medical Examiner tests in order to transfer to American schools, their rate of failure is topped only by American students in Spain.

A second expanding market for training American students is Italy. Again, with rejection rates for admission to American schools reaching as high as ten to one, students are flowing to the twenty-seven medical schools in Italy. Some fifteen hundred American students are now enrolled. Six hundred Americans are immersed in the Italo-American Medical Education Foundation, which helps Italianize the American students and then re-Americanize them after their education. At a three-day symposium in Rome, students and doctors discussed the means of closing differences between American and Italian medical education. It was agreed that American technology gave Americans a clinical edge, but the main gap was largely due to the overcrowding of the Italian medical-school system. Italians are now graduating twelve thousand physicians a year, or four times the number that Italy needs.[32]

Military ventures have also had an influence on the domestic supply of FMGs. Following the Cuban crisis, the substantial inflow of Cuban physicians could not be readily absorbed. Many worked as waiters and cab drivers while they studied the English language and American medical texts. Some 300 of South Viet Nam's 1500 physicians—including the entire staff of the Saigon University School of Medicine—turned up at American refugee centers, along with 60 dentists and pharmacists. Most are studying for the Educational Council for Foreign Medical Graduate (ECFMG) examinations, which require command of English as well as knowledge of clinical medicine. In the winter of 1975, only 7,000 of the 19,000 doctors who took these examinations passed. Since the organization of the ECFMG in 1958, its network of 178 examination centers has

[31] "The Mexican M.D.'s," *Newsweek*, July 8, 1974, p. 49.
[32] "Many Future Doctors Are Training in Italy," *Alton Telegraph*, February 23, 1976.

given 313,885 examinations, with an overall pass rate (including repeaters) of 67 percent. On the first try, only 45 percent obtain a passing score. Interestingly, American FMGs have a similar if not greater failure rate in the ECFMG examination than foreign-born FMGs, suggesting that language difficulties are not a major factor in success with the examination.

There has been a sharp shift to Asian rather than European sources of supply. In 1972, some seventy percent of the emigrating flow came from Asian countries.

FMGs in this country are distributed by specialty in much the same way as American-educated physicians and also tend to favor metropolitan areas for practice. The first criticism raised is that we have a dual standard for entry into the medical field that might undermine American standards. A second criticism, implicit in the above narrative, is that the FMG is not willing to practice in underserved areas. Once certified, the foreign graduate acquires the tastes, aspirations, and lifestyle of his American counterpart. Third, it is charged that we are grossly abusing the educational facilities of foreign countries. By our tacit encouragement of this brain drain, we deny other countries the service of critically required professional talent at home, where uniformly the ratio of population to physicians is much higher. The *American Journal of Psychiatry* noted that if the 3,016 foreign doctors permanently licensed in the United States in 1970 were trained here, this would require construction of 30 new medical schools. The cost of each medical school would be at least $50 million, and its annual operating budget about $3.8 million. In effect, the stock of 3,016 foreign doctors would require an outflow of $1.6 billion. This was equivalent to over one-half of the total foreign-aid program. Proponents of the foreign inflow point out that the costs of training M.D.s at home are undoubtedly much higher than foreign costs. *The Wall Street Journal* editorializes:

> About one third emigrated from the developing world, chiefly from India and the Philippines, and if all of them returned they'd make hardly a dent in the health problems of those nations, which stem from poverty rather than a health-manpower shortage. There are as many trained doctors in the Philippines who are working at other trades, for example, as there are Filipino doctors working in their profession in the United States.[33]

The major criticism involves speculation about oversupply. Medical schools are now graduating about 10,000 a year, compared with 7,500 in 1965. The anticipated number of graduates will reach 15,000 annually by 1980. If we add to this about 3,000 FMGs a year, the 1974 stock of 360,000 physicians will increase to 440,000 by 1980. That increase is about 4 times

[33] "Our Foreign-Trained Doctors," *The Wall Street Journal*, February 22, 1974, p. 8.

the rate of population growth and should ease the persistent problems of access to medical services.

A RECAPITULATION AND SOME POLICY ISSUES

Our interlacing of statistics with descriptions of attitudes throughout the chapter does not leave us with a crisp definition of values or a sharp profile of postures. It remains true that the physician has unprecedented authority and influence in determining the quantity, quality, and directions of medical services. We have identified a social "dissonance" of attitudes of the public and patients: some hold to the godlike father figure of the physician, while others display unguarded contempt for the hypocrisy implicit in Hippocratic pretensions. Even a casual reading of the outpouring of literature on the medical field suggests that the mantle of professional authority is slipping. Speculation about future change is clouded. Let's review a few key issues of the conflicting value systems.

First, it is widely held that the American public is beguiled by the remarkable breakthroughs in medical technology. These are reported in the daily press, the Sunday newspaper supplements, TV news, and the like. We can find both assurance and pride in the brilliance of our medical scientists. Life-sustaining equipment seems able to deal with just about any contingency. This is a mischievous misconception, which sets the stage for many problems of credibility facing the medical sector today. The problem emerges most explicitly in the malpractice issue.

Technical advances in medicine have, of course, provided prevention, cures, and remedies for many illnesses considered fatal a few years ago. Hospitalization for tuberculosis has virtually been eliminated through drug therapy; death from bilateral kidney failure or destruction has been reduced by kidney transplants and hemodialysis; previously inoperable cerebral tumors can now be operated upon by cryosurgery; and so on. Even so, these sweeping triumphs of science and technology have created unrealistic expectations of what medical intervention can, in fact, produce. We have tended to forget the long way we must go to ameliorate or cure cancer and heart disease and to deal effectively with stroke victims. In effect, the widely heralded triumphs have tended to obscure the new risks involved with new drugs, techniques, machinery, and operations.

The human response to this has been a tendency to neglect the delicate and fragile structure of the human system. We are no longer willing to accept illness as a usual or expected event in our lives. We are less willing to accept sickness as an act of God. As noted above, the success stories, supported with glowing accounts of the effectiveness of miracle drugs and sophisticated technology, have shifted faith from the diety to the doctor. And if the doctor fails, we do not revert to religion: we file charges for human negligence.

Most citizens lack an appreciation for both the complexities and the risks of contemporary medical practice. Even so, consumer-rights movements are insisting on quality care and insisting, too, on the right for product evaluation. And they are increasingly insisting on recompense for negligence.

> . . . the press and broadcasting media fostered greater public interest in medicine and particularly in its "miracles," leading the public to develop many unrealistic expectations about medicine's capabilities. Many Americans regard good health as though it were a commodity, something that the doctor can dispense at will. But good health is not a purchasable commodity. It is a matter first of heredity and, above all, a matter of personal responsibility, choice, and self-governance. Unfortunately, the failure to achieve ideal health has caused great disappointment with the results of treatment on the part of some patients, and they turned with greater and greater frequency to the lawsuit as a means of resolving their disappointment.[34]

In a similar vein, Congressman James F. Hastings reported to Congress:

> The medical-care system has made great advances . . . but it has created patient expectations which are often beyond the capacity of the system to fulfill, a system with risks associated both with the nature of the treatment itself and the possibility of human error, and a system which is more impersonal than that which existed 30 or 40 years ago. When a patient experiences an unfavorable outcome of his treatment in this climate, the stage is set for a malpractice claim.[35]

In a paper presented to a national malpractice conference, Robert Maplis made the point with similar force:

> The miraculous achievements of modern medicine, and the doctor's image which has been so tremendously improved on TV, are fine. But they are also leading the public to believe that virtually any condition can be cured by one of the wonder drugs, some fantastic new operation, or some form of medical treatment. . . . There is an almost universal overexpectation by the patients of possible results. Also, it is almost universally true that any drug (or indeed any operation), however beneficial, is almost always dangerous in proportion to its potential efficacy.[36]

34 *Report of the Secretary's Commission on Medical Malpractice*, Department of Health, Education and Welfare, January 16, 1973, DHEW Publication No. OS 73-88, GPO, p. 3.
35 *An Overview of Medical Malpractice*, Staff Report for the Committee on Interstate and Foreign Commerce, U.S. House of Representatives, 94th Cong., 1st Session, March 17, 1975 (Washington, D.C.: GPO, 1975), p. 7.
36 *National Conference on Medical Malpractice*, p. 3.

At the same conference John E. Linster described the public perception of the physician as one with the physical prowess of Superman, the practical wisdom of one who has been attending patients for fifty years, and the familiarity with medical skills of the most recent graduate from our best medical school.[37]

Optimism, then, about the consequence of medical intervention may help explain the individual's neglect of his personal health as an implicit attempt to shift to the medical profession responsibility for all afflictions. An angry and exasperated AMA representation responded: "We are dealing with the same old fat patients who smoke or drink too much. . . ."[38] In his view, it is unfair for the judicial system to expect medicine to compensate patients for failure to be cured when patients so often contribute to their own injury through carelessness, by failing to follow instructions, or through poor personal habits.[39]

This charge raises a second and closely related policy issue: most individuals appear unwilling to alter their lifestyles in any major way to avoid affliction or prevent disease. Those who admonish the public to improve its lifestyle probably have simplistic notions about the rationality of human response. Advertising the incontrovertible fact that cigarette smoking is injurious to your health has been associated with more, rather than less, smoking. We have yet to probe fully to discover and implement an educational strategy that is capable of changing human behavior.

John Ruskin's aphorism is relevant to this issue: "Education is not that one knows more, but that one behaves differently." The more thoughtful students of the subject realize that information and knowledge does not, in itself, lead to recommended actions, particularly if the change conflicts with existing motives, attitudes, beliefs, and values. Resistance is most conspicuous if guidelines for good health are not consonant with existing social and group norms.

The seriousness of resistance to change can only be appreciated when we enumerate the kinds of threats more injurious to health. N. David Richards makes the point with appropriate force:

These new conditions, the "diagnoses of civilization" (chronic degenerative diseases such as cancer, heart disease, and arthritis), have assumed critical importance as reference to morbidity and mortality will show. Together with changes in age patterns, dependency ratios, and the duration of disease, they have occasioned a transfer from sudden to routine

[37] Ibid., p. 17.
[38] Testimony by John Coury, of the AMA Council on Legislation, ibid., p. 24. Coury also testified: "No longer can providers of medicine be expected to solve society's psychological and socioeconomic problems. Doctors cannot be expected to continually finance society's ills. We are willing to accept our responsibility. We expect the public, the legal profession, and the judiciary to accept theirs" (p. 22).
[39] Ibid., p. 22.

episodes of sickness. The association of behavioral pattern of disease has led to the concept of *disease being self-afflicted or socially induced, and a realization that a large and increasing proportion of contemporary morbidity is man made.* Research into the role of cigarette smoking in lung cancer, dietary factors and physical activity in heart disease, oral hygiene practices and peridontal and gingival conditions, . . . has furthered this concept. . . . Nonetheless, and despite the cognitive recognition of health information, people are still dying from ignorance or want of knowledge relating to the risks they are taking.[40]

But are health-care providers responsible for spreading information about the threats to health from drinking, overeating, reckless driving, and other forms of merriment? Is the current trend one toward liberalism, toward the emancipation of youth from parental authority, toward wider sexual freedoms and liberation of the spirit from all forms of moral and political authority that are considered oppressive? Will these set the stage for a renewed discipline commensurate with good health? If man is now not only the host but also the agent of disease; if the threat is not found in the bacteria of the external environment, but in the quest for pleasure within the internal environment, then the question of intervention involves the profound issues of free will and breaches of individual autonomy. It is a strange and discomforting hypothesis that man may be the agent of many of his own afflictions, that his health is more likely to be determined by what he does to himself rather than by what some germ or viral infection can do to him. But is it realistic to expect individuals to willingly reduce their exposure as "hosts" of disease caused by smoking, drinking, and stress? Does our culture encourage a shift to a health-promoting mode? Most of the evidence leads to a negative response.

Many traditionalists within the medical fraternity caution about the involvement of medical personnel in seeking to promote remedies for self-inflicted impairment. The reasons for caution are obvious. First, there is little prospect that the public will change its behavior pattern, no matter how persuasive or sophisticated the educational program. Second, intrusions into questions of value and lifestyle raise moral issues that are beyond the scope or responsibility of the medical-care provider. In an ultimate sense, the provider respects the individual's right to die, his right to knowingly destroy himself. Third, the current educational program requires an already-demanding number of obligatory courses. To introduce the sociology or philosophy of medicine would burden the schedule and threaten the scientific core of medical education. We may end up with uncertain methodologies for changing lifestyles, while eroding the core of

[40] N. David Richards, "Methods and Effectiveness of Health Education: The Past, Present and Future of Social Scientific Involvement," *Social Science and Medicine,* Vol. 9 (Elmsford, N.Y.: Pergamon, 1975), p. 143. Italics added.

well-tested scientific technique responsible for so many of our past advances.

A third major attitudinal issue is the appropriate focus for medical education itself. Public pressure is growing to have physician training synchronized to serve the human needs of the population as well as the intellectual curiosity of the laboratory scientist. Its major thrust is the cautious revolution calling for "comprehensive" care. It is seen, too, in the government's formal request to have medical students receiving federal assistance serve a portion of their time in the medically underserved areas.

By way of contrast, let us describe the elements of comprehensive care and family practice. First, it is care that is person- and family-centered. There is a functional integration of supporting services that are accommodated to patient and family problems, rather than the other way around. Comprehensive care is personalized and compassionate. Beyond this, it involves birth-to-death attention that stresses preventive, advisory, and rehabilitative activities. This contrasts with the episodic and impersonal care that involves a single shot of attention to single problems. Comprehensive care acknowledges the importance of both the emotional and environmental components of good health. It combines the services of the generalist with those of the specialist. In its refined form, it is likely to be a team effort, with team experts sensitive to issues of family structure and environment that have major influences on both the causes of affliction and recovery from disease. The medical team will be made up of persons trained in primary or family care, in psychiatry, internal medicine, pediatrics, preventive medicine, and relevant elements of the behavioral sciences, including economics, sociology, and psychology.[41]

We have noted that because of the 1910 Flexner report, medical schools have cultivated the scientific disciplines. The schools represent federations of diverse disciplines with a strong research orientation in anatomy, physiology, biochemistry, microbiology, and the like. From World War II until very recently, government subsidies to medical schools have had the effect of furthering this research orientation. In 1969, for example, over 272,000 students attending medical schools were not medical students in the traditional sense. They were involved in research projects, often sponsored by the National Institute of Health. Indeed, at that time, non-M.D. students outnumbered student physicians by about three to two.[42] The most recent perception is that medical schools are now weighted down by the fruits of their own creative research energies, with a growing dichotomy between medical research and its applications.

---

[41] For a fuller discussion, see Darley Ward and Anne R. Somers, "Medicine, Money and Manpower: The Challenge to Professional Education," *The New England Journal of Medicine*, Vol. 276, no. 23 (June 8, 1967), pp. 1291–96.

[42] Rosemary Stevens, *American Medicine and the Public Interest* (New Haven: Yale University Press, 1971), p. 349.

The massive infusion of federal funds helped raise average medical-school income from $3.7 million in 1958 to $15 million in 1968–69, an increase by a factor of 4 in only 10 years. Federal funding reinforced the tendency for medical schools to become research enclaves, concentrating on the biology and chemistry of disease. It is not widely appreciated that the National Institute of Health served as the feeder mechanism for the infusion of funds to medical education. By 1968, the NIH had a full-time staff of over 13,000 and a budget of $1.6 billion, of which $254 million was spent on its own operations. As early as 1955, one-third of medical-school income was secured from research grants, and by 1960, there were about 120 full-time faculty members per medical school, with 1 in 7 receiving more than half of his salary from federal sources. By 1969, the average faculty size was 250 per school, with more than 1 full-time faculty member for every 2 medical students. A substantial number of this newly acquired faculty were involved not in instruction but in research. Indeed, just under half of the faculty received some of their funds from federal research grants. As Rosemary Stevens explains:

> While the AMA had been opposing federal aid for medical education, using as one argument distrust of increased governmental control over a traditionally professional responsibility, the medical schools had de facto become extensively dependent on the government through the back door of research subsidy.[43]

In the early 1970s this interest in biomedical research, though filled with sparkling potentiality, began to wane as interest shifted to an increased effort to produce more physicians. The focus on laboratory research was somewhat deflected by the realization that research efforts were not providing direct services to the population. It was hoped that additional physicians would close the gap between research and its applications. The AMA expressed reservations about heavy federal subsidies to encourage the growth of medical schools, but the deans of medical schools were less wary.

On reflection, can we conclude that the benefits of the Flexner standards have run their course? Can we have too much research, after all? The issue is expressed with impressive authority by Rosemary Stevens:

> The average doctor has been transformed in sixty years from an incompetent physician, whose strength lay in the "bedside manner" of his mystique, to a specialist internist, surgeon, or endocrinologist whose own competence is buttressed by an array of diagnostic and treatment aids and techniques. American doctors are among the best-trained, perhaps the best-trained technological physicians in the world. Together, however, they are not providing optimal medical care; and it is this

[43] Ibid., p. 359.

factor which has become the education paradox—the manpower crisis —of the 1970s. Traditional goals of professionalism are no longer enough. If the medical schools are to meet their role as public-service corporations, the inbuilt conflict between the goals of professionalism and the improvement of health services has to be resolved.[44]

But is it, in fact, now possible to humanize and integrate medical services through the redesign of medical education? Can we provide patients with a systematically integrated care system? One senses that we dare not forego the research orientation and its result, specialization. Modified systems will more likely require an integration of skills in service teams than they will mandate that greater number of physicians become generalists.

SUGGESTED READINGS

CHASE, ROBERT A., "Proliferation of Certification in Medical Specialties: Productive or Counterproductive?," *The New England Journal of Medicine,* Vol. 294, no. 9 (February 26, 1976), pp. 497–99. A critique of the university's emphasis on specialization for health-care personnel.

"Datagram," *Journal of Medical Education,* Vol. 49 (March 1974), pp. 302–7. An examination of enrollment in medical schools, breaking down the students in terms of race and sex.

EBERT, ROBERT H., "The Medical School," *Scientific American,* Vol. 229, no. 3 (September 1973), pp. 139–48. A survey of the influence of the medical school on students.

FEIN, RASHI, and GERALD I. WEBER, *Financing Medical Education,* A General Report Prepared for the Carnegie Commission on Higher Education and the Commonwealth Fund (New York: McGraw-Hill, 1971). A discussion of the costs of medical education and its sources of financing.

GROBE, JAMES L., "How to Pick a Family Doctor," *U.S. News and World Report,* September 10, 1973, pp. 42–45. An interview dealing with the lack of information available to assist the consumer in choosing a physician.

HAGGERTY, ROBERT J., "The University and Primary Care," *The New England Journal of Medicine,* Vol. 28, no. 8 (August 21, 1969), pp. 416–22. A commentary on the university role in encouraging specialization.

HAUG, MARIE R., "The Erosion of Professional Authority: A Cross-Cultural Inquiry in the Case of Physician," *Milbank Memorial Fund Quarterly,* Vol. 54, no. 1 (Winter 1976), pp. 83–106. Discusses the revolt of the client against the authority of the physician.

"How to Find a Doctor for Yourself," *Consumer Reports,* September 1974, pp. 681–91. A guideline to assist consumers in physician selection.

LICCIONE, WILLIAM J. and SUSAN MCALLISTER, "Attitudes of First Year Medical Students Toward Rural Medical Practice," *Journal of Medical Educa-*

[44] Ibid., p. 374.

tion, Vol. 49, no. 5 (May 1974), pp. 449–50. Explores the reasons that most medical students prefer urban rather than rural practice.

MITCHELL, WAYNE D., "Medical Student Career Choice: A Conceptualization," *Social Science and Medicine,* Vol. 9, no. 11/12 (November/December 1975), pp. 641–53. A comprehensive analysis of the way in which the educational experience influences student choice of specialization.

REZLER, AGNES G., "Attitude Change During Medical School: A Review of the Literature," *Journal of Economic Education,* Vol. 49, no. 11 (November 1974). Surveys the literature on the medical school's influence on student attitudes.

ROGERS, PAUL, "Congressional Perspectives on Government and Quality of Medical Education," *Journal of Medical Education,* Vol. 51 (January 1976), pp. 3–6. A critical essay warning the medical academy that public patience for the medical sector's response to poor distribution of health care is wearing thin.

"Trouble for 'Ted Terrific,'" *Newsweek,* November 17, 1975, p. 75. A discussion of malperformances within the medical sector.

WILLIAMS, KATHLEEN N. and ROBERT H. BROOK, "Foreign Medical Graduates and Their Impact on the Quality of Medical Care in the United States," *Milbank Memorial Fund Quarterly,* Vol. 53, no. 1 (Fall 1975), pp. 549–81. A comprehensive survey of the case of the foreign medical graduate practicing medicine in the United States.

5

THE DEMAND
FOR MEDICAL CARE:
SOME INSTITUTIONAL AND
SOCIOLOGICAL INFLUENCES

We have placed the issue of demand on center stage, for it reflects the multifaceted dimensions of human welfare. In this enormously complex area, we are confronted with contradictions of philosophy and empirical analysis. Some economists attribute the shortcomings of the medical market to interventions that are inadequate to support demand, and others to the excess of intervention. The ubiquitous concern of the latter is that removal of budget and price constraints in providing free health services would invite the inundation of the health-care system. Public pressure for health care has been dubbed the "moral hazard" of nationalized systems. But the question has been raised: "What is, in fact, immoral about wanting more health services?" As Brian Abel-Smith explains:

> How many of us are such chronic hypochondriacs that we are likely to camp out on our physician's doorstep, take our vacations in hospitals, or beg for prescriptions we can fill? Or are we worried that people may make hats out of gauze and suture? Is this immorality or a special form of sickness?[1]

Do we, in fact, have firm evidence of an indiscriminate demand for health services, simply because it is there? The evidence for the surfacing of a vast reserve of unmet needs when a system offers service to all comers is not conclusive. But economists are quick to note that if the rationing of services does not cost the consumer money, it may well cost him the time required by the queuing process, as people await their turn for attention.

In this chapter, we shall explore three major issues. First, we shall briefly identify some of the peculiarities of the demand for medical serv-

[1] Brian Abel-Smith, "Value for Money in Health Services," *Social Security Bulletin*, July 1974, p. 17.

ices. If we are to apply market calculus as a measure of performance for the medical market, what are the novelties of structure that must be considered in any fair accounting process? Second, we will briefly review the cultural influences in medical-care demand. The third issue (related to the second) is the relationship of work satisfactions to health. The sociological information provided in this chapter will complement the discussion of the patient–physician contact reviewed in the last chapter.

MEDICAL DEMAND: A SUMMARY OF NOVEL FEATURES

Let us briefly review some of the most noteworthy features of medical-demand analysis. First, as we have noted previously, the typical consumer is often a poor judge of the care or medical intervention he receives, either before or after the fact. Second, the physician serves as an agent on behalf of the patient in the treatment regimen. He is the patient's surrogate in the purchase of goods that could benefit the patient's welfare and the physician's pocket. Third, the physician, by training, has a technologic reflex to "buy the best rather than find the best buy."[2] In functions two and three above, the physician is confronted with commercial influences. Abel-Smith has noted:

> After training he [the physician] is exposed to conflicts between his conscience and his pocket and conflicts between interests of his paymaster and those of competing commercial interests. His doormat is piled high with drug-firm literature, and his doorstep is shaded by drughouse detail men. Over his shoulder looms the risk of malpractice litigation. His hospital, rather than any other, is his preferred workshop. Nearly all of his decisions are of financial consequence to him as well as to his patient or the third party paying the patient's bill.[3]

Fourth, the typical patient-consumer suffers errors of optimism about what can be accomplished by medical intervention and, as a consequence, is often insensitive to his personal responsibilities for maintaining good health:

[2] Ibid., p. 18.

[3] Ibid., pp. 18–19. Most physicians are undoubtedly offended by any intimations that commercial incentives transcend professional obligations. Paul Feldstein acknowledges that as the physician is making choices for the patient (customer), he does so with the "necessary assumption" that the physician is familiar with the patient's financial resources as well as his medical needs. Thus, he acts in a manner consistent with the way the patient would behave if he were able to make the decisions. Feldstein verifies such physician "awareness" by noting the numerous studies relating hospital use to the patient's economic resources, including insurance coverage. Paul Feldstein, "Research on the Demand for Health Services." In John B. McKinlay (ed.), *Economic Aspects of Health Care* (New York: Prodist, 1973), p. 133.

Cigarette smoking, overeating, underexercise, alcoholic consumption, manner of automobile driving, family crisis and many more environmental and social hazards are essentially very personal life styles that have a major bearing upon one's health and will be improved only to the extent that the person affected feels enough responsibility for, and pride in, his power to change his way of life.[4]

Fifth, the determination of "adequate" or "quality" medical care is confounded by differences of opinion between professionals and the public. There are many influences of the environment and the home that also affect recovery. In one colorful analogy, evaluating outcomes is about as troublesome as attempting to put a river bank on a swamp.

A sixth reality is that social class is strongly correlated with the prevalence of disease. There is some risk, in all of this, of blaming the ship for the weather, but we must note that climatic and cultural forces interact with biological structures in peculiar and mysterious ways, a mystery compounded by the traditional isolation of biological and sociological studies. It is clearly illogical, of course, to conclude that social class is in itself a "cause" of pneumonia, any more than we can say that it is a culture, and not individuals, who paint their fingernails. But we can identify some incidence of morbidity by class. Further,

> We know that there are enormous variations in the perceptions of illness and [in] what people do about it in different groups and that these differences are not all related to differences in the frequency of illness. Merely providing care or removing financial barriers, as important as these steps are, does not ensure its proper use.[5]

A seventh major policy issue of demand analysis is how to deal with individuals who are denied access to health-care facilities because of their meager resources. Most contemporary societies have avowed that the medically indigent should have access to health care. In the liberal view, the problem is resolved by elevating the economic status of the poor. But until that goal is attained, we are confronted with awkward problems of consumer sovereignty. As Kenneth Boulding explains:

> In the case of medical indigency . . . the temptation is to deny consumers sovereignty as the price of the relief of indigency, and to say that the poor must have what the professionals think is good for them whether they want it or not. This is part of a very old and still unresolved question as to whether the grants economy should content itself with grants of money, leaving the recipient to spend it as he will, or should consist essentially of grants in kind, supplying needs as defined by the professionals. Those who are somewhat liberal are in-

---

[4] Robert J. Haggerty, "The University and Primary Medical Care," *The New England Journal of Medicine*, Vol. 281, no. 8 (August 21, 1969), p. 416.
[5] Ibid., p. 418.

clined to emphasize demand even in the case of the indigent, and to give them at least some freedom to reject medical care if they prefer a short life and a merry one, though the liberty to preach against such behavior should also be preserved.[6]

Grants, such as food stamps, can be given to the indigent on the demand side of the market. In this way spending is confined to those things society believes "ought" to be desired. Those opposed to outright payments never tire of pointing to system abuses, including the purchase of luxury commodities with stamps, loss of incentives to work, and so on. Similarly problems apply to grants offered to suppliers. Again, Boulding notes:

. . . certain casual administrative regulations in the social security system have stimulated a profitable practice of keeping indigent patients in nursing homes in bed, simply because the nursing homes are paid an extra amount for keeping people in bed. Hence, nursing homes make more money on bed patients than on ambulatory ones. As a result of the strong financial pressure, patients are kept in bed, in spite of the fact that this may be quite unwarranted medically and may contribute to the already bad enough miseries of old age and incompetence.[7]

The present Medicare–Medicaid system, instituted since Boulding's discussion, limits the sovereignty of users to a prescribed package of health benefits. And it also limits reimbursements to charges that the government considers "reasonable." Complications quickly develop when definitions of reasonableness established by the providers do not coincide with those of the government. For example, J. Alexander McMahon, president of the American Hospital Association, has rejected the charge that the inflation of health-service costs can be attributed to hospitals: "Let them tell us what services they don't want us to provide and what patients they don't want us to take care of. . . . If you expect hospitals and doctors to control costs when you promise to pay for any service, then you've forgotten the history of the United States. . . . You cannot control costs in the face of unlimited demand."[8] If the medical market were to behave as other markets, however, one would expect that the enlarged demand for services would set in motion the expansion of facilities. In time, the demand pressure should pull sufficient resources into the medical sector to moderate price and cost inflation.[9]

[6] Kenneth E. Boulding, "The Concept of Need for Health Services," *Milbank Memorial Fund Quarterly*, October 1966, p. 19.

[7] Ibid., p. 19.

[8] Reported by John Cunniff, "Hospitals Fighting Bad Image," *Edwardsville Intelligencer*, May 13, 1976, p. 11.

[9] For an interesting discussion of the market response to demand pressures, see James R. Jeffers, Mario F. Bognanno, and John C. Bartlett, "On the Demand Versus Need for Medical Services and the Concept of 'Shortage,'" *American Journal of Public Health*, Vol. 16, no. 1 (January 1971), pp. 46–61.

An eighth aspect of the demand question is what ceiling to place on expenditure appropriated for the purchase of health care. Clearly, the goal of securing perfect health for everyone is both biologically and economically unattainable. Avedis Donabedian draws an appropriate analogy between health and the advance of public education. In both cases, how much is enough?

> Medical-care needs are so extensible that prohibitively large sums of money can readily be swallowed up by the health-care system, if clients and professionals are given a free reign to consume and to provide services, respectively. If the restraints of the market are removed, how are we to decide what is enough medical care? The answer seems to be: in the same way that we decide what is enough public education— through a political decision that sets a limit on the total resources to be made available. This being done, we would expect that this total is reallocated within the system as productively as we know how. In this way, everyone has equal access to medical care that is equally good or, for that matter, equally bad. It is possible, of course, to give special attention to groups that now carry a disproportionately large burden of unmet need, so that they can be made to catch up with the rest. It is also possible to favor any other segment of the population, depending on who holds political power, and what the values and objectives of the powerful are. Thus, the switch from the market to another method of rationing holds for many the terrifying prospect of a loss in present privilege, even though, in the end, the roster of those who are favored may be seen to have remained remarkably unchanged.[10]

The political determination of the appropriate spending limits must be made. The social values of health-care need must be reconciled to the competing interests of society. Ideally, a rational allocation for health should take account of cost-benefit ratios for all alternative public investments. And allocations within the health-care sector would follow comparative ratios as well. The conceptualization is obvious enough: the measurement of alternative streams of benefits requires a valuation process that cannot help but bring into sharp focus the conflict of values endemic to our society.

A ninth feature is the differentiated services, reflected in the fact that the physician must treat each case individually. As noted above, the cost of treatment is often not fully known before the fact, nor can we readily make estimates of cost effectiveness since the output (good health) reflects concurrent influences.[11]

---

[10] Avedis Donabedian, "Issues in National Health Insurance," *American Journal of Public Health*, Vol. 66, no. 4 (April 1976), pp. 349–50.

[11] Paul Feldstein points out that "without considerations of all the components of care used in a particular treatment, conclusions cannot be drawn regarding the "proper" amount of care received from one component." Feldstein, "Research on the Demand for Health Services," p. 128. More specifically, it is difficult to identify the

Related to this are varying levels of intensity of need. Even if the cost of life-sustaining services increases, there is little reduction in the demand for those services. Most of us do not ponder probability tables dealing with various afflictions; we simply feel that illness—particularly serious illness—is a random event. We may, for that reason, have little impulse to anticipate the reality and thus have little interest in insurance designed to protect us from these contingencies. We optimize our investments in medical care when the cost of not having services available is equal to the cost of providing such care. If a person is incurably optimistic about "escaping the law of averages," he may not want to purchase insurance: "Never bet against yourself." But those concerned with health planning are likely to substitute their own definitions of need, based on probabilistic estimates of morbidity.

Some studies have attempted to identify the emergency aspect of medical care. One hospital study found that "emergent" patients, classified as those admitted immediately, and "urgent" cases (admitted within twenty-four to forty-eight hours) represented less than twenty percent of total admissions. Another study found that (excluding maternity cases) thirty-two percent of admissions were "same-day emergency" episodes. Some thirty-three percent of admissions were for illnesses present for more than a year.[12] Potential patients are now stopping to consider whether they need certain services and whether these could be postponed. Such discretion would also be likely to increase as preventive examinations and diagnostic techniques improve.

When we move to a second category of need, involving nonserious and curative medical services, price elasticities will increase.

> There are many substitute products that compete with medical services when the consumer seeks alleviation of a nonserious problem: Various proprietary drugs and medicines, home remedies, alcohol, nonprofessional advice, and so on. The lowering of the price of medical services makes these alternatives less desirable and hence more medical services are demanded.[13]

More specifically, nonserious medical services compete with the full range of other options for spending money. This reduced sense of urgency is even more conspicuous in the demand for preventive medical services. Here, we are confronted with consumer apathy, along with a conven-

---

effectiveness of one component of care unless all other components are specified. Most indices of care received by individuals do not comprehend the entire range of services, and thus damage our efforts to impute the effectiveness of any single service.

[12] These data are reported by Feldstein, "Research on the Demand for Health Services," p. 137.

[13] Richard M. Bailey, "Why We Need to Plan." In Mary F. Arnold, L. Vaughn Blankenship, and John M. Hess (eds.), *Administering Health Systems: Issues and Perspectives* (Chicago: Aldine, 1971), p. 236.

tional attitude of "letting well enough alone." There may be both hidden fears that a thorough physician may uncover difficulties and an exaggerated faith in nature's restorative capacities. The apparently limited "taste" for preventive medicine is a reality that may well require considerable education, advertising, or the application of other Madison Avenue techniques to tease public interest. There may be some aversion to checkups because of the queuing problem, particularly in group plans.

A tenth market feature is the absence of competition, as traditionally defined by the economists. Exigencies of emergency care require that the patient hurriedly seek access to facilities, and in any event the physician will want to assign his patient to a facility in which he has staff privileges. It is often difficult to determine whom one should go to see, especially since there are no "bargains" to be had. The use of price adjustments to attract patients is frowned upon by the industry, and the physician enjoys an unusual measure of influence and power.

An eleventh market feature is the question of the market response to increased demand and, more particularly, of whether the "invisible hand" will guarantee that the physician's economic gain will ensure the patient's greater well-being. Bailey views with skepticism the physician's comfortable assumption that this is so:

> We have assumed that there is competition and, therefore, as the consumer enters this marketplace to buy medical services, he does so in a setting where the resources supposedly are allocated effectively. Many statements in medical publications are based upon these ideas. Accordingly, physicians are encouraged to act in their own best economic interest, feeling that consumer well-being also will be served well. Personally, I do not believe we can say that if the physician acts in his own economic interest this will benefit the consumer. . . .
>
> . . . an overview of the medical-practice industry reveals that the producers are in a very strong bargaining position relative to the consumers. Over the last twenty to twenty-five years, as demand for medical care has grown for a variety of reasons, the power of the physician-producers in the marketplace has been strongly evident. Because consumers have not been subjected to pressures to be more efficient in their productive activities. This strong demand, moreover, has made it easier for physicians to raise their prices rather than increase efficiency and reorganize the production process which would work to the consumer's advantage, not to the advantage of the producer.[14]

A twelfth market feature is that demand influences comingle with supply influences. This is not unique to the medical market, but what is unusual is the statistical evidence that the supply variables have such a strong influence on use of services.

The nature of interaction between demand and supply can be seen

[14] Ibid., pp. 241–42.

in Figure 5-1. We start, with the left panel, by showing increased levels of spending over time, from X to Y to Z. To what extent does this increasing index show demand or supply influences? Instinctively, one would attribute increased spending to increased demand, for the former would seemingly reflect the latter. This case is illustrated in the top panel on the right side of the figure. Total spending is found by multiplying the average cost of medical services times the volume of services supplied. Thus the rectangle OAXC in the righthand panel is equal to the vertical height EX. The demand schedule shifts to the right from D_1 to D_2 to D_3 in the top right figure, resulting in a larger rectangle of expenditure as we shift from X to Y to Z.

Figure 5-1

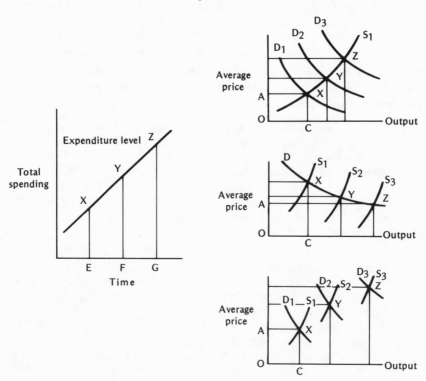

But supply shifts alone may account for the increase in expenditure, as seen in the middle figure. Here we shift the supply schedule increasingly to the right. This results in successively lower prices for health care, which prompts a considerable increase in the volume of services purchased. If the quantity response is greater than the price reduction, the levels of expenditure have actually increased. But there is no shift in demand; rather, consumers "slide down" a given (elastic) demand schedule.

In the more frequent situation, both demand and supply schedules are shifting concurrently. We have drawn three points of intersection in the bottom panel, and as we move from the origin to the right, spending has increased. The task is to untangle the concurrent forces in order to isolate variables most likely to account for changes in spending.

A final feature of the medical market is the difficulty of penetrating the money illusion through which we seek additional services through additional expenditures. This involves measurement of "real" services, along with qualitative measures of their effectiveness. The problem is twofold. As noted above, the increase in the expenditure flow may largely be met with price and cost adjustments, thus offsetting the "real" advance of services patients are seeking. The second and much more complicated issue is the measure of quality. We will soon review the shift of morbidity patterns from generation to generation. The system's effectiveness in dealing, for example, with tuberculosis has added to life expentancy, and with the extension of life, the aged are confronted with a new set of chronic afflictions. The switching of affliction patterns in this context does not reflect the failure of contemporary medicine so much as the triumphs of yesterday's medicine. There are, in effect, improvements in the quality of care, reflected somewhat paradoxically in the heavy incidence of chronic afflictions that threaten the aged. The identification of reasonable performance standards for health suppliers represents one of the most neglected and yet critical issues in the field.

In the search for quality standards, we cannot slip into the comfortable assumption that increases in supply must necessarily be preceded or followed by increased expenditure. For example, in the top panel of Figure 5-2, we introduce a supply shift from S_1 to S_2 and find that levels of spending have diminished because of the limited price elasticity of demand for health services. It is the hope of all that the stimulus of demand in the purchase of health services will lead to a supply response that might, in time, provide for reductions of the expenditure flow.

Similarly, reduced supply need not be associated with reduced spending. As we see in the lower panel of Figure 5-2, the demand increase from D_1 to D_2 has been associated with sharp price increases. The net effect has been to increase the dollar value of expenditures, while reducing the real level of medical services available. While somewhat simplified, the top panel represents the idealized market response, the bottom panel a very discomforting market response. In brief, we cannot simply identify demand as equivalent to the expenditure flow. Stated in other terms, we cannot assume that all changes in the levels of expenditure reflect the autonomous choice of a sovereign public to buy more or less service. Further, we cannot always predict just what the market response will be when we decide to spend more for health.

Figure 5-2

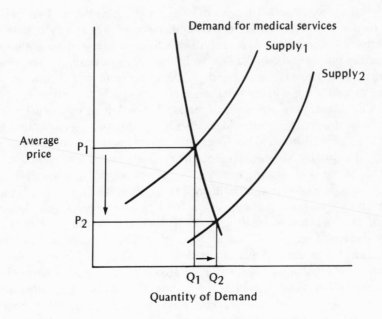

Demand for medical services

Supply₁

Supply₂

Average price

P₁

P₂

Q₁ Q₂

Quantity of Demand

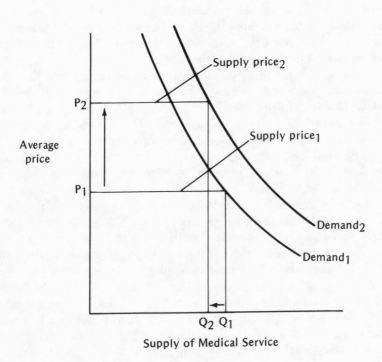

Supply price₂

P₂

Average price

Supply price₁

P₁

Demand₂

Demand₁

Q₂ Q₁

Supply of Medical Service

CULTURAL DETERMINANTS OF THE DEMAND FOR MEDICAL SERVICES

There is no magic in constructing a demand schedule to represent how varying levels in the price of medical services might influence the volume of health care purchased. There is magic, however, in blending considerations of price with the vast range of cultural forces that influence the consumers' taste for medical services. Such analysis involves going behind the demand schedule to identify some of its more compelling determinants. Here we enter a world of perception, rituals, mythologies, with a startling array of value structures that are only dimly perceived by health-care providers. It is vital to uncover individual perceptions of the origins of illness, views about personal responsibility for health, the availability of information about diet and lifestyles, and the effectiveness and cost of medical intervention. The value-set may, in some cases, represent a subset of cultural beliefs. While we speak frequently of the "melting-pot" influences on homogenizing values in the United States, in the medical field it is more appropriate to speak of the Mulligan stew of attitudes. We should acknowledge the risk that the following abbreviated view of cultural influences may improperly stereotype ethnic groups or imply an unwarranted uniformity of outlook. The mischief caused by such stereotyping includes our possible intolerance of people's "eccentric" responses to their own health problems.

A central issue in cultural analysis is the prospect of little convergence between the professional's and the individual's determination of conditions requiring attention. In reality there is a large measure of self-screening, and it is probable that the treated population may not be fully representative of the larger population requiring help. Paul Feldstein notes:

> An actual need for care may not be perceived in some instances while a nonexistent or imaginary "need" may be perceived in others. Also, a recognized health deficiency may not be translated directly into expenditure because of variations in disposition toward risk-taking and differences in belief in the effectiveness of medical treatment.[15]

One study points out that definitions of a "good" response to illness are embedded in a middle-class Anglo-Saxon ethic, with the importance it attaches to functioning with maximum effectiveness. As Talcott Parsons has observed, illness is bad because it interferes with the capacity of the individual to achieve economic success. We tend, as a consequence, to be impatient with deviant behavior, or perplexed by individuals who ap-

15 Feldstein, "Research on the Demand for Health Services," p. 139.

pear lazy, indifferent or casual in regard to their health problems. To the white-collar and professional worker, investments in health can be amortized over a lifetime. But to members of subcultures with uncertain employment, the prospect of lifetime earnings may not be that clear. One study contrasts the white-collar and blue-collar attitudes, with the latter heavily represented by the poor and minorities:

> It is possible that in some measure the lack of preventive health orientation is another dimension of a general lack of future orientation that characterizes blue-collar workers. The problem is not wholly financial, although it may be aggravated by it. For example, regular checkups of automobiles to detect incipient repairs are not in the general value system of blue-collarites. In similar fashion, household objects are often worn out and discarded rather than repaired at an early stage of disintegration.

> The body can be seen as simply another class of objects to be worn out but not repaired. Thus, teeth are left without dental care, and later there is often small interest in dentures, whether free or not. In any event, false teeth may be little used. Corrective eye examinations, even for those people who wear glasses, are often neglected, regardless of clinic facilities. It is as though the white-collar class thinks of the body as a machine to be preserved and kept in perfect functioning condition, whether through prosthetic devices, rehabilitation, cosmetic surgery, or perpetual treatment, whereas blue-collar groups think of the body as having a limited span of utility; to be enjoyed in youth and then to suffer with and to endure stoically with age and decrepitude. It may be that a more damaged self-image makes more acceptable a more damaged physical adjustment.[16]

One sample of patients attending the clinics of the Massachusetts General Hospital found statistically significant differences between the working-class Italian and Irish patients. The Irish tended to deny many aspects of being ill, including denial of pain and denial that their illness had any serious by-products other than limiting physical behavior. They were specific about the terms and location of their impairment. In contrast, the Italians did not localize symptoms, described their pain fully, identified a general malfunctioning and described how their symptoms interfered with their daily functioning, making them irritable and difficult to get along with.[17] Zola contends that the Anglo-Saxon view is more like that of the Irish, with illness defined as an ailment of recent origin interfering with one's vocational and avocational activities. "They seem to involve a more impersonal and emotionally neutral decision-making process

16 Daniel Rosenblatt and Edward A. Suchman, "The Underutilization of Medical-Care Services by Blue-Collarites." In Arthur B. Shostak and William Gomberg (eds.), *Blue-Collar World* (Englewood Cliffs, N.J.: Prentice-Hall, 1964), p. 344.
17 Irving Kenneth Zola, "Illness Behavior of the Working Class: Implications and Recommendations." In ibid., p. 353 .

than do the others, and emotional neutrality is a characteristic commonly attributed to the Protestant middle class."[18]

Let us return to the risk that we may infer characteristics of the general population from those who enter hospitals or clinics for treatment, without fully appreciating the self-screening mechanism. In an extreme example, it was formerly believed that Buerger's disease was prevalent in Eastern European Jews, until it was later realized that this evidence was due not so much to the nature of the disease as to the fact that Dr. Buerger made his observations at Mount Sinai Hospital.[19] The morbidity patterns represented by the hospital census may, in fact, be a highly biased sample unsuitable for generalization to—or even treatment of—the larger population.

Another compelling consideration is the prospect that cultural or ethnic considerations may well influence the amount of information the patient elects to give the physician. If the patient does not define certain types of discomfort, the physician may err in his diagnosis. In the Navaho culture there is no terminology (and thus no way to conceive) different types of pain as being sharp, dull, searing, and so on.

A further related problem is the reluctance of minority patients, already self-conscious about being afflicted and with low self-esteem, to admit confusion about medical instructions they have been given. In many of the so-called low-class patient groups, there is a habit of acquiescing in the authority of the medical staff and pretending to understand all instructions. "Many of our working-class patients professed a general reluctance to inquire about anything, since they felt that the physician did not want to be asked 'foolish' questions, and that he was really 'too busy' to be bothered." This perception can, of course, affect the impulse to demand medical services and impair the prospect of successful medical intervention.[20]

Zola has extended the search in medical sociology to uncover the complex forces that might account for people's delayed attention to medical care. Traditionally, studies have found that the late respondent had been exposed to limited health education, and had obsessive guilt feelings and an inordinate fear of what the diagnosis might reveal. Or others might simply be too busy or too lazy. Zola contends that there are at least five separate trigger mechanisms that can induce an individual to seek medical attention. The first is an "interpersonal crisis," in which stress brings into sharp focus the nature of the affliction. In this category, the illness does not induce the crisis; rather, the crisis makes the illness explicit.

[18] Ibid., p. 354.

[19] Noted by Melitta Schmideberg, "Social Factors Affecting Diagnostic Concepts," *International Journal of Psychiatry*, Vol. 7, Fall 1961, pp. 222–30 and noted by Zola, p. 356.

[20] Zola, "Illness Behavior of the Working Class," p. 358.

The second trigger is represented as "social interference," in which the affliction threatens to impair a lifestyle or even participation in an enjoyed social interaction. A third trigger involves "sanctions"; an individual surrenders to the counsel of an authority figure who simply tells him to secure medical care. The fourth, the "perceived threat," is the appreciation that the lack of attention may jeopardize one's vocation. The fifth circumstance is a realization of the similarity of one's symptoms to those of a friend. He draws an inference about his prospects by reflecting on the experiences of a person who has similar problems. This listing is not, of course, exhaustive. Nor can we identify the statistical significance of each element. But it is believed that there are many considerations that compel action, all reflecting the socioeconomic status of individuals.

Individuals living in the subculture of poverty often have perspectives that vary considerably from middle-class norms. The characteristics of slum dwellings have frequently been documented, but some aspects that affect health include:

> high rates of disease and mental illness, high rates of homicide, criminal and juvenile delinquency, high rates of alcoholism, drug addiction, prostitution, desertion, illegitimacy and venereal disease, high rates of people on relief, high rates of dropouts from school, low rates of belonging to voluntary associations and so forth. In sum, all of the standard patterns of social disorganization are present as an obligation to the theme of urban poverty.[21]

The war on poverty has had little influence in changing this scene. In one account, government and private agencies made their triumphal entry into the core city in the manner of a colonial power determined to save the population from themselves. Such benevolent intervention would transform its populace into healthy and grateful citizens of a new world. Leonard W. Cronkhite of Children's Hospital Medical Center in Boston draws a portrait of the medical aspirations of the native population:

> The one clear voice was that of hundreds of thousands of individuals asking to be served medically in a fashion which did not destroy their sense of personal dignity and worth. They asked simple things: a medical setting which insured privacy, cleanliness, cheer, and order; medical explanations and directions delivered in an understanding vocabulary; delivery of care with an attitude of concern, promptness, courtesy, and the same air of light formality which characterizes the relationship between the personal physician and his own patients. None of these pleas could possibly be construed as outrageous or threatening, but many went unheeded, especially in the crowded outpatient services of the large urban hospitals. Here medical care is often delivered to the poor in the same basic style as in the early 1800s. The community clinic in a housing

21 Rosenblatt and Edward A. Suchman, "The Underutilization of Medical Care Services by Blue-Collarites," p. 341.

development or a shabby storefront offered few improvements, with the one exception that the staff, having largely selected itself for the task, was more likely to show evidence of real concern than its compatriots at the base hospital.[22]

There are cultural reflexes causing suspicions about medical care provided within this environment. For some poverty groups, a lay-referral system steers them toward pseudomedical healers, such as fortune tellers, mediums, faith healers, and persons with a reputation for concocting their own brews. Further, ghetto residents sometimes suffer from anomie, a condition of normlessness characterized by an excessive withdrawal from the social fabric, isolation, self-estrangement, a feeling of powerlessness and meaninglessness.[23] Such individuals are easily intimidated by complex hospital structures, in which their sense of helplessness is increased by obligations to be passive. "He expects to be a tiny cog in a big, fairly impersonal structure, and he knows that in many instances the doctor and nurse will be more interested in his chart or his temperature than they are in him. . . . His self becomes reduced at the same time that he becomes subject to the rules and regulations of a large-scale, rationalized, bureaucratic organization."[24]

William R. Rosengren, in a study of the behavior pattern of women during pregnancy, found sharply different roles played by the affluent and the poor. The poor tend to enact a "sick role," treating pregnancy more as an illness than a condition. (Social-class position of the women was specified by income, education, and occupation.) The poor also tend to seek dependence and support and a deference from others, inherent in the "role" of being sick. They subscribe to superstitions, such as "if a mother craves sweets, it is a sign the baby will be a girl," "shocking experiences to the mother tend to leave birthmarks," and so on. They not only regard themselves as sick, but also experience more difficulties and complications during delivery. This reflects the dictum that if a situation is defined as real, it is real in its consequences. They have longer labor periods, often accompanied by earaches, headaches, nausea, dizziness, and so on. One physician explained that when a middle-class woman wants to try natural childbirth, it is usually because she wants to experience having a baby. When a lower-class woman wants to try, it is because she is afraid she won't wake up from anaesthesia.[25]

[22] Leonard W. Cronkhite, Jr., "What Are the Conflicts Involved in Community Control?" In John C. Norman and Beverly Bennett (eds.), Medicine in the Ghetto (New York: Appleton, 1969), p. 284.

[23] Rosenblatt and Suchman, "The Underutilization of Medical Care Services by Blue-Collarites," p. 346.

[24] Ibid., p. 346.

[25] For an elaboration of the study, see William R. Rosengren, "Social Class and Becoming 'Ill.'" Shostak and Gomberg (eds.), Blue Collar World, pp. 333–40.

Rosenblatt and Suchman divided a sample of working-class individuals living in upper Manhattan into white-collar and blue-collar groups. They validated the hypothesis that the white-collar worker had much more knowledge of illness than their blue-collar counterparts. The blue-collar workers had a higher skepticism of medical care and a perception of low physician interest in patient welfare. Blue-collar workers found it more difficult to participate in the "sick role." They replied affirmatively, "I find it very hard to give in and go to bed when I am sick, and I usually try to get up too soon after I have been sick." The writers conclude:

> It is quite clear from our findings that, as compared with white-collar workers, blue-collar workers are less informed about illness, more skeptical of medical care, are more dependent when ill, and experience greater difficulty in internalizing the sick role.[26]

One of the most complete surveys that systematically contrasts the views of the wealthy and poor and the white, black, and Spanish segments of society was undertaken by Louis Harris for the Blue Cross Association. Although a 1968 publication, it reports patterns of perceptions that may not have shifted markedly since that time. The title of Harris's segment, "The Living Sick: How the Poor View Their Health," is taken from the words of a Negro sharecropper in Columbia, Mississippi: "People just didn't used to be sick as much as they are today. They died when they got sick and didn't live sick." What evidence was uncovered by indepth interviews with 145 blacks living in urban ghettos and 140 Appalachian writes living in rural areas?

First, the poor feel less healthy than other Americans and place a higher importance on trying to achieve health. It is even more important than having a job. A twenty-seven-year-old black in Bedford Stuyvesant explained: "When you have no learning, you don't know if you can't learn, then you can't learn nothing. And after a while, you want to give it all up. But if you're feeling down and sick all the time, you can't get started to learn or earn." Seventy-five percent of affluent Americans consider that their health is better than it was for their parents, but this consideration is reversed for poor whites and blacks. This was attributed to chemicals in food, the loss of access to good land, clean air, and water, and limited income that restricted consumption to starchy and fatty foods.

The Harris report found no difference in the desire of the poor whites, blacks, and the larger affluent sample for high-quality care. There was constant concern about illness: "I always got a visitation from the miseries."

---

[26] Daniel Rosenblatt and Edward A. Suchman, "Blue Collar Attitudes and Information Toward Health and Illness." In Shostak and Gomberg (eds.), *Blue Collar World*, pp. 324–33.

Some fifty-three percent of all homes in the country reported a specific current ailment, but this figure was forty-four percent for the affluent. Among the inner-city blacks, this increased to sixty-five percent; among Appalachian whites, it soared to seventy-two percent. The poor reported they suffered more from heart trouble, arthritis, back trouble, ulcers, kidney trouble, high and low blood pressures, and "nerve ailments." Commonly reported ailments also included bad colds, nervous tension, sore throats, indigestion, exhaustion, shortness of breath, bad coughs, insomnia, and "sores that don't heal."

The Harris report found that the poor are much more likely to believe that visiting a doctor was essential and beneficial. They maintain their faith in the technical skills of the specialist, including his capacity to cure such maladies as arthritis. But they are much more concerned about paying for these services.

A major concern of the poor is access:

> The doctors charge more money and there's no money to pay for the doctor. If you have no money, you can't buy medicine either. To get it free, you have to go through red tape, and after everything it just isn't worth the bother. So people can't get the right care, so then people are sicker and sicker.

A North Carolina sharecropper explained: "A lot of time you can't get a doctor. If you get your throat cut on Saturday or Sunday, you might as well sew it up yourself. You just can't get a doctor soon enough. They're too busy and there is no hospital here." A poor white North Carolinian explained: "You have to wait too long when you go to a doctor. You could die in the meantime." A housewife in Siler, Kentucky, explained: "Our clinic is always all filled up. It is so hard to get to see the doctor. Sometimes you will sit all day and then be turned away and have to go back." A haunting anxiety is the problem of waiting for care in an emergency clinic: "You might pass away before they get to your turn in line."

It is puzzling that although the poor have more faith in the healing powers of physicians, they are much likelier to charge that many who go to hospitals seek unnecessary attention and that physicians are likely to prescribe more medication than is necessary. This may reflect resentment of the queuing problem and the tendency to be given a prescription. Because of limited income, there is a much higher sensitivity to the inflation of all aspects of medical care. The poor are more anxious that their insurance will not cover major medical bills.

In a separate subsample of a Spanish-speaking poverty group, some rather startling contrasts in perceptions of the medical profession surfaced. First, the Mexican-American and the Puerto Rican are much less inclined to believe he is less healthy now than he was a generation or so ago. He does not see access to medical service in such critical terms, believing that having a good job was the key to a steady income, the purchase of health care, and securing good food for children. The line of causation was: a good job provides a good income, which allows a good education, which reassures the good job.

They are less inclined to complain of health problems, with forty percent saying they had "no trouble," compared with twenty-eight percent of the Appalachian whites. They acknowledge colds, diabetes, and uterus infections but are less frequent in reporting heart trouble, arthritis, ulcers, and kidney ailments. They acknowledge tendencies to obesity but are less inclined to view this as a health hazard. While sixty-seven percent of other poverty groups indicated that it was "important to rest when feeling tired," only forty-four percent of the Spanish-speaking group felt this was necessary. In contrast to poverty groups, they are less concerned with avoiding tension, with the importance of "relaxing when eating," overexertion, "getting enough sunshine," and getting enough exercise. They are also less concerned about access to medical services and about their cost. And still in contrast to other poverty groups, they are less persuaded that physicians can be trusted and more likely to believe they will be overcharged if they go to a doctor. These characteristics suggest a much stronger feeling of self-reliance, an imbued work ethic, and a tendency to look to the family rather than the hospital for comfort and care during illness. There appears to be a higher level of expectation that they can make it economically if given an opportunity to work. The absence of psychological scars (which can so often lead to adverse physiological consequences) may reflect the ready contrast to less adequate health-care services back home.[27]

WORK, HEALTH, AND THE DEMAND FOR CARE

One of the prime determinants of health is the work environment. Thus, the needs for health care are largely a by-product of the job environment. When we speak of the job environment, we are not simply concerned with the more obvious health hazards, such as industrial accidents. We are concerned with the vast range of influences that account for stress, frustrations, and anxiety. In most instances, the threats to health do not originate with demanding physical activities. For example, the Abkhasian people of the Soviet Union survive beyond the age of ninety by a factor twenty-five times greater than all other Russians. The major explanation is lifelong work: Abkhasians at the age of one hundred

[27] The data in this section are drawn from the Blue Cross Report, *Sources: A Blue Cross Report on the Health Problems of the Poor and a Louis Harris Survey* (Chicago: Blue Cross Association, 1968), pp. 21–26.

or more still put in as much as four hours a day on their farms. As the Abkhasians say, "Without rest, a man cannot work; without work, the rest does not give you any benefit."[28] Clearly, the challenges to health posed by one's job are much more pernicious and pervasive than indicated by physical activity.

One fifteen-year study on aging found work satisfaction and happiness to be the most important determinants of longevity. Statistically, these proved much more important than physical functioning, the use of tobacco, or genetic inheritance.[29] It is the forced retirement of workers from useful employment that appears to have the most serious physiological consequences. The Commission on Work emphasized the "absurdity" of a society investing millions of dollars on physiological and chemical research aimed at retarding the "aging process" while simultaneously encouraging the early retirement of workers.[30] Further, we impose a culturally sanctioned "sick role" on the retired population by encouraging their admission to nursing homes. This role requires dependency, which often leads to degeneracy of health and related psychosomatic illnesses.

One medical study undertook the medical control of the presumed causes of heart disease, such as cholesterol, blood pressure, smoking, glucose levels, and serum uric acid. But even when these physiological variables were controlled, they appeared to account for only about one-fourth of coronary heart disease. The remaining seventy-five percent of the risk factors might well be caused by unidentified biological problems, but perhaps are to be found in factors external to the treatment process.[31] Does the advance of good health require that we shift attention from medical-care institutions to the qualities of the external environment, including the job itself? Rick J. Carlson believes so:

> The greatest single predictor of longevity is not the fidelity of a patient to a physician, but job satisfaction. The amount of debilitation from job dissatisfaction is staggering.[32]

Because heart disease is the major cause of death in this country, it is important to identify the high-risk factors accounting for it. As noted above, we know that abnormal blood pressure, cholesterol, blood sugar, and body weight are factors. But the commission that prepared *Work in*

[28] Sula Benet, "Why They Live to be 100 or Even Older, in Abkhasia," *New York Times Magazine*, December 26, 1972, and cited in the Special Task Force Report, *Work in America* (Cambridge, Mass.: MIT Press , 1974), p. 77.
[29] Erdman Palmore, "Predicting Longevity: A Follow-Up Controlling for Age," *Gerontology*, Winter 1969.
[30] *Work in America*, p. 78.
[31] John R. P. French, Jr., and Robert D. Caplan, "Organization Stress and Individual Strain." In A. Morrow (ed.), *The Failure of Success*, quoted in *Work in America*, p. 79.
[32] Rick J. Carlson, *The End of Medicine* (New York: Wiley, 1975), p. 109.

America noted that other forces also appeared to be major influences, including job dissatisfaction, tedious work, lack of recognition, poor relations with coworkers, and poor working conditions. Occupational stress— extraordinary workloads and responsibility and conflict or ambiguity in occupational roles—are part of a high-risk job environment.

> The stress of work overload appears to result from the feeling that one does not have enough resources, time, or ability and hence may fail. Responsibility, especially for other people rather than things, has been pinpointed as a risk factor among managers, scientists and engineers in NASA, as well as among executives. Retrospective studies of heart-disease patients also found this factor to be highly significant. Certain occupations, such a air-traffic control and railroad-train dispatching, share the extraordinary stress of having to make life-and-death decisions minute after minute, with considerable tolls in heart mortality. Stress was indicated in a variety of blue-collar and white-collar jobs, as well as among several categories of practice in fields of medicine, dentistry, and law.[33]

Other forces accounting for stress are continuous change of employment and the incongruity between present job status and the expectations of status engendered by high educational attainment. Individuals who have invested heavily in education but find themselves with low job status are often consumed with anger, frustration, tiredness, and depression. Excessive aggressiveness, ambition, and competitiveness, including a sense of urgency about time, are high-risk personality traits.

Looking at the issue more positively, an individual is likely to enjoy good physical and mental health if he has various sources of gratification, if he has an understanding view (and yet respect) for his own capabilities as these might be constrained by his present circumstances, and if he sets realistic goals for himself. As one might infer from this, individuals confronted with prolonged periods of unemployment are haunted with the specter that they are indeed of little value to society. The erosion of self-esteem and self-confidence may lead to depression, psychiatric hospitalization, or even suicide. In brief, a person who feels good about his job and has a job to feel good about is far likelier to be a person in good health.

These descriptions, while perhaps self-evident, have enormous implications for a strategy to promote health. They are particularly supportive of evidence of vast amounts of employee dissatisfaction with work. Assembly-line workers believe their jobs to be dull, repetitive, and unchallenging, and have a sense of helplessness. They escape to passive, nonwork activities such as television for the fantasy of fulfillment. Any

[33] *Work in America*, p. 80.

persistent pattern of failure can erode an individual's self-respect and encourage such a retreat or withdrawal.[34]

There is, in this, some point at which the obligation to acquiesce in the external environment in order to preserve health and peace of mind involves a pragmatic surrender to arrangements that are themselves far from healthy. As has been observed, there may be madness in adjusting to the pathologies of the organization.[35] But unhappily, individuals who "take on" their organizations as a matter of personal conscience and health often find themselves crushed in spirit and health. As Kornhauser testifies:

> The unsatisfactory mental health of working people consists in no small measure of their dwarfed desires and deadened initiatives, reduction of their goals, and restriction of their efforts to a point where life is relatively empty and only half meaningful.[36]

This brief excursion into the sociology of work does not give us direct explanations of the demand for medical services, but it does help explain the origin of need for such service.

SUGGESTED READINGS

AUGER, RICHARD and VICTOR P. GOLDBERG, "Prepaid Health Plans and Moral Hazard," *Public Policy*, Vol. 12, no. 3 (Summer 1973), pp. 353–93. An examination of whether patients will make unreasonable demands on the delivery system if the costs are covered by prepaid insurance.

BOULDING, KENNETH E., "The Concept of Need for Health Services," *Milbank Memorial Fund Quarterly*, Vol. 44, no. 2 (October 1966). A study of the demand issue in more general, nonempirical terms.

CULYER, A. J. and J. G. CULLIS, "Some Economics of Hospital Waiting Lists in the NHS," *Journal of Social Policy*, Vol. 5, Part 3 (July 1976), pp. 239–64. Discusses the effect of national health insurance on the demand for medical service.

[34] In his study *Automobile Workers and the American Dream*, Eli Chinoy found that employees denied opportunities for advance rationalized their disappointment by concluding that those advanced to foremen enjoyed only modest income gains and that promotions tended to reflect the accidents of events and neglected considerations of merit. With the help of consumer credit, such employees could capture the trappings of success (a new television set or new car) without its occupational substance. And they speculated that they might open a tackle shop or a gas station when they retire. *Automobile Workers and the American Dream* (Garden City, N.Y.: Doubleday, 1955).

[35] *Work in America*, p. 84.

[36] Arthur Kornhauser, *Mental Health of the Industrial Worker* (New York: Wiley, 1965).

FREIBERG, LEWIS and F. DOUGLAS SCUTCHFIELD, "Insurance and the Demand for Hospital Care: An Examination of the Moral Hazard," *Inquiry*, Vol. 13, no. 1 (March 1971), pp. 54–60. A discussion of price elasticity of demand for health services as related to out-of-pocket costs.

GARFIELD, SIDNEY, MORRIS F. COLLEN, ROBERT FELDMAN, KRIKOR SOGHIKIAN, ROBERT RICHART, and JAMES DUNCAN, "Evaluation of an Ambulatory Medical-Care Delivery System," *The New England Journal of Medicine*, Vol. 294, no. 8 (February 19, 1976), pp. 426–31. An examination of the belief that when medical services appear costless to potential consumers, there is little limit to levels of service demanded.

JEFFERS, JAMES F., MARIO F. BOGNANNO, and JOHN BARTLETT, "On Demand versus Need for Medical Services and the Concept of 'Shortage,' " *American Journal of Public Health*, Vol. 61, no. 1 (January 1971), pp. 46–62. Offers alternative conceptualizations of demand and need.

JOSEPH, HYMAN, "Hospital Insurance and Moral Hazard, *Journal of Human Resources*, Vol. 7 (Spring 1973), pp. 152–61. A discussion of patients' excessive use of what they consider to be a "free" service.

MCCREADIE, CLAUDINE, "Rawlsian Justice and the Financing of the National Health Service," *Journal of Social Policy*, Vol. 5, Part 2, (April 1976), pp. 113–30. An application of Rawls's standard for distributive justice to health-care policies in Great Britain.

MITCHELL, BRIDGER M. and CHARLES E. PHELPS, "National Health Insurance: Some Costs and Effects of Mandated Employee Coverage," *Journal of Political Economy*, Vol. 84, no. 3 (June 1976), pp. 553–71. A more technical approach to the demand for medical service. Includes a review of the economic costs of a national insurance system as this influences demand.

"Munchausen's Syndrome," *Newsweek*, November 5, 1973, p. 66. A description of individuals with a psychological compulsion for medical service.

PAULY, MARK V., "The Economics of Moral Hazard: Comment," *American Economic Review*, Vol. 59 (December 1969), pp. 906–8. An analysis of the cost of overuse of health-care services.

6

PATTERNS OF ILLNESS: A PROFILE AND PROGRESS REPORT

The document setting the stage for the American experience proclaims our claim to "life, liberty and the pursuit of happiness." None of these can be realized without good health. Indeed, the success of the American system is more properly measured by the quality of life and health enjoyed by individuals than by the growth of the national product. In chapter 3, we identified the enormous expenditures we are making in pursuit of good health. In chapters 4 and 5, we identified some of the links between this burgeoning health system and our population. In this chapter, we attempt a report card of performance, based not on the subjective assessments of patients and population, but on the objective evidence of good health. We begin with a brief overview of the patterns of morbidity and causes of death, comparing the year 1900 with contemporary experience. We move swiftly to a compressed essay on physiology, intended to emphasize the complexity of the interdependence of intricate organic structures, along with commentaries on the consequences of their malfunctioning. The third portion of the chapter provides the survey of our contemporary health status by age category, using measures of both morbidity and mortality. The final section deals with chronic afflictions and the problems we have in dealing with the realities of death.

THE QUALITY OF HEALTH IN AMERICA

Measuring health presents substantial analytic and conceptual difficulties. Some view good health in broad terms, encompassing mental and physical qualities and a successful interaction with the environment and culture leading to a positive outlook, if not a euphoric or joyous experience of daily activities. More modest definitions of health measure, in essence, the absence of affliction and the avoidance of accidents or disease that impair one's capacity to function, either in the home or in the labor market. Two measures of health are identified in these narrow terms: life expectancy, on the assumption that afflictions inadequately cared for can lead to death, and absenteeism from work. We have been attracted to measures of health that focus on life expectancy, simply because it is much easier to distinguish life from death than health from sickness. As we have emphasized in the previous two chapters, social, economic, and psychological variables interact with physiological experiences to determine whether individuals "permit themselves" to play the sick role.

Morbidity data will reflect the subjective elements of diagnosis, and be biased toward opportunities for patient examination and facilities to deal with medical problems. Such data can be influenced by the timing and form of the reporting procedure itself. Because of these problems we are attracted to the relative simplicity of death rates. This mortality index serves as a direct—although admittedly imperfect—measure of health. It also, we should recognize, permits the inference that extensions of life are the most desired goal, while perhaps unconsciously detracting attention from the quality of life. This latter consideration is important because our success in increasing longevity has greatly increased the incidence of chronic diseases. In many cases, as noted, we have developed the technical capacity to postpone death, without the capacity to cure the disease that has threatened life.

For most of man's history, the greatest amount of illness in the human body has been caused by a small number of harmful strains of microorganisms (bacteria, viruses, fungi, etc.). Until very recently, these harmful microorganisms, known as pathogens, have been more significant as causes of human diseases and death than have such occurrences as accidents or heart attacks. Our major illnesses and their causes have, however, been changing in the last one hundred years or so.

At the beginning of this century, the major killers were diseases like pneumonia and influenza (11.8 percent of all deaths), tuberculosis (11.3 percent), diarrhea and enteritis (8.3 percent), nephritis (a kidney disease, 5.2 percent), and diphtheria (2.3 percent). All of these diseases are caused by microorganisms. Some are communicable, and can result in epidemics. Significantly, diseases of the heart accounted for 8 percent of all deaths, cerebral hemorrhage (stroke) for 6 percent, and cancer for about 4 percent.[1]

[1] David L. Dodge and Walter T. Martin, *Social Stress and Chronic Illness: Mortality Patterns in Industrial Society* (Notre Dame, Indiana: University of Notre Dame Press, 1970), p. 6.

Statistics on mortality and morbidity are always somewhat suspect, even from "advanced" nations like the U.S., largely because of reporting and diagnostic uncer-

By the mid-1960s, the death-dealing power of these illnesses had changed dramatically. By 1965, tuberculosis resulted in only slightly more than 4 deaths per 100,000, and death from diarrhea, diphtheria, and nephritis were almost nonexistent. Deaths from pneumonia and influenza were down from almost 12 percent to slightly more than 3 percent. On the negative side, diseases of the heart resulted in 39 percent of all deaths, while deaths from cancer were almost 17 percent, and from stroke, 10.9 percent. Circulatory diseases increasingly accounted for mortality. These killers have increased both the absolute and the proportionate numbers of people they strike.

Cancer, heart disease, and stroke (now grimly referred to as "the big three") are really general labels for numerous afflictions that share common characteristics. Cancer is the growth and spreading of abnormal body cells. It can occur in almost any part of the body and appears to have numerous causes. Heart disease and stroke indicate some type of malfunctioning of the heart, the veins, the arteries, or other passages through which blood and similar fluids pass. Again, the causes and locations of the interrupted blood flow are numerous.

There are marked differences between these diseases and those dominant during the beginning of this century. Except for the possible role of virus in some cancer occurrences, these diseases are not caused by pathogens. And they are not communicable. The risk of their occurrence is at least heightened by psychological stress. Indeed, some contend that stress is a major cause of modern illness, not just a contributing factor.[2]

---

tainties. Relatively reliable information, however, can be obtained from the World Health Organization, Annual Epidemiological and Vital Statistics Report. For this reference, see the 1965 report. Some secondary sources are also useful, e.g., Bruce Wallace, *Disease, Sex, Communication, Behavior: Essays in Social Biology*, Vol. 3 (Englewood Cliffs, N.J.: Prentice-Hall, 1972), p. 87.

[2] Dodge and Martin, *Social Stress and Chronic Illness*, chapter 3, "A Theory of Social Stress and Chronic Disease." Interpreting absolute and relative growth of various afflictions can cause some misconceptions unless one takes account of age-adjustment factors for the population. A government study emphasizes that the prevalence of major cardiovascular diseases in this country has grown rapidly. In 1969, about 27 million Americans suffered from major cardiovascular diseases, and this had increased to 28.4 million by 1972. But even though the rate of incidence was increasing, the death rate from heart diseases did not rise if one takes account of the change in the age composition of the population. Without those adjustments, the death rate from heart diseases increased from 356.8 per 100,000 in 1950 to 366.1 in 1969. With adjustments, it dropped from 307.6 in 1950 to 262.3 in 1969. "It is generally considered unlikely that changes in medical practice during the last few decades could account for this drop. Even the current enthusiasm for exercise and dieting seems an inadequate explanation. Those have come too recently to affect the basic process responsible for most heart-disease deaths. It is generally assumed that heart disease is a slow process, so that the death trends of the 1950s and 1960s would have to have their roots in factors that began to work at least five to ten years earlier." Even without age adjustment there has been a drop in the death rate from other major cardiovascular diseases—high blood pressure, strokes, and

They also frequently include both a short-term, serious (acute) episode and long-term (chronic) periods. Cancer, cardiovascular illness, diabetes, kidney failure, and similar illnesses that can last months and years are now the cause of the vast majority of hospitalizations and deaths in our society.

THE PHYSIOLOGY OF ILLNESS

A brief discussion of the human body and its major illnesses is useful here. Medical textbooks vary in their discussions of the body and its systems. Gray's anatomy is something of a classic, however, and has been quite influential.[3] That book lists ten systems: nervous, digestive, respiratory, vascular, urogenital, endocrine, skeletal, muscular, joints, and external covering. The notion of "system" here stresses the fact that the organs and processes of these systems significantly affect one another.

It is often helpful, though slightly oversimplified, to think of human illness as having direct causes and predisposing factors. The former includes pathogenic organisms, malnutrition, physical and chemical agents (such as those involved in accidents), congenital and genetically related illnesses, degeneration (usually related to "aging") and neoplasms (cancer and other types of tumors).[4] Factors that predispose us toward illness include: aging; lifestyle characteristics, particularly those that are stressfull; deprivation and diet; environmental factors, such as pollution; occupation and its hazards; preexisting illness. The trilogy is the human body and its systems, the causes and predisposing factors for illness, and the illnesses themselves.

When man's major diseases were primarily those caused by germs, the causes (etiology) of illness were relatively simple. The infection appeared, and the victim became sick, recovered, or died. Modern diseases, however, require increasing attention to personality factors, economic class and other cultural elements, and conditions in our environment. Bodily illness and its course are influenced greatly by how we live.

Let us briefly outline the functioning of the system:

---

arteriosclerosis. See *Trends Affecting U.S. Health Care Systems*, Health Planning Information Series, prepared by the Cambridge Research Institute for the U.S. Department of Health, Education and Welfare, DHEW Publication No. HRA 76-14503 (January 1976), pp. 46–47.

[3] Henry Gray, *Anatomy of the Human Body*, 29th ed. by Charles Mayo Goss, M.D. (Philadelphia: Lea and Febiger, 1973).

[4] Ruth L. Memmler, M.D., *The Human Body in Health and Disease* (Philadelphia: Lippincott, 1962), chapters 1–3; or William Boyd, *An Introduction to the Study of Disease* (Philadelphia: Lea and Febiger, 1971). For discussions of the body and its diseases intelligible to the layman, see these references.

1. The vascular system contains approximately sixty thousand miles of veins, arteries, capillaries, and the like, which carry food and oxygen to the body cells and carry waste away. The heart is the force behind this activity, and the blood supply is its major form of transportation. As noted earlier, cardiovascular disease is now the greatest cause of all deaths in this country. By 1970, more than one-half million American citizens were dying annually from this cause. Some forms of the illness are coronary heart disease, in which the blood supply to the heart is disturbed; heart ailment due to high blood pressure, or what is called hypertension; and degenerative heart disease, encouraged by obesity, aging, improper or insufficient exercise, or other chronic illnesses. Disease of the veins and arteries, such as arteriosclerosis (hardening of the arteries), are also common.

Although vascular diseases result from some malfunctioning of the heart muscle, its valves or the arteriovenous networks, numerous other factors play a major role. Some persons are born with heart defects, and thus have received their illness through heredity. Many books warn readers of the vascular risks of overweight, the benefits of reducing coronary occurrences through regular and vigorous exercise, and the importance of avoiding cigarettes, heeding the heart-trouble danger signals, and having periodic medical examinations.[5]

The nature and frequency of vascular diseases appear to illustrate some rather strange and conflicting beliefs about our health and health care. Heart disease is the major killer of our citizens, but few of us know much about it. Except for inherited heart disease, we can significantly reduce its risk to us by changing our lifestyles; yet overindulgence continues. We often seem to mix a fascination with our bodies and its afflictions on the one hand, with ignorance and disregard for these realities on the other. We are often content to clean, groom, and feed (more often, "stuff") our bodies, only becoming aware of their basic processes when major illness occurs. This may well be based on a pervasive belief that we are essentially free to treat ourselves as we desire, leaving medical technology and physician abilities responsible for curing anything that develops as a result.[6]

2. The nervous system is frequently the victim of debilitating and deadly illnesses. The main components of the nervous system are the brain, the spinal cord, and the nerves, which "reach every millimeter of skin surface, every muscle, every blood vessel, every bone . . . every part of the body,

---

[5] For example, see Wesley P. Cushman, *Reducing the Risk of Noncommunicable Diseases* (Dubuque, Iowa: William C. Brown, 1970).

[6] Alan E. Nourse and the editors of *Life, The Body* (New York: Life Science Library, Time, Inc., 1964), chapter 1. For an interesting discussion of attitudes and changing views of the body, and an instructive discussion of the body's systems, see this reference.

from tip to toe.[7] The basic function of the nervous system is to receive, filter, and send messages. Some of the messages pertain largely to occurrences within our body, such as when the nervous system is coordinating our digestion of food. Other messages relate more directly to factors in our environment, such as cold, heat, or significant emotions in our social world. The cerebral cortex of the brain is the seat of our emotions and our "rational" thought processes.

The major illness to affect the nervous system is stroke, or what is technically called cerebrovascular disease. Broadly speaking, there are two types of stroke. The first, accounting for sixty percent of all strokes, occurs when there is brain damage due to blockages in the cerebral blood vessels. The other occurs when an artery breaks and there is intracranial bleeding.

While men are more susceptible than women to heart disease, stroke occurs in either sex at about the same rate. In addition, both heart disease and stroke occur more frequently with age. We should note that our increasing life expectancies, due in part to the decline of the infectious diseases, means that we are now living long enough to experience heart disease and stroke. Stroke is related to hypertension and cholesterol deposits. But, unlike other health problems, it is only moderately related to overweight.

A stroke can lead to continued severe physical and psychological disabilities. We have mentioned that the brain is the basis of emotion and thought processes. The arteries of the neck and brain provide nourishment to cells that control almost all human functions. Sometimes stroke is rapid and severe, resulting in coma and death within a few hours or days. But the majority of stroke victims are still alive from three to four weeks after the occurrence. Others live much longer. Prolonged loss of consciousness and age are factors encouraging rapid death from stroke.

The stroke victim who survives the immediate occurrence often has residual symptoms, which are apparent and constant. The most frequent is hemiplegia, paralysis on one side. Aphasia, the partial or total loss of the ability to use and understand words, is also common. The loss of ability to communicate can be a severely traumatic experience for both the patient and many of those around him.

Since many stroke victims survive, but are somewhat disabled, care of the patient becomes the immediate problem. Care and rehabilitation is a growing socioeconomic and medical problem for the health-care system in all long-term illnesses, including stroke. One physician explains the human agony and dilemma for stroke survivors:

> The hemiplegic who loses all or the greater part of his physical independence has a right to be unhappy not only because of his helpless-

[7] Ibid., p. 142.

ness, but because he is a burden to others as well. If in addition he is aphasic, he cannot express his concerns, cannot apologize to or thank others for their trouble and this saddens him further. It may be called "fortunate" that in some patients mental deterioration is so advanced that the patient is unable to worry about such niceties. Some patients who were fastidious before their illness will drool or become incontinent and this makes them more miserable. What was a loved father only a short time ago may become a "dirty old man." A significant number of wives and families resist suggestions that they accept once more the hemiplegic into what was his home. He contributes nothing to the operation of the household, he cannot be left alone, bedrooms and furniture must be rearranged, he may become "another person." The family does not always know how much he understands. They must be careful not to upset him by letting him know how much he has disrupted their lives. If the victim was deeply loved before the attack, if the home is architecturally adequate and the income sufficient, the patient is welcomed back into the bosom of the family. When this happens, it is a "break" for the patient, for he will probably live a little longer than he would have at a nursing home.[8]

3. The digestive system, by which food is processed for fueling the body, begins in the mouth and ends at the anus, involving over 30 feet of coiled and twisted organs. After leaving the mouth, what we ingest enters the part of the throat (pharnyx) that is common to both the digestive and breathing (respiratory) systems. From here, it goes through the esophagus, the stomach, the small intestine, the large intestine (colon), and finally is eliminated as waste. Other organs involved in the digestive process are the liver (one of the most versatile and critical organs of the body), the pancreas, and the gall bladder.

Cancer frequently attacks some part of the digestive system. About twenty-five percent of all cancers occur in the stomach, but the disease also occurs in the throat and colon. Some people chronically suffer various forms of indigestion and heartburn, which usually is not serious, though debilitating. An ulcer, the disintegration and loss of tissues in the mucous membrane, can occur in the esophagus, stomach, or duodenum. The liver, without which we would perish within twenty-four hours, is frequently the victim of cancer or cirrhosis. The latter is a chronic disease, common to alcoholics, in which inactive scar tissue takes over for active cells.

The digestive system in general, and its common illnesses in particular, again illustrate the involvement of social and psychological factors in our ailments. After we swallow, little of the digestive process is voluntary. But we can choose what goes into our mouths. In addition to the demonstrated relationship between overweight and cardiovascular occurrences, cancer of the throat may well result from heavy drinking of al-

[8] Sidney Licht, M.D. (ed.), *Stroke and Its Rehabilitation* (Baltimore: Waverly Publications, 1975), p. x.

cohol and is certainly encouraged by smoking. The rationalizations many people use for continued abuse of the throat and stomach would challenge the skills of the best psychologist.

Although what occurs once food leaves the mouth is largely beyond voluntary control, it is controlled by the brain. In addition, we have mentioned that the brain is the seat of our emotions. Thus, emotional upset frequently affects our digestion, as might be expected. In 1965, about one-fifth as many of our citizens died of ulcers as of automobile accidents.[9] Ulcers are sometimes fatal, always chronic, and frequently debilitating. Psychological stress plays a major part in their occurrence. With some individuals, ulcers are a source of pride rather than concern, symbolizing the essence of the harried executive, frustrated housewife, or dominated son.

4. The respiratory system begins with air entering the nose (sometimes the mouth), moving through the pharnyx to the trachea (windpipe), and from there into the lungs. Its basic function is to provide oxygen to the body cells and remove unneeded carbon dioxide.

Tuberculosis, which (as we have noted) is of dramatically reduced importance as a cause of death in this country, is caused by a pathogenic strain of bacteria. It can attack any body organ, but it usually occurs in the lungs of adults. At one point in our history, its occurrence was so widespread that we maintained a large number of hospitals primarily for the care of its victims. Unlike polio, which was defeated through immunization, tuberculosis has been limited largely through effective sanitation and treatment. It is probably true that low-income farm workers continue to experience the disease at an unusually high rate.

Although the lungs are increasingly safe from tuberculosis, cancer in these organs is fearful. Only about three percent of male lung-cancer victims survive longer than five years.[10] On the bright side, we have two lungs just as we have two kidneys, and we can survive after one of either of them has been removed.

The majority of our fatal illnesses occur in these four body systems. The other six systems, however, do experience ailments resulting in long-term illness, disability, or death.

5. The urogenital system contains organs and processes that eliminate body waste through urination and that are significant to sexual reproduction. The kidneys, a pair of approximately five-inch-long organs through which we filter more than forty gallons of water daily, experience numerous illnesses. Chronic nephritis, once a major killer in this country, leads to uremia, an accumulation of urinary constituents in the blood. Kidney

9 Howard E. Freeman, Sol Levine, Leo G. Reeder (ed.), *Handbook of Medical Sociology,* 2nd ed. (Englewood Cliffs, N.J.: Prentice-Hall, 1972), p. 66.
10 Ibid., p. 69.

malfunctions can also occur from tuberculosis, tumors, and kidney stones.

Kidneys aptly demonstrate man's ability to survive major illnesses. We have noted that because we have two of these organs, one can become totally useless and even be removed with the patient surviving. Illustrative of our technical advances is the use of mechanical "artificial kidneys" for the treatment of uremia. The patient with nonfunctioning kidneys periodically spends several hours attached to a machine that literally cleanses his five or six quarts of blood. Nonetheless, the acceptance of the necessity of this procedure for a lifetime is traumatic for most chronic sufferers of uremia.

Both the female and male reproductive systems experience illnesses with which most of us have some familiarity. Uterine and breast cancer are common in the female. Elderly men are particularly susceptible to tumors in the prostate gland. Various forms of venereal disease are now epidemic. Both chronic impotence and sterility can be caused psychologically or physically or by a combination of physical and mental factors. Treatment of diseases of the reproductive systems almost always seems to cause the patient major embarrassment.

6. The endocrine system is the anatomical phrase used to describe the few scattered organs and glands that produce internal substances known as hormones, dispensing them through blood and lymph systems. Hormones regulate many body functions, including growth and food use. Two glands most common to laymen are the thyroid and the pituitary. The thyroid, which is located in the neck, produces a hormone that (thyroxin) regulates the production of body heat and energy, and is sometimes blamed by fat people as the cause of their obesity. The pituitary gland, which is located near the brain, promotes growth and sexual development.

Because glands are so involved with basic changes in human physiology, glandular diseases can have bizarre consequences. Cretinism, resulting in dwarfed idiots, is caused by underactivity of the thyroid gland. Giantism, caused by a tumor in the pituitary gland, produces extremely large and weak humans.

Tumors occur in all of the basic systems of the body. Because the words "tumor" and "cancer" produce such fear and aversion in our society, some clarification of their characteristics might enhance understanding of these diseases. Tumors are the abnormal growth of new body tissue, occurring independently of the surrounding body structures and having no beneficial physiological functions. Many tumors are benign: they have not spread, have fixed boundaries, and their limits can be identified. When tumor cells break off (metastasize) and spread to other parts of the body, they are malignant. At this point the tumors are called cancerous.

Diabetes is a chronic disease that illustrates many of the tragic characteristics of serious chronic illnesses. The glands of the pancreas, which is located behind the stomach, produce insulin, a hormone necessary for normal use of sugar in our system. Sometimes the pancreas fails to produce enough insulin, and we get an overabundance of sugar, which usually appears first in the urine. Hence, the importance of urine tests for "sugar diabetes."

In 1970, about 2.5 million people were known diabetics, with an estimated 1.6 million being undetected diabetics.[11] Diabetes is a life-long illness, requiring major adjustments in lifestyle. Restricted diets in the minor cases is minimal therapy. Injection of insulin to achieve the appropriate chemical balance is frequently required. Insulin cannot be taken orally because it is destroyed in the digestive process, an occurrence in which bodily processes work against the treatment itself. Major diabetics are thus faced with a daily routine of shots, which they often administer to themselves. Diabetes also frequently causes heart disease, hypertension, and blindness.

7. The skeletal and muscular systems and the joints, listed separately by Gray, are often discussed together as the musculoskeletal system. The skeleton, serving as the framework of the body with 206 bones in the adult, also protects vital structures like the brain and spinal cord and produces blood cells in the marrow. Tumors can originate in the bone tissue; this is somewhat more common in younger people than cancer originating from other types of tissue. As bones age, they become harder and even brittle, making the healing of fractures more difficult and providing a constant health danger for aged adults.

Joints are found at the union of two or more bones. Arthritis, an inflammation and pain in the joints, is a chronic disease. Rheumatoid arthritis is often crippling. Gout and the degeneration of joints due to aging are other related illnesses.

We have about six hundred skeletal muscles, and their primary function enables us to move part or all of the body. Muscular strain, bursitis, and lumbago are wide-spread, though seldom serious disorders.

Serious disorders of the musculoskeletal system are frequently highly traumatic to the victim and those around him. The psychological reaction to amputation due to cancer or to some severe violence such as an automobile accident may well result from the esteem lost by no longer being a "whole person." The various forms of paralysis are anxiety-producing, and few are untouched by the sight of children with leg braces, common to fund-raising efforts to combat diseases like muscular dystrophy.

8. Three layers of skin comprise the final physiological system. Skin diseases, even skin cancer, are usually less serious than other forms of illness, though vanity can make them trying. Abnormal skin coloring provides

---

[11] Cushman, *Reducing the Risk of Non-communicable Diseases*, p. 29.

physicians with a valuable diagnostic tool. It is probably also true that the unattractive nature of aging skin contributes to our aversion to older people.

AFFLICTIONS BY MAJOR AGE CATEGORY

The dramatic improvement in life expectancy we have experienced since 1900 reflects the substantial reduction of death for the very young.[11] It is here that medical technology's triumph in avoiding death is most conspicuous. For example, the death rates in 1965 were, for all ages, thirty-two percent the death rates of 1916. But when we view the decline of the death rate over the age spectrum, we find that for those under one year of age, the decline of the death rate was seventy-eight percent; for those one to four, the decline was an even greater ninety-one percent. Percentage gains in mortality reduction were sustained at levels above sixty-six percent for those to age forty-four. For the fifty-five-and-older categories, there is a sharp decline in our capacity to reduce mortality. We can acknowledge, therefore, that only a limited "stretching" of the life span has been made for the older age categories. Under the mortality conditions prevailing in 1910, one of every ten boys died before reaching his twenty-ninth birthday; in 1965, only about one in twenty would not attain that age.[12]

In 1940, little more than half of all births occurred in hospitals, and nearly 9,000 mothers died in childbirth. In 1973 there were fewer than 500 such deaths. In 1940, the infant mortality rate was 46 per 1,000 live births; in 1974, this had declined to 16.5. There is considerable range in the death rate by socioeconomic status. Seventy-five percent of white women receive prenatal care the first 3 months of pregnancy, compared with only 52 percent of women of other races. The United States ranks only 15th among nations in the category of infant mortality, the rate being higher by two-thirds for black infants. Such rates increase sharply if the birth is illegitimate or if the mother is economically poor or poorly educated. They increase, too, when the mother is under the age of 20 or over 35.

Once the child has survived his first year, he remains, to age 14, in the category with the lowest overall death rate. As we have noted, the infectious diseases, which previously had such a lethal influence on children, have largely been brought under control. The major killers, such as cholera, plague, typhus, yellow fever, and smallpox, are rarely experi-

[11] The data and analysis of this section draw heavily on *Health: United States, 1975,* DHEW Publication No. (HRA) 76-1232, GPO, 1976, esp. pp. 152–599.
[12] *Modern-Day Capitalism: Progress, Problems, Potentials* (New York: National Industrial Conference Board, 1966).

enced today. Even here, the advances have been dramatic in recent years. In 1950, tuberculosis, diphtheria, poliomyelitis, and measles claimed the lives of 2,729 children; in 1973, these diseases claimed only 43 childhood deaths. In 1950 there were 3,245 deaths from influenza and pneumonia; in 1973, there were only 1,345.

Although we have been able to control infectious childhood diseases, we have not been able to control death rates resulting from violence and accidents. Those aged 1 to 14 experienced a total of 12,448 accidental deaths in 1973. Half of these were caused by motor-vehicle accidents. Those under 17 years experienced 25 million accidental injuries in 1973, with about half of these requiring inpatient hospital care. Unhappily, some 435,000 of these injuries caused life-long impairments.

Other problems for the earliest age group are defective vision and poor dental health. By age 11, 17 percent have defective distant vision, and 10 percent defective near vision. By the age of 17, 19 of 20 youths have decayed, missing, or filled permanent teeth, averaging about 9 such teeth per person. As we move to the youth and young-adult categories, the death rate for both sexes increases, but more rapidly for the male. Here again, death rates from traditional causes—tuberculosis, heart disease, influenza, and pneumonia—have been sharply reduced. Afflictions of heart disease, for example, were 27,200 in 1940, and these were reduced to 17,700 in 1973. Such improvements are all the more dramatic when one appreciates the rapid population growth in the interval.

But again, as disease control proved effective, there were offsetting changes in lifestyle that proved destructive. In 1973, there were 77,575 deaths of persons aged 15 to 44 from accidents, suicides, and homicides, a figure almost equal to the number of deaths from all other causes. For the younger age category, 15 to 24, the increase of death from violence was even more dramatic. From 1950 to 1973, death rates from motor-vehicle accidents increased by one-third, while those from suicides and homicides more than doubled. Apart from the loss of life, many of these episodes caused impairment of function, handicapping individuals in their studies, jobs, or homemaking duties. Venereal disease is also displaying a resurgence, with an estimated 2.7 million cases of gonorrhea and 81,000 new cases of infectious syphilis occurring each year. An estimated 450,000 persons presently need treatment for syphilis.

One of the emerging problems for the age category of 18 to 44 is obesity. This problem appears more of a concern for women than men. The highest incidence is for black females (30 percent), followed with white females (19 percent). The incidence is 16 percent for white males and only 11 percent for black males.

The use of inpatient and outpatient psychiatric facilities is highest at ages 18 to 44. While overall use has more than doubled in the previous 20 years, they have increased even more rapidly for young adults.

As we move to the 45 to 64 age group, we find that the chronic diseases begin to take their toll and have an influence very much greater than accidents. Diseases of the heart emerge as the major killer. In 1973, there were 404 deaths per 100,000 for those 45 and older. Heart afflictions are the leading cause of inpatient hospitalization and the cause of more long-term limiting activity than any other condition. Even so, there has recently been a decline in the death rate from heart conditions, as well as from strokes, arteriosclerosis, kidney diseases, and gastric ulcers.

What afflictions have, on the other hand, increased in recent decades? First, there has been a rapid growth in the second most significant cause of death: malignant neoplasms. The death rate from cancer increased from 269 per 100,000 in 1950 to 292 in 1973. In 1973, 125,914 persons aged 45 to 64 died of cancer. Death rates also increased from cirrhosis of the liver (associated with alcoholism) from 23 to 45 deaths per 100,000 between 1950 and 1973. Death rates from bronchitis, emphysema, and asthma, (aggravated by smoking and air pollution), increased from 7 to 18 per 100,000.

Through interview data from among the 43 million persons in this age group, it was found that 8 million reported some chronic limitation of activity, including 1.8 million unable to work or do housework and 4.6 somewhat limited in their ability to carry on regular duties. One and one-half million were limited because of heart problems, 1.3 million because of arthritis, 620,000 because of impairments of the lower limbs or hips, 420,000 by hypertension, and 400,000 by diabetes. If we add the toll of disability from chronic diseases to the toll of acute short-term conditions, we find a billion days of restricted activity, including one-third as many bed days for this age category. This means the loss of some 180 million work days each year (or an average of 6.6 days for each employed person).

We turn, finally, to the most elderly segment of the population, those 65 and older. It is well known that we have improved our life expectancy. In 1900 only 41 percent of the newborn could expect to reach the age of 65. In 1973, about 73 percent reached that age. For the female who reaches the age of 65, life expectancy is greater by some 4.1 years than for men. She has an average life expectancy of 17.5 more years. The man reaching 65 can anticipate, on the average, 13.4 more years of life.

The male–female survival gap has been widening steadily ever since 1900, with women outliving men. Why? Hereditary and environmental factors are reasons, of course, but probably the single most important factor lies in the relative biological basis. Women are stronger than men. At present there are only 69 white males for every 100 white females 65 and over in the U.S. Forty years ago their numbers were almost equal. Among blacks, 65 and over, there are 73 males per 100 females, and for those of Spanish origin, the ratio is 87 males per 100 females. In short, the average white American male, for whatever reason, drives himself into the grave at a more rapid pace than his fellow men of black and Spanish origin.[13]

In 1900, we had only 3.1 million persons 65 and older; by 1970, that number increased to 20.2 million. Those in this age category are increasing by 300,000 to 400,000 per year, with an anticipated total of about 29 million by the year 2000. Not only are there more aged persons in the country, but their proportion has now increased. As of 1973, they made up 10 percent of the population.

Because retirement is usually compulsory at age sixty-five, the extensions of life create genuine economic problems for the retirees and their families, particularly when serious levels of inflation have a tendency to erode retirement benefits. Affording care and dignity for this aging segment presents major challenges to our society, and is particularly difficult to realize because of the youth orientation of our value structure. While only one percent of the American population is institutionalized, five percent of those sixty-five and over are residents of institutions. By age eighty-five and older, the percentage jumps to nineteen. There has been some shift in the nature of such institutionalized care. As recently as 1950, thirty-seven percent of those in institutions were in mental hospitals. The 1970 census revealed that only eight percent of the institutionalized older population were residents of mental institutions, while sixty percent were in homes for the aged and dependent.

The most commonly diagnosed illnesses among the aged are hardening of the arteries, senility, strokes, and mental disorders. Half of those who are institutionalized cannot see well enough to read a newspaper, even with glasses. One-third cannot hear a telephone conversation. There is little therapy provided for nursing home residents: only fifteen percent are offered recreational therapy, ten percent physical therapy, and six percent occupational therapy. For those who have been residents over a year, thirteen percent had not seen a physician for at least six months, and almost nine percent had not seen a physician for at least a year. But ninety-five percent of the elderly are living in their own homes or with relatives; a few share apartments or boarding houses with each other in communal arrangements. Two-thirds of this group regard their health as good or excellent compared with other people their age.

The aged are the least likely to use either outpatient clinics or emergency rooms, but some twenty percent of physician care for the minority-group aged is still provided within these hospital-based facilities. The rate of hospitalization for the elderly is highest in the North Central region, which has more hospital beds per one thousand persons than any other region. This age group made over twice as many short-stay hospital

[13] As noted by Lloyd Shearer, *Parade*'s Special Intelligence Report, August 8, 1976, p. 10.

visits than the forty-five to sixty-four age group. These visits were usually for heart conditions, hypertension, and cerebrovascular diseases. Heart diseases, cerebrovascular diseases, and cancer account for about two-thirds of all deaths in this age group. Even though the death rate from heart disease has been dropping in recent years, it still accounted for forty-six percent of the deaths in this age group in 1973.

THE UNIQUE CHALLENGE OF CHRONIC ILLNESS: SOME SOCIAL PERSPECTIVES

If we make the improbable assumption of an unchanging medical technology, about two-thirds of everyone living in the United States today will eventually die of cancer, some form of cardiovascular illness, or stroke. Most of the remainder will die of influenza or pneumonia, ulcers, diabetes, or accidents, including those in automobiles. The following paragraphs summarize the shift in morbidity patterns in the past century:

> In the old days, people who died from diseases contracted them quickly, reached crisis shortly thereafter, and either died or pulled through. Modern medical researchers have changed this dramatic pattern by taming many once-devastating ailments. Improved conditions of living, along with effective medical skills and technology, have altered the nature of illness in scientifically advanced societies. While patients suffering from communicable diseases once filled most hospitals, treatment centers now serve mainly those afflicted with chronic ailments.

> Many who would have died soon after contracting a disease now live and endure their affliction. Today most illnesses are chronic diseases . . . slow-acting, long-term killers that can be treated but not cured.[14]

We should note that many episodes of such diseases as strokes and heart attacks have both an acute stage, in which the patient is quite ill for a number of days and his life in danger; and, for those who survive, a chronic stage, often with residual effects, recurring illness, and disability. This has led many authors to use hyphenated categories, such as "acute-chronic." We will use the term "chronic" to signify an illness that will remain with the patient, though it may be abated, for the remainder of his life; his life, under the circumstances, may reasonably be expected to last a number of months or years. Some confusion arises from the fact that "chronic illness" was once used largely as a label for the various degenerative illnesses related to aging. We use the terms "chronic" and "long-

[14] Anselm Strauss, "America: In Sickness and in Health," *Society,* Vol. 10, no. 6 (September/October 1973), p. 33.

term" interchangeably, since few truly long-term illnesses end with total cure.

Some long-term or chronic illnesses end by causing death; some are not fatal but can be debilitating; others are only irritating. Epilepsy, which results from an abnormality of brain function, demonstrates some of the variables and uncertainties of serious chronic illness. Seizures can be harmful or even result in death, usually from choking or other forms of accidental self-harm. But the illness is also often controllable by drug therapy, and many epileptics have few or no overt symptoms. Reduction in the medicine, for whatever reason, can lead quickly to seizure. Diabetes is another serious chronic ailment that can usually be controlled medically. By comparison, such chronic ailments as skin rash, flat feet, or lumbago take their toll in human discomfort, but tend to ask little of our health-care system.

The economic costs to society and the patient of serious chronic illnesses are staggering. Economists sometimes distinguish between direct and indirect costs. Direct costs are those expenditures made by the patient or his representative for the physicians, drugs, hospital rooms, and the like directly involved in the treatment of the illness. Indirect costs are the loss of income by the patient because of disabling afflictions or death. Another perspective comes from looking at the total health expenditures by age, with particular attention to those costs that are directly related to chronic serious illness.

Nursing-home care almost always involves patients with chronic illness, since their function is to provide long-term health services.[15] The nation spent $5.7 billion in 1974 for such care, an increase of 12 percent from the previous year.[16] The issue of costs relative to long-term institutions will undoubtedly continue to grow dramatically in importance, due both to the increasing numbers suffering from chronic illness and the growing governmental role in supporting institutional care for those so afflicted. There are more than 1 million patients currently in nursing homes and other long-term care institutions.

An increasing amount of medical research is oriented toward the cure and prevention of the major chronic illnesses, especially cancer, stroke, and heart disease. We now have "The President's Commission on Heart Disease, Cancer and Stroke," which is influential in setting health-delivery, planning, and research priorities for the nation. In fiscal year

[15] Hospitals, nursing homes, and extended-care facilities are discussed fully in chapter 10. The fact that some long-term rest homes or nursing homes are more like hotels, providing personal maintenance and very little medical care, is indicative of society's method of dealing with the chronic condition known as aging.

[16] Nancy L. Worthington, "National Health Expenditures, 1929–1974," *Social Security Bulletin*, February 1975, p. 4.

1972–73, for example, we spent about $2 billion on medical research, much of it oriented toward the major chronic illnesses.[17]

There are some occurrences and consequences of serious chronic illnesses that are alleviated through publicly funded programs. In 1973, we spent $9 billion on health insurance for the aged, $63 million on temporary-disability insurance, and $1.2 billion on medical benefits under workmen's compensation. More than 60 percent of all nursing-home expenditures are publicly supported.

Massive efforts at seeking out and treating illness, rather than waiting for the patient himself to seek care, are enormously expensive. One study estimated the costs of discovering cancer in various locations.[18] The cost per case of discovered uterine-cervix cancer was estimated at $913, while the costs for discovered head and neck cancer exceeded $13,000. Estimated costs per deaths averted ranged from $2,217 for uterine-cervix cancer to an excess of $46,000 for colon-rectum cancer. Both of these cost levels are related to the frequency of the cancer occurrence and to the treatment prognosis. Uterine-cervix cancer is quite common, and death aversion through treatment relatively favorable.

Our best estimate is that between 40 and 50 percent of all American citizens suffer from some form of chronic illness, and that about 25 percent of that total lose days at work due to the illnesses. The direct financial costs to the patient, when he is not covered by insurance, can create a serious economic crisis. During the early stages of the illness, whether severe or not, there is often an accumulation of medical expenses as efforts are made to stabilize the patient or, in potentially fatal illnesses, to take all steps to be sure he survives. If the patient stabilizes, long-term and expensive treatment is often required, and the cost obligations can be life-long.

Chronic kidney failure illustrates many of the financial traps in modern illness. As we noted earlier, a primary function of the kidney is the elimination of body waste through urination. A person whose kidneys have ceased functioning has four choices. One is to die, and some have chosen this alternative to avoid financial ruin. A second option is to seek kidney transplantation. If a suitable donor is found, costs for this surgery are astronomical, ranging from $30,000 to $45,000. Even after this expense, the body may reject the new kidney. One author roughly estimates

[17] Richard A. Ward, *The Economics of Health Resources* (Los Angeles: Addison-Wesley, 1975), p. 21.

[18] Many economists argue for the importance of economic considerations in a cost-benefit framework as part of health-policy considerations. For an interesting discussion of cost-benefit analysis in the health field and a brief review of such studies, including some mentioned in this text, see Ward, *The Economics of Health Resources*, p. 21.

that 30 percent of all kidneys taken from live donors are rejected, and that 50 percent or more of those taken from cadavers are rejected by the host.[19] The small percentage of patients having identical twins have the greatest opportunity for success if their donor is that sibling.

The third and fourth options for sufferers of chronic kidney failure are even more ironic. One is to purchase a dialysis machine and undergo attachment to and treatment from the apparatus two or three times a week. A home dialysis machine can cost $5,000 or more, and the expense only begins at that point. Achieving stabilization of the patient and conducting the training necessary for home use of the kidney machine are costs that double the price of the apparatus. From then on, the yearly expenses for operating the machine at home are about $3,000. The cost for receiving treatment in a clinic or hospital, the fourth choice, averages between $20,000 and $30,000 per year. There are about 24,000 persons in this country known to be suffering from chronic kidney failure.

One study identified the interpersonal factors between the home dialysis patient and his assistant-spouse that affect success in training and treatment.[20] Generally, older couples do not do as well in adjusting to the rigors of treatment and training. Couples that have similar methods of dealing with stress, particularly when they share methods of excessive denial, dependency, and regression, are also less apt to do well in home dialysis. The authors found evidence that the display of "good old-fashioned hostility," in which the patient's spouse shows anger, can enhance patient adjustment to the routine.

The impact of large medical expenses is frequently deemphasized because it is assumed that most of us have public or private health insurance. The dilemma is that most private health insurance covers costs for acute illness and therefore have maximum amounts they will pay. Public support under Medicare and Medicaid also have limits on services covered and amounts to be paid, as illustrated by the fact that forty percent of all nursing-home costs are paid by sources other than government. This means that the victims of chronic illness frequently find their private health insurance and the public-support programs inadequate to meet their financial obligations. Financial ruin from serious chronic illness is all too common.

The various disease entities referred to as "leukemia" further demonstrate the interplay of factors affecting the treatment of chronic illness. Leukemia is essentially cancer of the bone marrow, which results in (among other things) an extremely high increase in the white cells of

[19] Barbara Suczek, "Chronic Medicare," *Society*, Vol. 10, no. 6 (September/October 1973), p. 48.
[20] John R. Marshall, David G. Rice, Mary O'Mera, and Weldon D. Shelp, "Characteristics of Couples with Poor Outcome in Dialysis Home Training," *Journal of Chronic Diseases*, Vol. 28, no. 7/8 (August 1975), Pergamon Press.

the blood. Its occurrence is probably related to radiation: citizens of Hiroshima and Nagasaki experienced a high rate of leukemia after the atomic bombs. Radiologists develop leukemia more often than other physicians. Some authors believe it may have a viral origin, others deny any proof of that cause.[21]

Leukemia during childhood is devastating to all concerned. It is almost always fatal, ranking as the second greatest killer of children between age one and fourteen, exceeded only by accidents. The physical signs of the disease are tragic, including easy bruising, a tendency to bleeding, nausea, vomiting, bone and abdominal pain.

The time aspect of the illness is significant to the family of children with leukemia. The child may die within a few days, but immediately following diagnosis the usual approach is to conduct chemotherapy in an attempt to achieve remission—essentially, a temporary reduction in the number of leukemia cells. This effort is invariably done in the hospital and often involves blood transfusions, numerous tests, and consulting physicians. Costs for the first hospital stay during early stages of leukemia are substantial, often totalling thousands of dollars.

If initial remission is achieved, the child returns home. Remission often leaves the afflicted child looking quite healthy and normal, and the frightened and grieving parents are encouraged to believe the doctors are wrong; or perhaps they think the child will beat the illness. But soon the child's body develops an immunity to the drug being used to maintain remission, and signs of leukemia return. Remission is sought again, and the cycle is repeated. If the repeated efforts are successful, the child survives until he has built an immunity to the various available drugs. This can mean two or more years of life. Before the development and extensive use of chemotherapy in the illness, fifty percent of all children with acute leukemia, receiving only supportive therapy, died within four months of the occurrence of the symptoms.

Physicians and the medical literature frequently allude to progress in the control or even cure of the illness.[22] For this reason, parents frequently do all they can to give the child time in the hope that a cure will be found while the child is alive. A belief commonly expressed by physicians treating the illness is that a cure for a significant proportion of leukemics may come any day and that some now being treated may survive.

The parents are caught in a tragic conflict. The reality is that almost all children afflicted with acute leukemia have ultimately died. Treatment is expensive, and much of it may not be covered by health insurance. On the other hand, progress is being made, and the best treatment might buy "enough" time for the child. The temptation for many parents to do every-

21 Andre D. Lascari, M.D., *Leukemia in Childhood* (Springfield, Ill.: Charles C. Thomas, 1973), p. 5 or Boyd, *An Introduction to the Study of Disease*, p. 74.
22 Lascari, *Leukemia in Childhood*, p. 5.

thing to keep the child alive for as long as possible may include finding ways to pay for trips to research and treatment centers in various parts of the nation. An adult may choose to let himself die rather than face financial disaster in paying for dialysis. He is much less likely to feel the same way if the choice involves one of his children and this dreaded disease.

The role and obligations of health providers, in particular physicians, are different when treating patients with long-term or chronic illness rather than with acute curable illness. Whether or not the illness is grave or potentially fatal, the physician is likely to have repeated contact with the patient with chronic disease. Thus, the physician must settle for the satisfaction of minimizing the impact of the illness, rather than curing the patient; and there is an obligation to keep current on the patient's involvement with the illness. This seems to encourage the physician's concern over matters of the patient's lifestyle that relate to the illness. Heart and ulcer patients, for example, are frequently chastized for their eating habits. Some physicians tell patients not to come back until they have lost weight, or quit smoking, or have found ways to rest more.

Thus, chronic illnesses require an educational and counseling role on the part of physicians as well as other health providers. The diabetic and his family must be told how to guard for insulin shock, and those living with epileptics are usually told what to do if a seizure occurs. Medical books for physicians often have chapters devoted to the emotional reactions to disease, recommending how the patient and family should be prepared for various stages in the illness. Health providers may be psychologically or educationally unprepared for this obligation, and can thus add to the patient's problems. The following describes some of the emotional conflicts physicians feel in dealing with terminal leukemic children:

> The physician is confronted with two antithetical emotional responses to the dying child. He is drawn by compassion to help the child at every level and is also repulsed by the threat of death and the impulse to move away to protect himself from the impending loss. To be most effective, the physician should understand his own fears and emotions about death and should avoid the extremes of overprotecting the patient and that of being totally uninvolved. He has a right to feel frustrated and angry as his treatment eventually fails, but he has no right to feel guilt as the basic objectives of the physician are thwarted by the death of his patient.[23]

Treatment of serious chronic illness often requires numerous physicians, other health providers, hospitals, and even nursing homes. This involvement is loosely alluded to as the "team approach." Again, a physician treating the diabetic may find that the condition encourages heart

[23] Ibid.

disease or blindness, and this can precipitate a call for involvement of various specialists. Rehabilitation of stroke victims or paraplegics also involves a wide variety of health professionals from medical and sociopsychological disciplines.

THE FEAR OF DEATH: SOME PSYCHOLOGICAL PERSPECTIVES

We have noted that the illnesses resulting in most deaths in the United States can result in the rapid decline of the patient. They also often have a chronic or long-term stage. We have noted, too, that there are common chronic illnesses that are not life-threatening but still exact their costs in time, expense, and discomfort. Illness of whatever severity has the potential psychological cost of reminding us that our bodies are fallible, our existence tenuous, and our status mortal. Thus, any sign of illness, however slight, produces in many people a morbid reminder of their own impending death (someday) and results in fears and anxieties often termed "death response."[24]

Fear of death is a realistic concern for patients suffering serious chronic illnesses. The dilemma of serious long-term illnesses is that the patient survives for a time but his biologic balance may be disturbed and his life could end suddenly. He thus has reason and time to worry about his own possible death. Some patients know their own survival is precarious, but they do not know if or how their death might occur. An example is patients who have undergone serious cancer operations and who are waiting to see whether it will recur. Here, the normal fears of death are heightened by not knowing with any certainty what the future holds. On the other hand, patients who have been told they "only have two months to live" have that grim reality to face.

One author argues that death fears should be seen as a kind of interaction between three types of such fear, and whether we or someone else is the one seen as dying. Our types of death are fear of what comes after death, fear of the event of dying, and fear of ceasing to exist. The characteristics and dynamics of these fears vary according to whether it is our own death or someone else's that we fear.[25]

It might be argued that fear of death is a, or even *the* basic human fear. It clearly seems to heighten and multiply our other fears. Patients with serious chronic illnesses also frequently fear pain, real, imagined, or expected. The ability to withstand pain and our psychological tolerance for it vary with the individual, but all have their limits. Chronic illness

[24] Robert Kastenbaum and Ruth Aisenberg, *The Psychology of Death* (New York: Springer, 1972), chapter 3.
[25] Lascari, *Leukemia in Childhood,* pp. 44ff.

often means recurring pain. The chronically ill are often disturbed also about the financial costs of their illnesses and their increasing dependence on family, friends, and medical providers. The fact that serious chronic illness often introduces handicaps—for example, in the stroke victim with hemiplegia—is itself a source of fear and depression to the patient.

Persons with chronic illnesses that may threaten their lives create discomfort and fear in many around them. Friends and family often isolate the patient and are highly agitated in his presence, and this adds greatly to his psychological burden. This desire to avoid the person with serious illness is particularly forceful when the disease is visible, such as with stroke, the final stages of terminal cancer, the various degenerative illnesses so common to the aged, and major amputations.

Our discomfort in the presence of an ill person has numerous sources. The obvious one is that illness serves as a reminder of our infallibility. Not knowing what to say to or how to act with a person suffering from fatal cancer, for example, is also agonizing. Related to this is fear of the unknown. How will the sick person act? What will he do in insulin shock? How frightening is an epileptic seizure?

Fear of our own death and anxiety resulting from contact with seriously ill or dying people speak to the psychology of death in our society. Ultimately, though, two major developments affecting society as a whole combine to create our social methods of coping with death. First, it is frequently noted that we live in a youth-oriented culture. The emphasis is on the young, and their thoughts are kept from mortality: the good jobs are for the young, most educational opportunities exist for them, and recreational activities emphasize youth. Second, modern medicine and sanitary measures have helped produce an unusually long life expectancy for our citizens. Most of us live twice as long as most of our ancestors, and decades longer than people currently living in underdeveloped nations. Most of us will live seventy years or more, though survival into the eighties is common and into the nineties is occasional. We encounter death less often than our ancestors until the "old age" of sixty years or older.

One of the consequences of these two factors is that the death of someone "young" is seen as particularly tragic. Children who die, from leukemia or automobile accidents, for example, are particular sources of grief and dismay for most of us. They have been robbed of their right to life. In fact death at an early age is now considered unnatural, and therefore particularly tragic.

At the opposite end of the age scale, we seem particularly resigned to the death of older people. She has lived "a good long life," and so grief or a sense of tragedy about impending death seems inappropriate. This undoubtedly encourages our tendency to "give up" on geriatric patients and is related to our tolerance of some "rest homes" that are poor and are even dangerous to their inhabitants.

The infrequency of the death occurrence in our lives has meant that our inclinations toward mourning have themselves died, or at least become severely weakened. Funerals are increasingly commercialized, handled by profitmaking companies and not by the family. Drive-up funeral homes now exist. Wakes are less common than in the beginning of this century. It seems that our long life expectancies and the infrequent occurrence of death during most of our lives means that the social institutions pertaining to death and mourning are less needed. This permits what one widely known author has called a "death-denying society."[26]

The magic of modern medicine has, ironically, helped us to deny the inevitable end we all must face. In this chapter we have traced the shift in the nature of illnesses in our society from the infectious-acute to the chronic. We have discussed the social and economic costs of those diseases, psychological reactions to them, and a few of their implications for medical providers. We also identified some of the personal and social implications of the death occurrence, affected as it is by chronic illnesses, longevity, and social changes.

Perhaps the best postscript to this report on health can be made by quoting from a *Time* centennial essay, "The Struggle to Stay Healthy," written by John H. Knowles, president of the Rockefeller Foundation and former general director of Massachusetts General Hospital:

> Where do we stand today, and what are our prospects for health beyond 1976? Gone are the scourges of small pox, yellow fever, tuberculosis, measles and infantile diarrhea. Life expectancy has increased from 47.3 years in 1900 to 72.4 years in 1975. Of the roughly 2 million deaths annually in the U.S., 37.8 percent are due to heart disease, 19.5 percent to cancer, 10.2 percent to strokes, 4.3 percent to lung disease (pneumonia, bronchitis and emphysema), 5.3 percent to accidents, 1.9 percent to diabetes, 1.7 percent to cirrhosis of the liver, 1.4 percent to suicide and 1.1 percent to homicide. But death statistics give only part of the picture. For every successful suicide, eight others (or 200,000 people) may have made the attempt. For every person who dies of cirrhosis—commonly related to alcoholism and malnutrition—at least 200 and probably 300 people can be classified as alcoholics (10 million Americans). For every accidental death, hundreds are injured, some permanently disabled. Twenty-four million Americans, 11 million who receive no federal food stamps, live below the federally defined poverty level, a level that does not support an adequate diet. Venereal diseases has been increasing annually, with nearly 1 million cases of gonorrhea and syphilis reported last year.
>
> Beyond death and disease statistics, there exist a steadily expanding number of the "worried well" and those with minor illness. *Has life itself become a disease to be cured in the American culture?* Some 80 percent

26 Elisabeth Kübler-Ross, Stanford Wessler, and Louis V. Avioli, "On Death and Dying." In *On Death and Dying* (New York: Macmillan, 1969).

of the doctor's work consists of treating minor complaints and giving reassurance. Common colds, minor injuries, gastrointestinal upsets, back pain, arthritis, and psychoneurotic anxiety states account for the vast majority of visits to clinics and doctors' offices. One out of four people is "emotionally tense" and worried about insomnia, fatigue, too much or too little appetite and ability to cope with modern life. At least ten percent of the population suffers some form of mental illness, and one-seventh of these receive some form of psychiatric care. Meanwhile, the figures for longevity are the highest, and for infant mortality the lowest in U.S. history, and the gap continues to narrow. We are doing better, but feeling worse.[27]

SUGGESTED READINGS

"The Annual Rip-Off," *Time*, July 26, 1976, p. 54. A critical commentary on the extravagance of annual checkups.

FUCHS, VICTOR R., *Who Shall Live? Health, Economics and Social Choice* (New York: Basic, 1974). Gives full attention to the interrelationships among environment, lifestyle, and access to medical services.

GLATT, M. M., "Today's Enjoyment: Tomorrow's Dependence: The Road Towards the 'Rock Bottom' and the Way Back," *The British Journal of Addiction to Alcohol and Other Drugs*, Vol. 70, no. 3 (March 1976), pp. 25–33. A discussion of the costs to one's health from alcoholism.

KNOX, A. E. HERTZLER and WILLIAM E. BURKE, "The Insurance Industry and Occupational Alcoholism," *Proceedings*, Industrial Relations Research Association, Spring meeting, 1975, pp. 491–507. A description of the implications of alcoholism for the work environment.

KREITNER, ROBERT, "Employee Physical Fitness: Protecting an Investment in Human Resources," *Personnel Journal*, Vol. 55, no. 7 (July 1976), pp. 340–44. A commentary on health-care management.

KÜBLER-ROSS, ELISABETH, "On Death and Dying," *Journal of the American Medical Association*, Vol. 22, no. 2 (July 10, 1972). An examination of the emotional problems of dying patients.

O'ROURKE, KEVIN D., "Active and Passive Euthanasia: the Ethical Distinctions," *Hospital Progress*, November 1976. A treatment of how the terminally ill should die and the misunderstanding surrounding active and passive euthanasia.

PENDER, NOLA J., "A Conceptual Model for Preventive Health Behavior," *Nursing Outlook*, Vol. 23, no. 6 (June 1975), pp. 385–90. A presentation of a preventive strategy for sustaining health.

POMERLEAU, OVID, FREDERIC BASS, and VICTOR CROWN, "Role of Behavior Modification in Preventive Medicine," *The New England Journal of Medi-*

[27] John H. Knowles, "The Struggle to Stay Healthy," *Time*, August 9, 1976, p. 62. Italics added.

cine, Vol. 292, no. 24 (June 12, 1975), pp. 1277–82. Deals with the effect of lifestyle on health.

RICHARDSON, DONNA RAE, "A Matter of Life and Death: A Definition of Death: Judicial Resolution of a Medical Responsibility?," *Howard Law Journal*, Vol. 19, no. 2 (Spring 1976). A discussion of the definition of death.

STRAUSS, ANSELM, "America: In Sickness and in Health—Chronic Illness," *Society*, Vol. 10, no. 6 (September/October 1973). A commentary on the increasing number of Americans afflicted by chronic illness.

SUCZEK, BARBARA, "America in Sickness and in Health—Chronic Medicare," *Society*, September/October 1973. Suczek illustrates the fear that results from changes within the family's social system, as she describes the life of a victim of chronic ailments.

Trends Affecting U.S. Health Care System (Washington, D.C.: GPO, DHEW Publication No. (HRA) 76-14503, prepared by the Aspen Systems Corporation of Germantown, Maryland, January 1976). A summary of each age group's morbidity patterns and differential rates of success in terms of the effectiveness of medical technology.

WALD, PATRICIA M., "Judicial Activism in the Law of Criminal Responsibility: Alcoholism and Drugs," *The Georgetown Law Journal*, Vol. 63 (October 1974), pp. 69–86. A consideration of the legal aspects of treating alcoholism.

WEISBERG, LILLIAN MIRO, "Casework With the Terminally Ill," *Social Casework*, June 1974. Discusses needs of those suffering from catastrophic illness and the need for a new approach to its management.

YONDORF, BARBARA, "The Declining and Wretched," *Public Policy*, Vol. 23, no. 4 (Fall 1975). Contends that the problems of the dying are not unique but are shared by the aged and hopelessly ill.

7

ETHNIC GROUPS, POVERTY, AND HEALTH IN THE UNITED STATES

In the previous chapter, we saw how the morbidity patterns in the United States have shifted during this century: in general, from acute and infectious diseases to those diseases such as cancer and cardiovascular illness, which are more directly related to lifestyle and can be chronic. We also discussed psychological and health-delivery aspects of these "new" illnesses. Astute readers probably recognized that morbidity patterns and medical technology have changed more rapidly than many of our cultural beliefs about health and illness, and that beliefs have much significance for our health and our medical care. When we add to this the recognition that many Americans participate in ethnic subcultures with their own health beliefs and practices, we come to understand the complexity of health delivery to the pluralistic population groups comprising this nation. We will begin this chapter with a general statement of the relationships between culture, subcultures, and health-care systems. We will then describe health characteristics of our various ethnic groups, relate what is known about poverty and health, and discuss some major characteristics of our health-care system with implications for minorities and the poor.

CULTURES AND THE HEALTH-CARE SYSTEM

The concept of "culture" is used extensively in anthropology and somewhat less in sociology. Some authors argue that anthropology is concerned with man's culture, sociology deals with society, and psychology with human personality.[1] A combined use of these very broad concepts,

[1] Ernest L. Schusky and T. Patrick Culbert, *Introducing Culture* (Englewood Cliffs, N.J.: Prentice-Hall, 1967).

however, provides the most comprehensive understanding of man and his major social systems, such as health.

Simply defined, culture is the beliefs and customs a society has developed in attempting to manage its shared problems, a part of which concern the occurrence of illness and the need for medical treatment. For our own purposes, we will view culture as an *orienting concept*—that is, a concept that helps us see the direction of a society's beliefs and practices as it attempts to meet sets of needs and manage social problems. Culture is an extremely broad concept, as these two interpretations from noted culture theorists demonstrate:

> Culture is that complex whole which includes knowledge, belief, art, morals, law, custom, and any other capabilities and habits acquired by man as a member of society.[2]

> A culture is a systematic and integrated whole. [It] . . . is an abstraction from the body of learned behavior which a group of people who share the same tradition transmit entire to their children, and, in part, to adult immigrants who become members of the society. It covers not only the arts and sciences, religions and philosophies, to which the word "culture" has historically been applied, but also the system of technology, the political practices, the small intimate habits of daily life, such as the way of preparing or eating food, or of hushing a child to sleep, as well as the method of electing a prime minister or changing the constitution.[3]

A society's culture has a number of characteristics that are significant for understanding the health-care system. First, beliefs and customs are cultural when they are quite commonly shared by the people of the society. Personal idiosyncracies or habits that deviate from the common practices are not considered part of culture. Thus, our faith in and acceptance of the medical superiority of physicians, a phenomenon that originated early in this century, has been an influential cultural belief, although there is ample evidence of its weakening.

Since cultural elements are those shared by a large group of people, we recognize that our society is multicultural: we have a majority culture with beliefs and customs (including those pertaining to health, illness, and treatment) shared by a great many of our citizens; and we have numerous subcultures (Mexican-Americans, Italian-Americans, Jews, blacks, etc.), large groups of peoples who share somewhat different cultural beliefs and customs.

We hedge by saying "somewhat different" for two reasons. First, any cultural subgroup will probably take on some of the larger culture's

---

[2] E. B. Tylor, *Primitive Culture*, 5th ed. (London: Gordon Press, 1871), Vol. I, chapter 1.
[3] Margaret Mead, *Cultural Patterns and Technical Change* (New York: New American Library, 1963), pp. 12–13.

elements. Thus, even in the most rural Mexican-American settlements in the Southwest, "Anglo" medical beliefs and practices have had some impact. Second, some persons in this country combine beliefs and practices from different cultures. Many studies, for example, have described the efforts of young Japanese-Americans to maintain various Japanese cultural traits while "fitting into" the majority culture.[4]

Culture is also cumulative: cultural customs and beliefs are developed, maintained, and passed on from generation to generation. We maintain our beliefs about health and illness, for example, in writing and in conventional wisdom, which is passed on from generation to generation. As an illustration, there remains a common belief that the predominant and best doctor–patient relationship is one in which the "family physician" supplies the medical services and patients meet their obligation by paying for services out-of-pocket. This belief appears to remain strong even though government and other forms of health-insurance payments make up the vast majority of fee payments to physicians. Students of culture have discovered that beliefs often lag far behind changes and progress in technical practices. They have termed this occurrence "cultural lag." To say that cultural elements are passed on from one generation to another is not to say that cultural change does not occur. It certainly does. We have, for example, discussed the increased use of hospitals as a health center in substitution for the older pattern of the home as medical center for the family. But cultural beliefs and habits often continue "beyond their time," seeming to have a survival power of their own that makes change quite difficult.

In brief summary, then, culture has the following characteristics. It is shared by a group of people. It is cumulative, a "storehouse" of beliefs and practices that are passed from one generation to the next. It is diverse in the sense that one population group may have one set of beliefs and customs, and another group living in the same country (or even city) will have another. Last, the components of a culture are interdependent; they rely upon interaction and sometimes change one another. Clearly, our beliefs about the family and its obligations to the elderly have changed in ways that help explain the enormous growth in rest homes and nursing homes as places to put the elderly. The availability of these institutions permits the family to avoid the burden of caring for aged parents, an obligation inconsistent with working wives, frequent changes in residence, and high divorce rates. Just as clearly, our commonly held belief that government is inept and insufficient, and that the "private sector" is more efficient, is partly the source of resistance to and resentment of growing government involvement in the health-care industry.

Our majority culture and the various subcultures, then, set the stage

[4] Donald Keith Fellows, *A Mosaic of America's Ethnic Minorities* (New York: Wiley, 1972).

for basic belief systems and customs, through which we interact with the health-care system. The general set of relationships between culture and the health-care system are lucidly described by Margaret Clark:

> Health, the prevention of illness, and the curing of disease constitute a major area of interest to the peoples of all cultures. No human group lacks an explanation of the conditions that must be fulfilled or maintained for the individual to enjoy good health, and no human group lacks explanations of the causes of illness. No human group is so simple but that it has social, religious, and clinical devices to cope with illness—ceremonies to frighten away demons, magical rites to recover a lost soul, herbal remedies to cure a variety of ailments, and physical and surgical manipulations to repair broken bones and other injuries.
>
> No medical system (that is, a complex of ideas about causes and cures of disease) is entirely rational, and none is entirely irrational. Any medical system, whether based on the scientific knowledge and practices of modern medicine or on the superstitions and empirical knowledge of primitive groups, is at least a reasonably coherent and unified body of belief and practice. Since curing practices are a function of the beliefs on the nature of health and the causes of illness, most curative procedures are understandable and "logical" in the light of those beliefs.
>
> Medical beliefs in all cultures are among those held to most tenaciously. Many of these beliefs become firmly ingrained in the minds of people during childhood, and the emotional quality attached to them is almost sacred. Moreover, the stress of illness and the ever-present fear of death are not conducive to "rational" action, if by "rationality" one means the abandonment of old and tried-and-true procedures of new and little-understood treatments. Since medical systems are integral parts of the cultures in which they occur, they cannot be understood simply in terms of curing practices, medical practitioners, hospital services, and the like. Medical systems are affected by most categories of culture: economics, religion, social relationships, education, family structure, language. Only a partial understanding of a medical system can be gained unless other parts of culture can be studied and related to it.[5]

THE SUBCULTURE OF POVERTY

It has long been recognized that whites in our society live longer and get sick less often than blacks, Mexican-Americans, or American Indians. In part, this is so because whites in this society are likely to be more highly educated and less desperately poor than the three ethnic groups mentioned above. The evidence is overwhelming that poverty is

[5] Margaret Clark, *Health in the Mexican-American Culture*, 2nd ed. (Berkeley and Los Angeles: University of California Press, 1959, 1970), p. 1.

unhealthy. One study, which included interviews with a sample of 1,057 adults across the nation, discovered that only 7 percent of respondents from affluent families reported having a family member seriously ill, while 24 percent of the inner-city black respondents and the same percentage of Spanish-speaking respondents reported a seriously ill family member.[6] The relationship of poverty to incapacity is dramatically illustrated by the fact that 31 percent of the Appalachian whites, one of the nation's poorest white populations, reported a seriously ill family member.

In the past, middle-income whites visited physicians more often than the poor or those from ethnic groups. The affluent have made substantial use of the physician working in an office-based practice as distinct from hospital emergency rooms. But there is evidence that Medicare and Medicaid, along with other changes in the system, have increased physician contacts with the poor and minority groups.[7]

The more affluent are almost always covered by some form of health insurance, almost never receive "free" care, and infrequently make out-of-pocket payments. In effect, they seldom need to seek the charity of a free clinic or the government-sponsored outpatient units so often used by the poor.

It is possible to outline a generalized (and therefore oversimplified) model of the majority culture's health-care delivery system. Severe illness or early deaths are relatively infrequent occurrences. Health care is delivered by family physicians based in an office or clinic setting. Emergency services are sought only when emergencies arise at nights or on weekends. The physician provides the services and is usually reimbursed through the patient's health insurance. There is a strongly shared feeling that medical science can do wonders.

Margaret Clark offers some insightful analysis on how the major culture, the subcultures, and health care are interrelated.

> Whenever individuals from one culture, with their particular beliefs about health, illness, and the prevention and cure of disease, come to live as members of a minority group within another culture which has a vastly different medical system, emotional and social conflicts often result when illness brings members of the two groups together. Conflicts resulting from culture contact are not, of course, confined to medical relations. Similar conflicts arise in other areas of life when people, in contact with a culture other than their own, find it necessary to make significant changes in many of their ways of living and thinking. Medical changes are merely one phase of the larger process of acculturation.

[6] *A Blue Cross Report on the Health Problems of the Poor* and *A Louis Harris Survey* (Chicago: Blue Cross Association, 1968), p. 24.
[7] Spyros Andreopoulos (ed.), *Primary Care: Where Medicine Fails* (New York: Wiley, 1974).

Sometimes, however, medical conflicts are particularly disturbing, and their resolution may require special attention. Immigrant peoples in the United States often find themselves without the full spectrum of medical resources they had in their native lands. They may have no access to traditional ways of dealing with illness, and the healing methods commonly practiced in the United States may seem strange and frightening. Yet if members of ethnic minorities do not follow the health rules imposed on other residents (compulsory vaccination, isolation of contagious diseases, environmental sanitation), they may become a health threat to the total community and may find themselves in conflict with law enforcement agencies.[8]

There are at least eight major ethnic groups in the United States, the number depending on what one means by "major." Our society is made up of "minority" groups with beliefs and customs different from "the rest of us." It is true, of course, that all of us (except the American Indian) are from families that were immigrants. But many immigrant groups and their members tended to lose their distinctive culture and have joined the mainstream of American life.[9] When members of a subculture have physical characteristics that are plainly different from those of the majority culture, they will probably experience racial discrimination. Many of our subcultural groups have quite distinctive physical features: blacks, Mexican-Americans, Filipinos, Japanese, Chinese, and Puerto Ricans. It is not a chance occurrence that all of these groups have experienced discrimination in such areas as employment, housing, and education. There is evidence that many of their members have also been subjected to violence by "the rest of us."[10]

The interactions in this country between the majority culture, our subcultural groups, and the health-care system can be summarized as follows:

[8] Clark, *Health in the Mexican-American Culture*, p. 2.
[9] We choose not to enter the esoteric debate about whether there is a majority culture or whether we are really nothing more than a loose conglomeration of subcultures including youth, college subculture, the aged, etc. The clear correlations between ethnicity, poverty, health, and longevity show that medically the majority of our citizens do better (illness rate, child mortality, etc.) than our two largest minorities (blacks and Chicanos) and than our indigenous citizens (American Indians). In addition, we will show later that various ethnic groups, even those not beset by abject poverty, show rates of illness occurrences that are quite different from the total population of the country.
[10] Richard Hofstadter and Michael Wallace (eds.), *American Violence: A Documentary History* (New York: Random House, 1971) and Rudolf Gomez, Clement Cottingham, Jr., Russel Endo, and Kathleen Jackson, *The Social Reality of Ethnic America* (Lexington, Mass.: D. C. Heath, 1974). See these references for in-depth studies of American minorities and their history in this country.

1. In addition to the majority culture, we have numerous subcultural groups who view health, illness, life and death, and medical treatment through attitudes and beliefs of their own. Examples of such viewpoints were provided in chapter 5.

2. The health-care system, dominated by majority beliefs and personnel is often inappropriate and probably sometimes biased vis-à-vis these subcultural groups.

3. Antagonism toward these ethnic minorities (as well as other factors, such as "education") is reflected in the impatience and even intolerance of health-care providers.

4. Poverty (particularly for blacks, Chicanos, and American Indians) increases the possibility of illness (from hunger, cold, etc.) and can limit the quality and quantity of medical care they receive.

THE HEALTH STATUS OF MINORITIES

Our four most populous ethnic groups are also the poorest. There are more than twenty-one million blacks in this country, our largest ethnic group. In 1973, more than thirty-one percent of blacks were listed below the "official poverty line," as compared with slightly more than eight percent of the white population.[11] Throughout the Southwest, where they are concentrated, about thirty-three percent of the Mexican-American families live below the poverty line. The poverty condition of an unusually high percentage of American Indians and Puerto Ricans is also well documented.

It is true that the majority of persons living in poverty in this country are white; more than two-thirds of the poor are not minorities. But a higher percentage of nonwhites experience poverty status. We have noted that less than 9 percent of the white population was poor in 1973; the figure for all nonwhites was 29.6 percent. It is clear that membership in an ethnic subcultural group and poverty are directly related for most of our minorities.

This direct relationship holds not only between ethnic status and poverty (at least for most of our ethnic groups), but also between illness and poverty. The health commissioner of New York has dramatically claimed that "poverty is the third leading cause of death in New York City."[12] His insight into the connections between poverty and ill health is

[11] U.S. Bureau of the Census, Current Population Reports, Series P-23, No. 48, "The Social and Economic Status of the Black Population in the United States," Table 16.
[12] Robert E. Will and Harold G. Vatter (eds.), Poverty in Affluence: The Social Political, and Economic Dimensions of Poverty in the United States, 2nd ed. (New York: Harcourt, 1970), p. 121.

supported by data. In 1968, thirty-three percent of those with incomes of less than $2,000 suffered chronic conditions that limited their activity. The same figure was seven percent for families with incomes over $7,000. The poor show dramatically higher mortality rates, especially during perinatal and early-infancy stages.[13] Tuberculosis, venereal disease, untreated dental conditions, and visual and orthopedic illnesses remain higher among the poor. The morbidity rates at each income level are higher for nonwhites than for whites, showing how ethnic status and income work together to produce ill health. Even the dreaded "crib death," a largely unexplained tragedy in which apparently healthy infants go to sleep and die for no apparent reason, seems related to low income.[14]

 ⁓ Poverty contributes to ill health and early death in a number of ways. Poor people usually do not eat well, and constant and severe hunger is unhealthy. An estimated twenty-five million of our residents lack sufficient money to keep themselves adequately fed. Some of the unhealthy consequences include illness associated with vitamin or protein deficiency; deaths attributable to severe diarrhea and starvation; anemia, blindness, and brain damage resulting from improper and inadequate food.[15]

Low income also produces living conditions that encourage illness. Pneumonia and influenza occur twice as often among blacks than among whites, partly because of inadequate housing and heating conditions. The incidence of tuberculosis is more frequent among the low-income, as is whooping cough. There were 14,000 known cases of rat bite in this country in 1965, again related to poor sanitation measures.

While conditions of poverty produce more illness and higher mortality rates, they also frequently discourage the proper and efficient use of medical services. Until recently the poor visited physicians less often than the wealthy or middle-income, but by 1969, Medicare and Medicaid appeared to have changed this situation. One study indicates that in 1969 the low-income had 4.6 physician visits per capita, while the middle- and upper-income had 4.0 visits.[16] But the picture is not as bright as these figures indicate. Many physicians will not treat Medicare and Medicaid patients, and it has been charged that the least capable doctor welcomes the "public" patients. It is also not clear that the care the poor receive

[13] Mary W. Herman, "The Poor: Their Medical Needs and the Health Services Available to Them," *The Annals of the American Academy of Policy and Social Science,* Vol. 399 (1972), p. 13.

[14] United States Department of Health, Education and Welfare, Public Health Service, "Sudden Death in Infants," NIH, National Institute of Child Health and Human Development, PHS publication no. 1412, 1963.

[15] Barbara Milbauer and Gerald Leinwand (eds.), *Hunger* (New York: Pocket Books, 1971).

[16] Andreopoulos, *Primary Care,* p. 163.

when their bills are paid by government is equal in quality to that of the middle-income citizen whose costs are supported by a health-insurance policy. Inferior care may be the rule. In addition, the 1969 figures on physician visits also show that poor youths under the age of fifteen and nonwhites over sixty-five continued to visit the doctor less often than their age counterparts of higher income. Finally, both Medicare and Medicaid will not pay for many types of treatment that may be medically necessary and desirable. Public programs do not permit the freedom of medical choice enjoyed by the more affluent citizens.

Partly for economic reasons, the poor suffer longer with their illnesses before seeking help. Of course, they are not as likely to have a family physician on call or one readily accessible through an office appointment. Thus, they are more likely to be quite ill when they do seek help. If they do not qualify for government payment for medical services they seek, they will probably continue to put off obtaining the needed care. Low-income families have less to spend on health, and they spend twenty-five percent less of the income they do have.

We also believe that perpetual poverty itself develops a set of health-related beliefs in those experiencing it. Oscar Lewis argues that under certain conditions, people suffering continual poverty develop and maintain certain habits, customs, social relationships, and attitudes that are predictable and significant for all aspects of their lives, including their health. This he described as the "culture of poverty." The many characteristics of poverty culture include a lack of contact with and segregation from the majority culture; hostility to basic majority institutions; feelings of helplessness and dependency, even inferiority.[17] The poverty-stricken Chicano who will quietly suffer the pains in his left arm rather than seek medical help may seem tragically foolish to those in the majority culture. But his actions are reasonable in light of what we know about the health implications of poverty and low income.

As mentioned above, subcultures experience rates of disease quite different from the rest of society. As noted in chapter 5, the subculture's ways of viewing and handling their own health, medical care, and illness often appear strange and even irrational to the majority culture, making the minority member ill-at-ease in hospitals and with physicians. If poor, they are sick more often and have limited access to care. If poor, they do not have private health insurance, although Medicare and Medicaid may be available. Because they often do not have a family physician, they make frequent use of emergency services in hospitals. The health-care system does not seem relevant to their needs except in emergency situations. Let us examine the patterns of morbidity and of the use of health services by blacks, Mexican-Americans, and American Indians.

[17] Oscar Lewis, *Five Families* (New York: Basic Books, 1959) and Lewis "The Culture of Poverty," *Scientific American,* October 1966.

BLACKS

There are more than twenty-one million blacks in this country, the majority concentrated in the South and East and West coasts. Their numbers easily make them our largest ethnic minority. For the reason of population size alone, our ability to improve the quality of life of black citizens will remain a critical issue for the foreseeable future.

Blacks in this country begin life with enormous health disadvantages. Senator Edward Kennedy, long concerned with the nature of our health-care system, has often alluded to "the stunted bodies, shortened lives, and physical handicaps of those who live in poverty."[18] Pregnant black women are less likely to seek adequate prenatal care, a treatment deficiency strongly related to children being born with nervous disorders and mental retardation. In urban areas, black mothers die during childbirth four times as often as white mothers, and black children die during the first year of life three times as often as white infants.[19]

Throughout life blacks experience illness more frequently. They are twice as likely to contract pneumonia and influenza as any white group. It has also been shown that blacks have unusually high rates of hypertension.[20] Sickle-cell anemia, at times a deadly killer, is characteristic of the black population.

Blacks clearly illustrate the complex interactions between various characteristics of a population group and the causes and occurrences of modern illness. Put simply and directly, blacks are biologically prone to illness not affecting nonblacks, such as sickle-cell anemia. A few other illnesses are also related to "racial type" rather than to cultures. But the most significant causes of morbidity pertain to lifestyle and cultural characteristics. We noted earlier, for example, that hypertension is encouraged by stress and anxiety, feelings quite common for blacks as a population group experiencing poverty, and frequently in relationships of anger and deprivation with the majority culture. It also seems reasonable to believe that "poverty and minority status" is a state of being that leads to such unhealthly expressions of frustration as excessive drinking and narcotics addiction.[21]

It is no wonder, then, that blacks have a shorter life span than those of the majority culture. A newborn black has approximately ten percent less life expectancy than a white infant.[22] The average black male can ex-

[18] John C. Norman and Beverly Bennett, *Medicine in the Ghetto* (Des Moines: Meredith, 1969), p. 270.
[19] Ibid., pp. 6–7.
[20] Howard E. Freeman, Sol Levine, Leo G. Reeder, *Handbook of Medical Sociology* 2nd ed. (Englewood Cliffs, N.J.: Prentice-Hall, 1972), p. 77.
[21] Ibid., p. 157.
[22] Ibid.

pect to live into his middle to late sixties, while the average white male survives into his early to middle seventies.

In this country, the number of years of completed schooling is strongly related to healthier and longer lives.[23] This is not surprising since schooling is directly related to higher income and also encourages the understanding of one's physiological and psychological processes. Our largest ethnic minorities, excepting the Japanese-Americans, have substantially less education than the average citizen.

One study of attitudes toward health care demonstrates additional cultural aspects of the black health status in the United States. As noted, blacks from the inner city are twice as likely as the rest of the nation to report that someone in their family is currently experiencing a major illness.[24] More significantly, only twenty-nine percent of the blacks surveyed reported that they were healthier than the previous generations, while fifty-one percent felt they were less healthy. This seems to indicate not only that blacks are ill more often and die younger than the rest of society, but also that they regard the health status of their own ethnic group to be deteriorating from generation to generation.

MEXICAN-AMERICANS

Since the late 1960s, Mexican-American spokesmen have frequently complained that Chicanos are ignored, misunderstood, and given low priority in social programs, at least in comparison with blacks.[25] An attempt to find adequate literature on the health status of this group supports that complaint: it is sparse at best.

Chicanos are the country's second-largest ethnic group. More than six million Mexican descendants reside in this country, although the inaccuracies of the census and the difficulty of assessing the number of Mexicans living "illegally" in the United States make the total a matter of speculation. The vast majority of all Chicanos are concentrated in the Southwest, and there is an additional large concentration in Chicago.

As with blacks, Mexican-Americans suffer poverty in comparison with the rest of society. The Census Bureau found that about twenty-nine percent of all Mexican-Americans in 1972 were low-income. They are also less educated, more often unemployed, and less frequently have white-

[23] David M. Heer, *Society and Population* (Englewood Cliffs, N.J.; Prentice-Hall, 1968), chapter 4.
[24] Gomez, Cottingham, Endo, and Jackson, *The Social Reality of Ethnic America.*
[25] Octavio Ignacio Romano-V. (ed.), *Voices—Readings from* El Grito, *1967–1973: A Journal of Contemporary Mexican-American Thought* (Berkeley: Quinto Sol Publications, 1971), pp. 16–23. The term "Chicano" is used interchangeably with "Mexican-American."

collar jobs.[26] In most Southwestern states Chicanos have lower educational attainment levels than blacks, although their average incomes tend to be somewhat higher than for blacks.[27]

Although their health status has not been thoroughly investigated, it is generally believed that Chicanos have an unusually high incidence of illness and early death. One observer notes that Mexican-Americans living in Colorado die ten years earlier than whites, and it is reasonable to believe that rural Chicanos have extremely high illness and low life-expectancy rates.[28] As with blacks, Mexican-American infants are about three times as likely to die at birth as whites.

Diet may be a major health factor for those Mexican-Americans who frequently eat Mexican meals. Many Mexican dishes make heavy use of carbohydrates and minimal use of protein. It is generally believed that Chicanos are quite prone to sugar diabetes, possibly because of their diet. They are, however, less likely than whites to have cancer, chronic heart disease, or vascular lesions. Since these are diseases common to advanced age, earlier death among Chicanos may help explain these lower rates.

A high percentage of Mexican-Americans die from accidents. About forty-three percent of all Chicano deaths in the age group of sixteen to twenty-five years result from fatal motor-vehicle accidents.[29] Chicanos also still die quite frequently from influenza and pneumonia, diseases that we have seen to be of rapidly declining mortality importance for the rest of society.

Chicano health habits and attitudes present a mixture both similar to and different from those of blacks. As is common with all low-income groups, they only infrequently have health insurance. Chicanos and Puerto Ricans, responding to the question of how many had "someone in the family now seriously ill," also showed an affirmative-response rate of twenty-four percent, more than twice as high as the nation as a whole.[30] But these Spanish-speaking peoples were much less likely than other poverty groups to believe they are less healthy than the previous generation.

---

[26] United States Department of Commerce, Social and Economic Statistics Administration, Bureau of the Census, Selected Characteristics of Persons and Families of Mexican, Puerto Rican, and other Spanish Origin: March 1972 (Washington, D.C.: U.S. Government Printing Office, 1972), Tables 4–7, pp. 5–8.

[27] Walter Fogel, Education and Income of Mexican-Americans in the Southwest, Mexican-American Study Project, Division of Research, Graduate School of Business Administration, University of California, Los Angeles, Advance Report 1, November 1965, p. 8.

[28] Joan W. Moore, with Alfredo Cuellar, Mexican Americans (Englewood Cliffs, N.J.: Prentice-Hall, 1970), p. 73.

[29] Ibid., p. 73.

[30] A Blue Cross Report on the Health Problems of the Poor and A Louis Harris Survey, p. 30.

Consistent with our earlier comments about Chicano morbidity patterns, the Spanish-speaking respondents said they had more cases of diabetes, colds, and uterine infections than other poverty groups, but also reported fewer instances of heart trouble, arthritis, ulcers, and kidney ailments. Significantly, the Chicanos and Puerto Ricans admitted to neglecting their diets and tending toward overweight, but relatively few believed that this was an important health consideration. Nor were they greatly concerned about avoiding stress and overexertion.

The availability of physician care to Chicanos is puzzling and ironic. Many of the country's agricultural laborers in the Southwest are Mexican-Americans or Mexican citizens. Yet the majority of the Chicanos in the United States live in urban, not rural, areas. Thus, many rural Chicano areas report little or no physician population. But in urban Chicano communities (usually called "barrios"), the physician presence is not much better. Few white doctors pick low-income Chicano communities in which to practice, and Chicano physicians are hard to find. As of the 1970 census, only five percent of all Los Angeles physicians, for example, was Spanish-speaking or Spanish-surnamed. This compared unfavorably with the fact that eighteen percent of the Los Angeles population was from this ethnic grouping. When Chicanos do complete medical school, they follow their white colleagues in moving to the richer white neighborhoods as places to practice.

AMERICAN INDIANS

In the 1970 census, about 800,000 respondents registered as Indian or of Indian descent. By moving from blacks and Chicanos to Indians, we turn from the poor to the poorest in this country. Indians have the highest unemployment rate, the lowest educational attainment, and the lowest median family income of all ethnic minorities. The following statement by one of this country's leading senators and his spouse is a lucid summary of the current status of Indians.

> Since health is closely related to economic and social status, no one should be surprised that American Indians are the least healthy major identifiable group in our society, because, by most measures of economic and social condition, they are the last Americans. Family disorganization and mental illness are far more common among them than among poor urban negroes, yet like negroes in our society, their opportunities are frequently restricted by prejudice and discrimination. In short, they have the least chance of all of our citizens to achieve the promise of America in their own lives.[31]

31 Ibid., p. 38.

The geographic distribution of Indians, blacks, and Chicanos shows some similarities. Some blacks and Chicanos have "escaped" neighborhoods composed primarily of members of their own ethnic groups, but the majority remain in the ghettos and barrios. Some American Indians, too, have left reservations and entered city life, but many remain, particularly in the Southwest. About eighty-five percent of the American Indian population live on reservations.

Illness is rampant in the Indian reservation. In the early 1970s, the infant-mortality rate on reservations was 23.5 per 1,000 live births while it was 16.8 for whites. Postneonatal death rates for Indian infants is 2.9 times higher than for white infants. The maternal death rate for Indian women has been about 1.9 times higher during this decade.[32]

The morbidity rates and patterns for American Indians are shocking. Disease rates in every reportable category are higher for reservation Indians than for any other group in the country. Their disease rates range from four to fifty-four times higher than for the rest of the nation. But the tragedy does not end here. American Indians continue to contract diseases so long ago cured for the rest of our society that we do not even bother to collect information on their occurrence. Reservation Indians still suffer frequently from typhoid fever, diphtheria, and trachoma. Cases of bubonic plague even now occur among the tribes. Morbidity occurrence is increasing in every reportable disease category except tuberculosis, and some illnesses, which the rest of us have long ago forgotten, continue to strike reservation Indians.

Not surprisingly, the life of deprivation experienced by most American Indians leads to unhealthy and even fatal behavior. Violence is an extremely frequent cause of hospitalization on the reservation, and homicide occurs among Indians nearly three times as often as for the country as a whole. Cirrhosis of the liver is also about three times more frequent for Indians. Among some tribes, the suicide rate is ten times that of the total American population, and many suicides are committed by men in their late teens.

Just as there have been efforts by government to provide resources and programs for the health care of other ethnic minorities, so the federal government has made some attempts at providing medical services to reservation Indians. There are about fifty-one hospitals, more than eighty health-care centers, and over three hundred health stations and clinics operated for Indians by the Indian Health Service of the United States Department of Health, Education, and Welfare. Nevertheless, a national debate continues over the adequacy of these government efforts.

[32] Hearings Before the Permanent Subcommittee on Investigations of the Committee on Government Operations—United States Senate, 93rd Congress, 2nd Session, *Indian Health Care,* September 16, 1974, p. 29.

The critics of the IHS programs focus on the quality of care provided. They note that as of the early 1970s, only sixteen of the fifty-one Indian hospitals met national fire and building-code standards. They also criticize the fact that many Indian children experiencing Otitis Media, an infection of the middle ear that can require surgery, do not get proper and immediate treatment. Some observers report that budget constraints on IHS hospitals mean that most of them admit only two types of patients: those ready for childbirth and those bleeding severely from accidents. Many physicians practicing in IHS hospitals believe that the needless death of patients often occurs because of inadequate medical personnel and equipment.[33]

The Indian Health Service sees the problems differently. They report "remarkable progress being made in elevating the health status of Indian people," and allude to data showing dramatic decreases in mortality at all ages, in the infant death rate, and in the occurrence of such diseases as tuberculosis and diarrheal illnesses. The IHS also points out that a substantial number of new medical facilities have been developed since 1955. Yet their greatest insight has been to recognize the importance of Indian acceptance of the services of their facilities, and they see progress in Indian willingness to use these services, particularly ambulatory care.[34]

OTHER ETHNIC GROUPS AND THE INCIDENCE OF MORBIDITY

Some scant information exists on morbidity rates and health-service use of other subcultural groups. We know, for example, that drug addiction is high among Puerto Ricans and alcoholism low among Jews. Alcoholism is high among the Irish, and low among Italian-Americans. Jewish women only infrequently suffer from cervical cancer, probably because of the traditional circumcision of the Jewish male. Japanese and Chinese living in this country develop coronary disease infrequently, but Japanese-Americans still die twice as often from heart disease as the Japanese living in Japan. Japanese living in their homeland have the highest mortality rate in the world from stroke; but Japanese-Americans fare substantially better. Polish-Americans have high rates of cancer of the esophagus and lungs. A few attempts have also been made at studying the interpretations of illness and pain, and the attitudes regarding various forms of

33 Ibid., pp. 1–29.
34 Department of Health, Education, and Welfare, *Indian Health Trends and Services*, Public Health Service, 1974, pp. 1ff. Also see, United States Department of Health, Education, and Welfare, *Indian Health Service Annual Discharge Summary, Public Health Service*, Fiscal Years, 1967–72.

medical services peculiar to these other groups.[35] Much more must be done, though, if we are to better the healthfulness and delivery efficiency for our subcultural population.

The key point to this topic is that our health system is most appropriate to white and middle- or upper-income citizens. It is inappropriate to the poor, in part because it maximizes the quality and quantity of care for those who can best afford it, and minimizes the quality and quantity of care for those who most need it. It is often inappropriate to ethnic groups because it is based on the beliefs and customs of the majority society, and it knows little of the health status or the beliefs and customs of our subcultures.

SUMMARY AND CONCLUSIONS

The politics of protest has given much attention to the data described above. Critics of the health-care system have emphasized that the problems of securing good health are distributional. Few now charge that we have an inadequate investment in health care; but there is a common charge that the benefits of such investment are distorted because of the tendency for professional specialization, and because these technical services are centered in population-dense, more affluent areas. In brief, the distortions are occupational and geographical. If we could find the means to ease both problems, the cost would be minimal. But how is this to be accomplished within the context of a free society?

As a nation, we have responded to the above statistics in two ways. First, we have increased our expenditures for the most seriously needy to a current annual rate of $32 billion. We have little data, as yet, to indicate just how this investment is paying off. We do have information that the poor are "seeing" physicians more frequently—indeed, more frequently than the affluent. This undoubtedly reflects attention to a backlog of needs.

It is now proposed that medical-school students receiving federal aid be obligated to serve in underserved areas. In 1967, Ward Darley and Anne R. Somers warned that "the American people have . . . given unmistakable notice to the health professions and to nonfederal institutions that their patience is not unlimited." The Regional Medical Program (Public Law 89-239)—intended to redirect and restructure portions of the medical-care economy to join together representatives of academic institutions, the health-care providers, public and voluntary health agencies,

[35] Stanley H. King, "Social Psychological Factors in Illness." In Freeman, Levine, Reeder (eds.), *Handbook of Medical Sociology*, pp. 129–47.

labor, and other consumer groups—was considered one of several attempts for reform.[36]

Ten years later, Paul G. Rogers (influential chairman of the Health and Environment Subcommittee of the House Interstate and Foreign Commerce Committee) pointed out that while the absolute numbers of physicians has increased substantially since 1963, the geographic distribution of those physicians has worsened. "The balance between primary- and nonprimary-care physicians is still badly skewed. Foreign medical graduates are flooding the country in ever increasing numbers." The House-passed health manpower legislation was designed to increase the number of medical-school graduates voluntarily serving rural and urban underserved areas in exchange for National Health Service Corps scholarships. But Rogers acknowledged: "I oppose mandatory service as unnecessary, of questionable constitutional validity, and as unwarranted social policy."[37] Again, however, he acknowledged the mounting pressures for reform:

> The Congress and the American people have been patient: we have waited for curricula changes; we have waited for the geographic imbalance to self-correct; we have waited for an expected upsurge in number of primary-care physicians. We cannot wait much longer. . . .[38]

Even more candidly, Senator Edward Kennedy issued a challenge to medical schools at a conference of the Association of American Medical Colleges:

> I am persuaded that the education of the men and women whose raison d'être is the provision of medical services to a society of more than two hundred million persons is too important to be left exclusively to you, your department chairmen, your academic vice presidents for health affairs, et cetera. This is especially true if you argue, as you quite appropriately have, that your institutions and their programs are national and not local resources. The taxpayer in Dayton, in Watts, and in Appalachia should not be expected to subsidize the education of the high-paid professional in America who then choose to practice on Park Avenue.[39]

The information recited in this chapter has done much to spark the demand for reform. If the outpouring of funds is not making significant inroads on the disparities of health treatment—a hypothesis, incidentally, that has yet to be fully verified statistically—we must come up with means

[36] Ward Darley and Anne R. Somers, "Medicine, Money and Manpower: The Challenge to Professional Education," *The New England Journal of Medicine*, Vol. 276, no. 23 (June 8, 1967), pp. 1294–95.
[37] Paul G. Rogers, "Congressional Perspectives on Government and Quality of Medical Education," *Journal of Medical Education*, Vol. 51 (January 1976), p. 4.
[38] Ibid., p. 6.
[39] Edward M. Kennedy, "Health Care in the Seventies," *Journal of Medical Education*, Vol. 47 (January 1972), p. 18.

for effecting the redistribution of services. This is no simple task. Paul Rogers has properly asserted that we should not have to choose between being sick in a free society and well in a controlled society. Or to repeat the popular aphorism: "These are not simple solutions, only intelligent choices."[40]

Our attention in this chapter to the "culture" of poverty and its unique sociological perceptions, while revealing the sharp disparities of health between the rich and the poor—or, between "mainstream" white America and its cultural enclaves—also drives home a fundamental truth: we cannot deliver health services in an imperial manner, with a caravan or convoy of trucks loaded with an armory of medical technologies (with persons riding "shotgun"), penetrating the unfamiliar terrain of restless, angry, or even hostile natives. The portraits of poverty cultures emphasize the necessity of improving contact through sensitive and sensible efforts, affording both provider and patient an opportunity for adequate personal contact; affording, in brief, a setting for cultivating mutual respect and concern. We have much evidence that health-care providers, serving in the ghettos, develop either an overwhelming sense of despair and frustration that causes them to quit or a protective layer of callous cynicism. They view the steady stream of persons who arrive with knife wounds, body punctures from homicide attempts, or strung out on narcotics, not as unfortunate accident victims, but as the inevitable consequences of the "perverse" lifestyles of other cultural jungles. All of this, of course, is a source of embarrassment and consternation, particularly when we realize we have one of the highest per capita incomes in the world, from which we spend one of the highest *proportions* of income for health care. We find that our health, by international standards, runs anywhere from tenth to twentieth, depending on the index of health being measured.

Clearly, if we are to solve the health-care problems of the nation, we will have to make a much more serious effort to study the dynamics of our subcultures and to develop a much-improved delivery system for care.

SUGGESTED READINGS

ALSTROM, C. H., ROLF LINDELIUS, and INNA SALUM, "Mortality Among Homeless Men," *British Journal of Addiction to Alcohol and Other Drugs*, Vol. 70, no. 3 (September 1975), pp. 345–52. A study of the homeless in Sweden. Estimated norms of morbidity and death are projected for the homeless and are compared with actual experiences.

ANDERSON, JAMES G. and DAVID E. BARTKUS, "Choice of Medical Care: A Be-

---

[40] As quoted by Richard W. Lyman, "Public Rights and Private Responsibilities: A University Viewpoint," *Journal of Medical Education*, Vol. 51 (January 1976), p. 12.

havioral Model of Health and Illness Behavior," *Journal of Health and Social Behavior*, Vol. 14, no. 4 (December 1973), pp. 348–62. An analysis of sociodemographic influences on the volume and form of medical care.

AUSTER, RICHARD, IRVING LEVESON, and DEBORAH SARACHEK, "The Production of Health, an Exploratory Study." In Victor R. Fuchs, ed., *Essays in the Economics of Health and Medical Care* (New York: Bureau of Economic Research, 1972), pp. 412–36. An attempt to untangle the influences of lifestyle, including alcohol and cigarette consumption, and other key variables such as income and education as determinants of health.

BERKANOVIC, EMIL and LEO G. REEDER, "Ethnic, Economic and Social Psychological Factors in the Source of Medical Care," *Social Problems*, Vol. 21, no. 3 (Fall 1973), pp. 246–59. Explores the cultural components of the demand for medical care as these relate to both ethnicity and income.

CANTOR, NORMAN, "The Law and Poor People's Access to Health Care," *Law and Contemporary Problems*, Vol. 35, no. 4 (Autumn 1970), pp. 909–22. Traces the formal legal obligation of both physicians and hospitals to treat "junk" cases.

CHAMBERLIN, R. W. and J. F. RADEBAUGH, "Delivery of Primary Health Care: Union Style," *The New England Journal of Medicine*, Vol. 294, no. 12 (March 18, 1976), pp. 641–45. The critical views of two physicians serving migrant workers.

HERMAN, MARY W., "The Poor: Their Medical Needs and the Health Services Available to Them," *The Nation's Health: Some Issues*, Vol. 399 (January 1972), pp. 12–22. An examination of both the sociology and economics of access of poor to medical systems.

HESSLER, RICHARD M., MICHAEL F. NOLAN, BENJAMIN OGBRU, and PETER KONG-MING NEW, "Intraethnic Diversity: Health Care of the Chinese-Americans," *Human Organization: Journal of the Society for Applied Anthropology*, Vol. 34, no. 3 (Fall 1975), pp. 253–62. An analysis of the health-care needs of the Chinese-American minority.

MILLER, A., "The Wages of Neglect: Death and Disease in the American Work Place," *American Journal of Public Health*, Vol. 65 (1975), pp. 1217–20. An examination of conditions in the early twentieth century and the evolution of public-health programs.

NAVARRO, VINCENTE, "The Underdevelopment of Health of Working America: Causes, Consequences and Possible Solutions," *American Journal of Public Health*, Vol. 44, no. 6 (June 1976), pp. 538–47. A survey of the health care of the working class.

REYNOLDS, ROGERS A., "Improving Access to Health Care Among the Poor: The Neighborhood Health Center Experience," *Milbank Memorial Fund Quarterly*, Vol. 54, no. 1 (Winter 1976), pp. 47–81. Discusses the fate of the neighborhood health center.

SHEPPARD, H. L. and N. O. HERRICK, *Where Have All the Robots Gone? Worker Dissatisfaction in the 70's* (New York: Free Press, 1972). Gives attention to job frustration and morbidity.

SMITH, DAVID E., JOHN LUCE, and ERNEST A. BERNBURG, "The Health of

Haight-Ashbury," *Transactions,* April 1970, pp. 36–45. A commentary on the health status of the indigent and homeless.

WELCH, SUSAN, JOHN COMER, and MICHAEL STEINMAN, "Some Social and Attitudinal Correlates of Health Care Among Mexican Americans," *Journal of Health and Social Behavior,* Vol. 14 (September 1973), pp. 205–13. A review of the health-care requirements of the Mexican-American population.

8

MEDICARE AND MEDICAID: TWO MICE THAT ROARED

We have shown throughout this book that the American health-care system (our ways of financing, organizing, and delivering medical services) assumes a particular model of patient that is realistic for only a portion of our citizens. Medically, it tends to focus on those experiencing acute illness, where chances of "cure" are high. In socioeconomic terms, the system assumes patients that are "white," middle-income with health-insurance coverage, educated, and capable of financing and managing their own passage through the health-care delivery system. We also demonstrated, in chapter 7, how the conditions of poverty common to our major ethnic minorities tragically combine a generally higher rate of illness and major disability with what has long been a diminishing use of health services.

The picture is no longer quite so bleak for the poor and others financially responsible for illnesses they cannot afford. We have alluded to recent studies demonstrating that our poor citizens may now visit physicians slightly more often than the middle-income—a fortunate occurrence if true, since their high morbidity pattern requires frequent physician contact. In the previous chapter, we also reviewed some evidence of progress with certain diseases that ravage the American Indian. Additional information supports the contention that the emergency and outpatient services of many municipal, community, and medical-school hospitals have become more attuned to the poor and aged as patients.[1] We have also seen some slight improvements in the percentages of minorities and women being recruited and trained in the medical professions.

The drive to make the health-care system more appropriate to the

[1] Mary W. Herman, "The Poor: Their Medical Needs and the Health Services Available to Them," *The Annals of the American Academy of Political and Social Science*, Sylvester E. Berki and Alan W. Heston (eds.), *The Nation's Health: Some Issues*, Vol. 399 (January 1972).

poor, although it has lost some of its steam, has made permanent changes in that system. We saw earlier that many minorities are poor and suffer ill health as a consequence. The same is true of those of the aged who live on a low fixed income. In this chapter we will discuss the two major public health-insurance programs significant for the poor and the aged, Medicare and Medicaid. It is the major thesis of this chapter that the establishment of these two programs in 1965 has had major consequences for the health-care system of the entire nation. The nation has experimented with the public provision of health services for the poor and aged, with results that form a basis for remodeling the health system for the entire population.

A LOOK AT THE 1960s

"Poverty causes ill health and earlier death." Few in our country today would disagree with this proposition, and most of us have heard and read statements like it. But this awareness of the plight of the poverty-stricken, and a widespread understanding of the health implications of poverty, are fairly recent phenomena. Our society's attention to and definition of the interplay between poverty and ill health occurred in the context of the civil-rights movement and a general concern about the plight of low-income citizens. A brief history of these occurrences is instructive.

The United States Supreme Court is an institution whose pronouncements have enormous policy significance and gain immediate national attention. Constitutional experts frequently marvel at the enormity of the Court's authority and influence, particularly since it has little formal power, such as control over the police or the military. Despite its lack of power, the Court has occasionally fought and won policy battles over our mightiest political official, the President. Its authority basically rests on our belief that the Court judges legislation and other forms of action by "correctly" interpreting the Constitution and voiding any actions or laws in violation of that basic governmental document. Their power to evaluate laws and actions is known as "judicial review," which was established by the Supreme Court itself in the famous case of *Marbury* vs. *Madison* in 1803. The willingness of other branches of government to accept Supreme Court decisions is known as "judicial supremacy" and is based on the "rightness" and authority of the Court rather than its formal power.

An early and enormously significant occurrence in the civil-rights movement during the second half of the twentieth century was the Supreme Court's decision in the 1954 case of *Brown* vs. *Board of Education*. In that case the Court ruled that segregation in public education was unconstitutional and that separate but equal was "inherently unequal." The public's attention to and concern with the decision was instantaneous. Black civil-rights leaders became extremely optimistic about the potential progress of their efforts, but the opposition of many Southern whites was stubborn. Direct confrontations, particularly in the South, began to occur almost daily, and they were often violent. In 1955 a bus boycott occurred in Montgomery, Alabama, following the arrest of a black woman who refused to give up her seat to a white. During the following year there was mob violence at the University of Alabama in opposition to the admission of a black student. There were sit-ins at lunch counters by blacks refusing to be denied service, frequent demonstrations by both blacks and whites, and violence resulting in numerous deaths. All of these occurrences were widely reported and analyzed by the mass media. People from all sections of the country and from all ethnic and economic groups followed the events and seemed to realize that something of enormous social importance was happening. The "black problem" just wouldn't go away.

We earlier described the concepts and usefulness of the "culture-of-poverty" theories of the noted anthropologist Oscar Lewis. During this period of turmoil he published *Five Families*, which systematically presents his ideas on the behavioral and attitudinal consequences of poverty. Three years later another book, significantly entitled *The Other America*, was published by Michael Harrington, and, "legend has it, introduced liberal America to the larger dimensions of poverty. . . . both books caught us all unaware."[2]

The year 1960 gave us the first nationally televised presidential campaign, including debates between the candidates. This meant, of course, that the issues and ideas presented by the candidates could immediately reach millions of people. The Democratic candidate, John F. Kennedy, decided to make poverty and society's obligation to help the poor and aged a major campaign issue. Kennedy as candidate caught the attention and imagination of many citizens, notably the younger segments of our society, and popularized a concern for ethnic minorities and the poor and disadvantaged generally. One of Kennedy's major accomplishments in this area was the acceptance of his insistence that Mexican-Americans as well as blacks were victims of poverty. Chicanos and their circumstances also became newsworthy and a focus for national attention. Many Mexican-American homes, restaurants, and other public places even today display large pictures of JFK, symbolizing the period when a President was attentive to their needs.

Kennedy as President had only limited success in initiating legislative programs to deal with the poverty he had so clearly described in his campaign. The Area Redevelopment Act (1961) and the Manpower De-

2 Charles Jack Rey, *The Political Economy of Urban Poverty* (New York: Norton, 1973), p. 7.

velopment and Training Act (1962) were his most notable successes. Kennedy's problems with getting legislation approved by Congress stemmed from the fact that a coalition of Republicans and conservative Southern Democrats could block virtually anything the Democratic, progressive President wanted. Kennedy had defeated his opponent, Richard Nixon, by the narrowest margin of any presidential election during the century, and thus had little ground for pressuring Congress with "the will of the people." In addition, he was the only President elected in the twentieth century whose party did not also gain seats in the Congress. Finally, since Congress passes laws through a series of committee actions that are usually more crucial than the vote of all the congressional members, the stubborn House Rules Committee and the House Ways and Means Committee were constant barriers to his legislative proposals.

Despite these congressional barriers, more legislation was approved and passed into law than at any time since the 1930s.[3] The problem for the new President was that much of what he had promised and been committed to during the campaign was unattainable with a hostile Congress. Particularly disappointing for Kennedy was his inability to achieve the passage of Medicare, a proposed program whereby working citizens could contribute to their own old-age health-insurance coverage through the Social Security system. In July of 1962, despite enormous pressure from Kennedy's administration, the Senate tabled the Medicare bill by a vote of fifty-two to forty-eight. Ironically, as one observer notes, that very Congress and the succeeding one "would in time pass more health legislation than any two Congresses in history—including landmarks in mental health and mental retardation, medical schools, drug safety, hospital construction and air and water pollution—but the President never got over the disappointment of his defeat [of Medicare]."[4]

Despite his setback, Kennedy's eloquence and personal magnetism had major impact on the country's attitudes toward various health policy issues. He had great concern for mental retardation, partly, no doubt, because one of his sisters was so afflicted. He publicly commented on the cost of his father's hospitalization, noting that he had come to understand how someone less wealthy might be financially destroyed by family illness. During his battle with Congress over Medicare, he addressed an enormous audience of senior citizens in New York's Madison Square Garden and was loudly applauded for his comments on the country's obligation to provide adequate health services to the aged.

Kennedy's assassination in late 1963 made many of his policy proposals and values almost sacrosanct and virtually guaranteed passage of a large number of federal programs. In addition, his successor, Lyndon B.

[3] For an excellent understanding of the Kennedy years and his health proposals, see Theodore C. Sorensen, *Kennedy* (Harper and Row, 1965).
[4] Ibid., p. 344.

Johnson, was a master at legislative politics. The Economic Opportunity Act was passed in 1964, and the entire "War on Poverty" was underway. In this context, President Johnson signed into law a bill establishing the Medicare and Medicaid programs. The American health-care system had been irreversibly altered.

A number of commonly held beliefs were articulated during the 1950s and 1960s that provided the background for the Medicare and Medicaid programs and that continue to influence our health-care system:

1. Our aged citizens who have worked throughout their lives should not be made destitute by ill health or forced to rely on charity for their health needs.

2. Poverty influences the poor in their attitudes, their family life, their housing, their education, and their health. The consequences of poverty occur in any and all of these areas.

3. The greatest number of poor are white, but a greater proportion of blacks and Chicanos are poorer than whites. Blacks and Chicanos (by 1970 we would add American Indians and Puerto Ricans) often face the dual disadvantages of poverty and ethnic discrimination. Many of the poor whites are elderly.

4. The health-care needs of our ethnic minorities, particularly those frequently experiencing poverty, are different from those of poor whites.

5. But poverty (regardless of ethnicity—e.g., Appalachian whites) results in higher morbidity, lower life expectancy, less physician contact, and inferior medical care.

6. The health-care system has some major characteristics that often make it of little help to the poor and aged.

7. Society has the obligation to assist the poor and the aged. Among the ways it should help them is by providing minimal levels of health-care services.

THE MEDICARE AND MEDICAID PROGRAMS

As noted earlier, Medicare is a program through which working citizens pay an earnings tax into the Social Security system, which forms trust funds for supporting medical services upon retirement. The program has two basic components: Part A, which is involuntary, provides coverage of certain inpatient services at hospitals, in extended-care facilities, and during need for skilled home health care; Part B, which is voluntary, provides "supplementary health coverage," such as physician services, outpatient hospital care, outpatient physical and speech therapy, additional home health care beyond that permitted under Part A, and other miscellaneous services not covered by Part A. It was estimated that in 1969–70, ninety-five percent of those enrolled in Part A had also opted for the voluntary Part B.[5] This high percentage of enrollees in both Parts A and B at first glance seems extraordinary, particularly since the individual pays fifty percent of the annual premium for coverage under Part B. In 1972, however, this payment by the insurer still only totaled $5.80 per month.

While Medicare is an insurance program for the aged involving premium payments by the insured, Medicaid is an aid program available to persons on public welfare and to a few other individuals having small enough incomes or personal assets to qualify as "medically indigent." Medicare is federally administered by the Social Security Administration; Medicaid involves a grant from the federal government to the participating states and their public-welfare programs. The Medicaid legislation requires that states establishing such a program provide monies for minimal medical services for their welfare recipients. States are not obligated to provide these minimal services for their "medically indigent," although more than half have chosen to do so. The indigent in nonparticipating states often rely on charity care or are ignored. State governments have often been unhappy with the Medicaid program, partly because the financing of Medicaid requires matching federal and state funds, a proposition that has proven expensive to states like California, with high numbers of persons on public welfare. In 1974, two-thirds of all federal Medicaid monies went into grants for only eight states (New York first and California second), which means, of course, that those states also had large financial obligations. In 1973, for example, $1,749,000,000 was spent for Medicaid benefits in the state of New York alone.[6]

Both programs have had operational difficulties, which seem related principally to the way they are structured. In the case of Medicare, medical institutions, usually hospitals, have the choice of either applying directly to the federal Social Security Administration for their payments or nominating an organization (subject to government approval) to function as a fiscal intermediary. Most institutions chose fiscal intermediaries, and as a result Blue Cross programs pay over ninety percent of all medical bills financed under Part A. Although government maintains programmatic and regulatory responsibility, the actual daily control of Medicare is with the "Blues." This has meant a kind of split between responsibility for Medicare and its operation. Medical institutions constantly express their unhappiness with the administrative structure of Medicare: the arrogance and high-handedness of Blue Cross officials, which is strength-

[5] John Krizay and Andrew Wilson, *The Patient as Consumer* (Lexington, Me.: Lexington Books, 1974), p. 73.
[6] Robert Stevens and Rosemary Stevens, *Welfare Medicine in America* (New Haven: Yale University Press, 1974), p. 366.

ened by the organization's control of the financial purse strings; the long wait medical institutions say they experience before payment of their charges; and the increasing tendency of Blue Cross to review and reject various claims submitted by these institutions. It should be recognized that these charges of "red tape" and official high-handedness are commonly expressed in these days of gigantic organizations, and are especially favored criticisms of the federal government. It does appear, however, that Medicare's use of fiscal intermediaries has resulted in an addition to the bureaucratic layer that is confusing and disconcerting to medical providers. It has also meant that important adjustments in the Medicare program have required decisions, policy formulations, and changes in two separate though related organizations: the federal Medicare structure and the Medicare intermediaries.

Some similar operational difficulties have occurred in Medicaid due to that program's reliance on both the federal and state layers of government. Federal law sets "minimal" standards for the program's eligibility requirements, medical-services provision, and administrative aspects. But beyond that, Medicaid is essentially a conglomeration of individual state programs, with medical benefits that vary enormously between states. We are not arguing that all programs should be centralized in the federal government, but the absence of strong federal regulation has permitted waste, fraud, and inadequate medical delivery in many states' Medicaid activities. In early 1976, federal officials estimated that ten percent of all Medicaid and Medicare dollars were lost in fraud and corrupt practices by medical providers.[7] The irony is that it has taken eleven years for federal officials responsible for the two programs to attempt to control corruption.

Despite the waste, controversy, and administrative-programmatic mistakes, there is no doubt that the Medicare and Medicaid programs have provided needed medical services. Virtually all Americans 65 years or older are covered by Medicare, and 90 percent of their hospital expenses are paid by that program. As early as July 1973, 23.5 million aged and 1.7 million disabled persons were insured under Medicare. The basic benefit of Medicare has been to provide medical services for the aged and disabled they might not otherwise receive and to keep them from having to seek those services through charity handouts. The same positive comments pertain to Medicaid, which provides medical services for a poverty group that otherwise would have little medical attention or would occasionally find it only on charity wards. By 1973, there were 23.5 million Medicaid beneficiaries, almost half of whom were children under 21 years of age.[8]

[7] "Billions in Medicaid Ripoffs. Can Anyone Stop It?" *U.S. News and World Report,* March 22, 1976, p. 18.
[8] Stevens and Stevens, *Welfare Medicine in America,* pp. 368–69.

PROBLEMS, ISSUES, AND CONSEQUENCES OF MEDICARE AND MEDICAID

At least four basic sets of problems have recurred throughout the history of the two programs. The first pertains to the enormous size and growth in the aggregate national expenditures required to finance them. In 1969, the public expenditure for Medicare was about $7 billion, and we were spending $4.5 billion for Medicaid. This seemed to be an enormous expense, particularly when compared with the *total public expenditure* for health care in 1960, which was only $6.3 billion.[9] But by 1976, annual public expenditures for Medicare and Medicaid were in excess of $32 billion. Government officials estimate the total will rise to $40 billion in 1977.

There have been numerous national reactions to this enormous growth in Medicare and Medicaid expenditures. One has been to tighten eligibility requirements for their benefits and cut back on the services offered, particularly those under Medicaid. By March 1976, twenty states were reducing reimbursement units, cutting back on benefits, and tightening eligibility in efforts to balance budgets.[10] Another reaction has been to search for waste and fraud activities. By 1976, public officials estimated that over $3 billion were annually being lost through fraudulent and corrupt provider practices. Still another reaction has been for government to become involved in experimenting with and controlling the delivery of medical services to Medicare and Medicaid beneficiaries. This is most obvious in the government's encouragement of HMO contracts for medical-service delivery to these recipient populations, and with their establishment of the PSRO program.

A second set of problems for Medicare and Medicaid relates to the mechanisms and procedures for payment. In Medicare the vast majority of payment to medical providers has been from Blue Cross (Part A) or Blue Shield (Part B), the philosophy being that such fiscal intermediaries are experienced in handling medical claims. We have already noted that the use of fiscal intermediaries has not satisfied the medical providers. It has had other ill consequences, as well. In the early years of Medicare and Medicaid, the "Blues" tended to rely strictly upon the word and billing accuracy of medical institutions and physicians. One result of this has been the fraud and corrupt billing activities mentioned earlier. Another was the great variation in the size of fees charged by physicians under Part B. Blue Shield chose to use the concept of "usual and customary" fees as a standard for establishing the amounts to be paid for physician

---

[9] Krizay and Wilson, *The Patient as Consumer,* p. 71.
[10] John Taft, "States Put Scalpel to Medicaid in Budget-Cutting Operation," *The National Journal* (May 1, 1976), p. 581.

services to Medicare patients. But "usual and customary" fees is at best a vague concept; it is not an efficient pricing mechanism. What is "usual and customary" for one town, county, or community may be much higher than the fee for the same service only a few miles away. The result has been irregular payments and a lack of cost control.

A third set of problems pertains to the service packages offered by both Medicare and Medicaid. Perhaps as many as twenty percent of our Medicare recipients live in poverty, and since Medicaid is for welfare recipients, poverty is the essence of that population group. This means that both populations have unusually high illness rates, and for Medicare, degenerative diseases combine with those resulting from low income. The medical services provided under both Medicare and Medicaid are specific and limited. Medicare in particular has been charged with being woefully inadequate in meeting the medical needs of the aged and disabled. It has also been particularly susceptible to charges that it is inadequate in dental benefits, ambulance-service coverage, and Pap tests for the detection of vaginal cancer. These services would appear basic to any adequate health program.

A final set of problems with both programs concerns the quality of their medical services. Some observers believe that only inadequate medical institutions and poorly trained and insensitive physicians cater to Medicare and Medicaid patients. Others argue that these patients are given inferior treatment. Still others contend that quality medical practice and service to Medicare and Medicaid recipients is impossible because of the unrealistic restrictions on services to be provided.

Lengthy analysis results in the conclusion that Medicare and Medicaid are mixed blessings. Clearly they have resulted in medical services for those who could not afford them on their own. We have noted frequently that the historic underuse of physicians by the poor probably no longer exists, largely because of the Medicare and Medicaid programs. But much of the money is wasted or lost because of fraudulent and corrupt activities by medical providers. The cost of the two programs is large and growing. The quality of medical care received by many of these beneficiaries is suspect, and they may need medical services not provided for in their benefits.

However one evaluates the successes and failures of Medicare and Medicaid, they have had major consequences for the health-care system. They have become the basis for an enormous growth in government involvement in the nation's health. The rapid growth in government expenditures in the health industry made its involvement in the system inevitable. It is ironic that the original legislation establishing Medicare expressly limited that program to a position of neutrality in the health-care system. Fiscal intermediaries rather than government agencies were to be used for bill payments. The standards used for paying claims and determining the amounts of reimbursement were taken largely from commercial health-insurance activities. Standards for evaluating the quality of care provided were essentially those used by the long-established Joint Commission on Accreditation of Hospitals. The following statement from the original Medicare law seems almost laughable in this day of heavy government involvement in the health-care system.

> The bill specifically prohibits the Federal Government from exercising supervision or control over the practice of medicine, the manner in which medicare services are provided, and the administration or operation of medical facilities.[11]

Medicare and Medicaid are significant for the future of our health system because they have helped legitimate the principle of government responsibility for providing medical services to large population groups. This is an enormously important step toward the country's acceptance of national health insurance. In fact, Medicare is national health insurance for the aged.

In addition, Medicare and Medicaid have also influenced the thinking of the nation's health policy makers on what form such insurance should take. One common occurrence is a growing anger at medical providers who appear willing to and untroubled about taking money not properly due them under these programs. The experience of Medicare and Medicaid has taught us that we cannot rely upon the private sector in the health industry to serve efficiently as a major disperser of public funds unless there are effective government regulations over those monies.

The difficulties of administration in Medicaid and Medicare, particularly the problems experienced by the states in Medicaid, has led many to pause in concern over the larger administrative problems that a national health insurance program would entail. The various proposals for national health insurance differ substantially in their ideas on the most effective way of organizing and administering it. Some see administration best done by the Social Security Administration because of its experience with Medicare. Some proposals want to maintain a strong role for commercial health-insurance companies; others virtually to exclude health-insurance firms. Some favor a major administrative role for the federal health agencies; still others support local and regional administration.

An additional implication of Medicare and Medicaid for national health insurance comes from the mere fact that they exist and have become entrenched. Each plan for NHI must wrestle with the knotty problems of either abolishing these established programs, or integrating them into the NHI proposal, or somehow amending them and relating them to the NHI. This treatment of the $32-billion programs will undoubtedly be

[11] H. R. Rep. No. 89–213, 89th Cong., 1st Session 21–22 (1965).

a major factor in the congressional evaluations of the alternative national health insurance proposals.

One of the greatest consequences Medicare and Medicaid have had for the health-care system has been their impact on the operation, funding, and visibility of health-maintenance organizations. It is not a matter of chance that the growth in the number of health-maintenance organizations was quite substantial from 1970 through 1973. There were about thirty operational HMOs before 1970, and that number had increased to more than ninety by mid-1973. This was also a period of critical financial dilemmas for Medicaid in particular, with numerous states having exhausted funds for the payment of medical bills before the fiscal year was complete.

When it became apparent that the cost growth for Medicaid was large and would continue, many states began to look for ways to control the increases. The federal government expressed the same interests regarding Medicare. Health-maintenance organizations were increasingly looked to as organizations that might be effective in controlling costs for both programs.[12] In the early 1970s, states began actively contracting with health-maintenance organizations for the provision of medical services to their Medicaid recipients, and the federal government was doing the same with Medicare. Rather than pay a multitude of medical providers on a fee-for-service basis, many government officials decided that prepaid contracts with HMOs for their beneficiaries had many benefits. First, it permitted the government agencies to predict more accurately the costs for Medicare and Medicaid recipients enrolled in HMOs. Budget forecasting is, of course, critical to government since it passes appropriations well in advance of expenditures. Prepaid contracts for recipients meant that the cost estimates involved a relatively simple calculation of monthly premium payments times numbers of beneficiaries enrolled in HMOs. The fee-for-service system required estimating the numbers of services that might be used by beneficiaries and what the payments for them would be.

Cost predictability was not the only benefit of HMOs that Medicare and Medicaid officials foresaw. Since the payment for medical services in an HMO is a fixed monthly fee per person, costs of services would not grow as rapidly as under the fee-for-service system. As early as March 1970, the U.S. Department of Health, Education, and Welfare proposed the development of contracts between the Social Security Administration and HMOs for Medicare services. During that same year, HEW issued a "Report of the Task Force on Medicaid and Related Programs," which attempted to articulate the benefits of HMO–Medicaid relationships and advantages. Finally in 1972, legislation was passed authorizing reimburse-

[12] Many of them were really only prepaid health plans, rather than HMOs having a consumer population from all socioeconomic groups.

ment to HMOs under the Medicare and Medicaid program. There was an immediate flurry in the development of HMO-like organizations (again, many were really prepaid health plans with limited populations), which were seeking Medicaid and Medicare contracts. This was particularly true in California, which experienced a rapid and exaggerated growth of Medicaid-oriented HMOs.

The growing interest in HMOs was not strictly a result of the problems experienced with Medicare and Medicaid. In his message to Congress in early 1971, President Nixon called for a national health strategy involving government encouragement of these organizations. But the difficulties with Medicare and Medicaid seemed to give HMOs a kind of urgency and a mission to accomplish.

While it was hoped that HMOs would benefit government agencies struggling with Medicare and Medicaid program problems, these medical-delivery organizations were also thought to have some advantages for the poor and aged. They were, after all, committed to providing comprehensive and planned medical services within a single organization. Once they contracted with the Medicare or Medicaid agency, they were also willing to treat these recipients, a willingness not shared by all medical providers. Their emphasis on preventive medicine also seemed admirably suited to the medical needs of the poor and aged.

Unfortunately, the promised benefits to government and Medicare/Medicaid beneficiaries of HMO participation has been inadequately realized. Many group practices, established only to acquire Medicaid contracts, proved to be inadequately conceived and even fraudulent. Various state and federal investigations found that these "fly-by-night" organizations tricked and lied to beneficiaries to get them to enroll into their HMOs, then failed to provide the services they had contracted to make available. HMOs received a bad reputation because of the corrupt activities of those few organizations seeking to hoodwink the Medicaid and Medicare programs.

The HMO experience with Medicare and Medicaid has taught us that these group-health plans are not automatically appropriate to the medical needs of the poor and aged. In fact, their inherent tendency to minimize the care provided, because they receive a regular monthly income rather than fees for service, makes them potentially disastrous for population groups needing a large amount of medical care.[13] By 1976, we had more than 180 HMOs, providing medical services to 6.5 million people. Many have chosen to deemphasize or ignore the Medicare and Medicaid populations because of their belief that the poor and aged require more services than HMOs can afford to deliver. In December of

[13] Andreas G. Schneider and Joanne B. Stern, "Health Maintenance Organizations and the Poor: Problems and Prospects," *Northwestern University Law Review*, Vol. 70, no. 1 (1975), pp. 97ff.

1973, the Federal Health Maintenance Organization Act became law. Although the legislation permitted HMOs to adjust their premiums and services to the specific requirements of Medicare and Medicaid, it required remarkably little of HMOs in servicing recipients of these two programs.

Throughout the history of Medicare and Medicaid, questions about the quality and medical necessity of their services have continuously been raised. Some of these questions have concerned the absence of medical services promised to Medicare/Medicaid recipients and fabricated services for which the programs were billed.[14] Other questions have pertained to inferior medical facilities and personnel and discriminatory treatment of the poor and aged.

We have noted that Medicare initially depended for quality control on the standards and policies of commercial health-insurance practices and the Joint Commission for Hospital Accreditation. In the early stages, quality control in Medicaid was even less stringent, depending upon the occasional interest of state department of health officials. By 1970 this had begun to change rapidly. Both because of increased costs for Medicare and Medicaid and because of complaints about the quality of care, Congress began to develop plans for reviewing medical services delivered under the two programs. A major result was the establishment of the Professional Standards Review Organizations, discussed at length in chapter 12. The principle of government noninterference in the delivery of medical services, expressed in the original Medicare legislation, was dead. It was a principle that had outlived its usefulness.

The history of Medicare and Medicaid raises philosophical questions that need answering as a basis for the future of our health-care system. Why the enormous growth in expenditures for the two programs? Corrupt and fraudulent charges by medical providers is only a partial answer to the question. It may be that we have only begun to measure and meet the medical needs of the poor and the aged. Perhaps medical needs for all of us are almost infinite; if so, then no society, not even one as wealthy as ours, can do everything that everyone needs for good health. How do we interpret the experiences of Medicare and Medicaid with reference to the services that should be covered under any expanded national health insurance plan? Where do the public's obligations for the health of our citizens end?

The two programs have also raised the possibility that some basic characteristics of the health-care delivery system must be changed completely. Medicaid and Medicare were efforts at "shoring up" the system rather than making basic changes in it. But the system has not responded well to the efforts. There is a major ethical conflict in a situation in which,

14 "U.S. Medicaid-Fraud Crackdown Slated to Focus on Massachusetts, Ohio Initially," *Wall Street Journal*, March 29, 1976.

on the one hand, public legislation seeks to support and guarantee medical services for the poor and the aged and, on the other hand, many physicians and hospitals either will not treat these patients or provide only poor-quality care. A ten-percent rate of payments resulting from fraud and corrupt billing procedures is shocking and points to a loose fiscal structure with an absence of control and of public commitment among the providers involved in these practices. One wonders whether our health-care system is not inevitably destined for large-scale remodeling of service delivery as a result of more than a decade of Medicare and Medicaid. But the spotty history of those two programs has made it seem that system remodeling may also be fraught with mistakes and costly errors.

SUGGESTED READINGS

"Billions in Medicaid Ripoffs: Can Anyone Stop it?," *U.S. News and World Report,* March 22, 1976, p. 18. Discussion of the program's performance.

CORBIN, MILDRED and AARON KRUTE, "Some Aspects of Medicare Experience with Group-Practice Prepayment Plans," *Social Security Bulletin,* March 1975, pp. 3–11. An exploration of the controversial uses of prepayment plans as a method for reducing Medicaid costs.

DAVIS, KAREN, "Equal Treatment and Unequal Benefits: The Medicare Program," *Milbank Memorial Fund Quarterly,* Vol. 53, no. 4 (Fall 1975), pp. 444–88. A summary of Davis's research on the benefits and costs of Medicare and Medicaid.

DENSEN, PAUL M., "Public Accountability and Reporting Systems in Medicare and other Health Programs," *The New England Journal of Medicine,* Vol. 289, no. 8 (August 23, 1973), pp. 401–6. Studies the conceptual and practical problems in establishing public accountability for government investments on behalf of the public.

"The Great Medicaid Scandal," *Time,* May 26, 1975, p. 55. An examination of Medicaid abuse.

Medicare and Medicaid Frauds (Washington, D.C.: GPO, Hearings before the Subcommittee on long-term care of the Special Committee on Aging, United States Senate, 94th Congress, 2nd Session, November 1975). A study by congressional committees on the problem of Medicare and Medicaid abuse.

Problems of Medicaid Fraud and Abuse (Washington, D.C.: GPO, Hearings before the Subcommittee on Oversight and Investigations of the Committee on Interstate and Foreign Commerce, House of Representatives, 94th Congress, 2nd Session, Serial No. 94–64). A critical commentary on the fraud surrounding the implementation of the Medicare and Medicaid programs.

STEVENS, ROSEMARY, "Shoring Up the System: Medicare," *American Medicine and the Public Interest* (New Haven: Yale University Press, 1971). A

survey of the institutional and political considerations that led to Medicare.

STUART, BRUCE, "Equity and Medicaid," *Journal of Human Resources*, Vol. 7,
no. 2 (Spring 1972), pp. 162–78. Analyzes the distributional influences
of Medicare and Medicaid.

STUART, BRUCE, "Who Gains from Public Health Programs?," *Annals of the
American Academy of Political and Social Science*, Vol. 399 (January
1972), pp. 145–50. Examines the modest benefits to patients and windfall
income to health-care providers that develop from the Medicare and
Medicaid programs.

VOGEL, ROBERT J. and ROGER D. BLAIR, "An Analysis of Medicare Administrative Costs," *Social Security Bulletin*, August 1974, pp. 3–23. Presents the
statistical dimensions involving the efficiency of the program.

WOLKSTEIN, IRWIN, "Medicare 1971: Changing Attitudes and Changing Legislation," *Law and Contemporary Problems*, Vol. 35, no. 4 (Autumn 1970),
pp. 696–751. A study of the political background for the legislation that
led up to the Medicare program.

9

MENTAL HEALTH
AND MENTAL ILLNESS:
WHERE BODY AND MIND MEET

The American health-care delivery system is largely curative; there is contact between medical provider and consumer when the belief exists that the latter is ill. Preventive activities, such as multiphasic screening, diet-control education, and the like, are quite minimal. The concept of physical health is an implication rather than a positive statement: health exists when there is an absence of illness.

In recent years, the field of *mental health* has struggled for a positive definition of what "mental health" is all about. The hope was that defining mental health might assist us in understanding how to achieve it, help in research and evaluations of treatment techniques, and serve as a basis for allocating resources in the establishment of delivery mechanisms. But precise and accepted definitions of mental health have not been forthcoming. A report issued in 1961 by the Joint Commission on Mental Illness and Health noted that the standards of what constituted mental health varied from time to time and place to place.[1] What one society or period of history regards as ill may be seen as quite healthy later on.

If what constitutes mental health is so relative to the times or even to the individual, is there any substance to the field? Mental health as a condition reveals positive emotional states and seems related to (though probably not synonymous with) such vague feelings as "happiness," "fulfillment," and "self-satisfaction." Viewed as a condition to be achieved, mental health must include positive relationships with other persons, particularly early in life. How one feels about one's self, including feelings of guilt or legitimacy, are additionally essential. Perhaps, then, the fact that "mental health" is different for different times, places, and people should not be surprising, since it is achieved or not by each person.

[1] Joint Commission on Mental Illness and Mental Health, *Action For Mental Health*, final report to the U.S. Congress, submitted to the Congress, Dec. 31, 1960 (New York: Basic Books, 1961).

171

If we have only inklings of the condition of mental health, we have some firm thoughts about how it is best attained.

> Mental health, it is conceded, stems from the fullest possible understanding of one's own motivations and actions; this concept is Freudian in origin. Mental health, the clinicals say, is the attainment of mental well-being by the early prevention of emotional disorders and, when these have occurred, through secondary preventative measures—detection, treatment, and rehabilitation of the mentally sick.[2]

This impressive statement clarifies some of the basic principles in recent mental-health activities. Self-understanding is an important value throughout the mental-health field and in such aspects of it as "need-psychology" and most forms of therapy. The mental-health providers also emphasize the importance of preventive activities, although, as is true for the medical field, prevention holds more promise than accomplishments. As Martin has emphasized, the field of mental health is principally involved with the detection, treatment, rehabilitation (and we would add "control") of mental illness.

THE DELIVERY SYSTEM

The basic outlines of the mental-health services delivery system are similar to those for the medical field, with a few significant variations. The majority of patients with mental difficulties are seen by providers in their private offices. In 1965, 1,300,000 patients were treated in private offices for emotional disturbance. Psychiatrists, M.D.s with psychiatric specialties, are at the pinnacle of mental-health service providers. Not surprisingly, many individuals use their family physician, even though he may have little or no training in mental therapy. Psychologists, professionals with a Ph.D. and special interest in clinical psychology, are also a large component of the mental-health manpower pool. In addition, any large community has numerous other providers, varying substantially in specialties and capabilities: family counselors, sex counselors, psychological social workers, and medical social workers interested in mental illness. One function of many churches in this country is having a clergyman, usually relatively young, who has training and interest in mental therapy and will provide counseling more psychological than religious to parishioners with emotional difficulties.

In the mid-1970s there has also been an enormous explosion in a

2 Lealon E. Martin, *Mental Health and Mental Illness: Revolution in Progress* (New York: McGraw-Hill, 1970), p. 58.

wide array of emotional "treatments" largely outside the more traditional therapies we discuss below. These include approaches like transcendental meditation, transactional analysis, massage workshops, the primal-scream occurrence, gestalt therapy, and the nude marathon exercise. We will not comment on the actual mental-health value of these approaches: this probably depends very much on the individual seeking their help and what is meant by value. The main point here is that these activities represent a multi-million-dollar business, which is related to, and yet outside of, the mental-health industry as traditionally constituted.[3]

The economics of the mental-health field is less complicated than for the medical field generally. Most patients seeing providers in their private offices do so on a fee-for-service basis. Mental-health services are often not covered in commercial health-insurance policies, although as of 1975, approximately fifteen million Americans were "covered by outpatient mental-health benefits as a consequence of collective bargaining between their union negotiators and their employers."[4]

There are numerous intriguing issues and attitudes about mental-health services and mental illness itself that have affected the financing of those services. The main reason that mental-health services are not included in many health-insurance policies is the fear that such a benefit would result in a stampede of the emotionally disturbed, of worried neurotics and of lonely people just needing to talk. "Contrary to the predictions of the insurance industry, there has been no stampede of ill-defined malcontents to the psychiatrist's couch and no escalation of costs."[5]

Commonly held attitudes about mental illness and disturbance also affect the delivery of these services and how they are financed. It is probably true that seeking and paying for mental-health services is something of a status symbol for many upper-middle-income citizens. Conventional wisdom has it that lonely wives of overly busy executives are a major source of patients for the private mental-health provider. In these cases, having a psychiatrist becomes a status symbol, just as having an ulcer is a badge of courage and suffering for others. But those who are severely ill mentally are disturbing to most of us. Mental illness itself is poorly understood by the average citizen and less well accepted as "natural" than physical illness. Thus, the fact that including mental-health coverage in health benefits has not caused a rush to use these services may partially result from the status of mental illness as a kind of taboo. Few want to admit that they are emotionally disturbed.

[3] Gloria Hochman, "The Therapy Vendors," *Today, the Inquirer Magazine*, August 22, 1976.
[4] Herzel R. Spiro, M.D., Guido M. Crocetti, Ph.D., and Iradj Siassi, M.D., "Fee-for-Service Insurance Versus Cost Financing," *American Journal of Public Health*, Vol. 65, no. 2 (February 1975), p. 139.
[5] Ibid.

A second major provider of mental-health services are psychiatric hospitals. There are more than 500 such hospitals, and over two-thirds of these are public. Of the public hospitals, by far the majority are state-owned institutions. In 1965 there were 161 private psychiatric hospitals; 73 of those were owned and operated by voluntary agencies, and 88 were proprietary.[6]

The dominant trend in mental-health service during the past decade has been a deemphasis on institutionalizing the mentally ill and an emphasis on their treatment as outpatients. This is not unlike the growing inclination in general hospitals toward the increased provision of outpatient services. The motivations are also similar. Psychiatric hospitals are expensive to build and operate, and since so many are public they are often seen as an undue burden for government budgets. Additionally, mental therapists usually contend that rehabilitation of the mentally disturbed is more effective if the patient can remain a member of the community. Living in a mental institution, contemporary theory says, breeds its own kind of illness and desperation, which is not conducive to improvement. Increasingly, mental institutions are considered desirable only for those mentally disturbed in ways making them dangerous to themselves, to others, or simply unable to function outside of an institution.

During his brief presidency, John F. Kennedy provided leadership in shifting treatment for mental illness from inpatient to outpatient care. In the case of mental-health services, he lived long enough to see actual programmatic achievements. In October 1963, Kennedy signed the "Community Mental Health Centers Act," which authorized $150 million for the construction of community mental-health centers. By 1975, more than $900 million had been spent or committed to the community mental-health centers program, and around 450 federally aided mental-health centers had begun providing the services. Some 86 million Americans live in the service areas of these centers.

One of the basic objectives of community mental health is to provide mental-health services for those with emotional disturbances too minor for hospitalization. The Community Mental Health Centers Act itself was supported politically by a series of studies concluding that mental disturbance was much more widespread than previously thought and that an enormous expansion in the delivery of these services was needed. To receive federal aid, the community centers must offer five basic services: inpatient, outpatient, partial hospitalization (either during the day or night), twenty-four-hour emergency services, and consultation and education for individual and group leaders in the community.

The Community Mental Health Centers have thus been based on the principle of providing diverse services within the framework of a sin-

[6] Martin, *Mental Health and Mental Illness,* pp. 109ff.

gle organization. They have also emphasized provision of these services on an outpatient basis whenever possible, and have even made use of hospitalization on a part-time basis. In addition, the community mental-health movement believes that therapy must go beyond the single thera-pist–single patient model and involve psychiatrists, psychologists, and other mental-health experts in concerns about the mental health of large groups of people and their social conditions. Thus, the objective is to apply these resources and personnel to the changing of society toward healthier conditions. Therapy is directed at social structure, not primarily or exclusively at the individual.[7]

The future of these federally aided mental-health centers is uncertain. It is conceivable that the federal government will terminate its role in these centers. The reasons for this are numerous. First, special programs of this type tend to come and go depending on the priorities of the particular presidential administration. More importantly, the "social-engineering" principle—applying mental-health knowledge to make a "healthier" society—is no longer popular and seems even naive today. If the Community Mental Health Centers are severely shortchanged or even eliminated from the federal budget, their demise will leave a major gap in mental-health services. One does not have to be totally committed to social engineering or accept the notion that "we are all a little sick mentally" to realize that many of us are occasionally in need of counseling, guidance, and therapy in a world fraught with pressures and tension.

Private practitioners, psychiatric hospitals, and the Community Mental Health Centers are supplemented by two thousand mental-health clinics throughout the country. These clinics vary greatly in size, therapy orientation, costs for services, and accessibility. About fifty percent are located in the Northeast. Few are found in the South, and they are rare in the West.

Certification for providing mental-health services is controlled by state law and, as might be expected, this leads to enormous variations in what it takes to be a provider. Generally, the psychiatrist is at the center of the mental-health professionals; he is the only such provider legally authorized to provide drugs as a part of therapy. In many areas, however, other mental-health therapists make arrangements with physicians, who are often not specialists in psychiatry, to give prescription medicine to the therapist's clients. A Ph.D. in clinical psychology, after passing the state requirements for certification in clinical treatment, may provide private therapy in his office. In addition, there are numerous settings where physicians, psychiatrists, psychologists, and psychiatric social workers form a treatment team. This is often found in the growing number of

[7] David F. Musto, "Whatever Happened to 'Community Mental Health'?" *The Public Interest,* no. 39 (Spring 1975).

general hospitals providing limited mental-health services. As noted earlier, the number of people who are not psychiatrists or Ph.D.s in psychology, but are providing some form of mental-health "counseling," is enormous. In most states, very little is required to be able to advertise as a "counselor," do whatever counselors do when clients come to their office, and collect fees. Clearly, many of these counselors are doing some good for people with specific problems, such as sexual maladjustment. Control and evaluation of these services, however, is almost nonexistent.

In 1973, the following was the distribution of inpatient and outpatient mental-health episodes. Forty-four percent of the episodes were conducted through outpatient psychiatric services, and an additional 20.7 percent were conducted by the Community Mental Health Centers on an outpatient basis. Thirteen percent were in state and county mental hospitals, 4.4 percent in Veterans' Administration hospitals, and 3.2 percent in private mental hospitals. General-hospital inpatient services accounted for 10 percent of the mental-health episodes. Relatedly, the number of resident patients of state and county mental hospitals has declined from slightly over 500,000 in 1950 to fewer than 300,000 in 1974.[8]

MENTAL ILLNESS: CATEGORIES, CAUSES, AND TREATMENTS

Despite the emphasis in recent years on "mental health" and the efforts to define it, the traditional emphasis of the collection of psychiatric hospitals, clinics, psychiatrists, and clinical psychologists has been on "mental illness." As with general medicine, we seem able to marshal resources for attempts at curing illnesses, but are seldom able to do much to avoid them.

There are many ways to categorize and define mental disturbances, but the following is widely accepted. Almost all systems begin with a distinction between organic and functional mental illnesses. Organic mental illnesses are those resulting from some form of brain pathology, as is true, for example, in latter stages of syphilis. Functional mental disorders involve no apparent brain pathology, and the illness is thus primarily personality-based. The distinction between functional and organic disorders, however, is recognized to be a matter of degree. Even in the case of syphilis, personality factors play a major role in the disorder. Body and mind go together in the human being.

Most theorists further divide organic mental illnesses into two categories: those that result from acquired illnesses and result in damage to

[8] *Health, United States, 1975,* DHEW Publication no. (HRA) 76–1232, U.S. Dept. of HEW, Public Health Service, Health Resources Administration, National Center for Health Statistics, Rockville, Maryland, pp. 317ff.

the brain (e.g., aberrant behavior resulting from a shortage of blood to the brain, which is frequent in the aged), and those that result from congenital defects—inborn damage that affects the brain (e.g., mental retardation in the newborn, probably due to the pregnant mother's insufficient diet). There have been some attempts to distinguish between hereditary organic illnesses and those that result from something in the environment of the fetus. This further distinction is subtle but important in understanding disorders like mental retardation.

There has been a long debate in psychological theory over the relative importance of mind versus body in mental illness, generally, and in various specific illnesses, particularly. This has been known as the "nature versus nurture" argument. Many clinical psychologists have opted strongly for "nurture," focusing on mental illness as a result of some environmental-personality interaction. Physicians, whom we have seen are often providers of mental-health services even if they have no specialization in psychiatry, are charged with being ignorant of personality dynamics and psychological principles important in illness.

Functional mental disorders comprise the bulk of those illnesses treated by the mental-health system, although organic mental disorders, especially those resulting from the aging process, are increasing. Most theorists recognize four major types of functional mental disturbance: psychoses, neuroses, character disorders, and psychosomatic illnesses. Again, these illnesses share the characteristic of being personality-based and of having no known involvement of brain pathology.

Psychosis is the most violent and severe form of functional mental illness. Psychotics often need hospitalization, and in some cases are dangerous to themselves or others. Psychosis is long-term and sometimes lifelong. The psychotic is greatly disturbed, usually unable to function in daily life, experiences feelings alien to himself, and often distorts reality. Victims of schizophrenia, a type of psychosis, commonly suffer hallucinations and delusions. Another major type of psychosis is depression. Symptoms include an enormous slowdown in the patient's mental and physical activity, slow response to others, self-isolation, and feelings of guilt and worthlessness. "Physiological difficulties also develop: he loses his appetite, and constipation sets in; he suffers from insomnia; and his physical movements become slower."[9] A majority of suicides result from the mental illness of depression. Manic-depression is a psychosis involving prolonged periods of excitement and depression in mixed or alternating occurrences.

While psychotics are the majority of the patients in our psychiatric hospitals, neurotics probably form the bulk of those using outpatient mental-health services. The central characteristic of neurosis is an overabundant anxiety. Unlike psychosis, however, neurosis does not involve

[9] Martin, *Mental Health and Mental Illness*, p. 23.

personality destruction and loss of reality contact. Acute anxiety in neurosis can lead to many bizarre behaviors. Irrational phobias—persistent fears of something despite the individual's knowledge that the fears are irrationally based—is a form of neurosis. Obsessive or compulsive behavior, in which the individual feels the uncontrollable need to say or do something repeatedly, is also neurotic behavior.

One of the most significant neuroses for our consideration is what psychologists have termed "conversion reaction." In conversion reaction, anxiety is channeled into functional symptoms of illness. This can mean, for example, that the patient suffers paralysis or loss of hearing or sight without any organic causes being present. Loss of sensitivity to pain can be another result of conversion reaction. Obviously this form of neurosis confuses efforts at medical treatment.

Textbook discussions of neuroses are always interesting for the self-insight, frightening as it may be, they give to their readers. Common phrases used to outline the characteristics of the neurotic are these: feelings of inadequacy and inferiority, high degrees of anxiety and fearfulness, tension and hypersensitivity, lack of insight and rigidity, disturbed interpersonal relationships, dissatisfaction and unhappiness. The point, of course, is that most of us occasionally experience some or all of these feelings. This is the basis of the common belief in our society that "we are all a little nuts."

A third major category of mental disturbances is personality disorders, or character disorders as they are sometimes labeled. Sufferers are usually engaged in antisocial acts, behavior regarded as undesirable or illegal by society's standards. Drug addicts, sexual deviants, alcoholics and criminals are common examples. Since sexual standards change, as do legal rules about what constitutes a crime, we can see that the behavior constituting character disorder also changes.

The fourth major category is the psychosomatic illness, those illnesses that have primarily physical symptoms, but in which emotional factors play a major causal role. We discussed some of these illnesses in chapter 6. Hypertension, which can also be described as a cardiovascular reaction to stressful living, is classic and tragically common. Many headaches are commonly produced by tension—by a musculoskeletal reaction to tension, to be exact. In fact, virtually all of the physiological systems described in chapter 6 can and do develop physical symptoms in illnesses where emotions play a major part. Emotional upset can produce chronic gastritis in the digestive system. Obesity can be emotionally based or at least reinforced. Ulcers and various skin diseases are also clear examples of illnesses with physical symptoms, pain, and discomfort accompanied by a major emotional upset.

Psychosomatic illnesses inevitably raise issues of the causal factors of mental disease. In some cases it seems quite clear. Cerebral arteriosclerosis in the elderly, brain damage, and intracranial tumor can all result in abnormal behavior. Personality factors influence the patterns of that abnormal behavior (for example, some may be hostile, others withdrawn), but the primary cause is brain pathology. In other diseases—for example hypertension—the personality and body seem to interact to produce the malady, almost is if they were partners in crime. In still other mental disturbances, personality and life occurrences seem primary, and physiologic difficulties follow the onset of mental illness. But the exact patterns of cause and effect are difficult to identify.

Other than brain pathology, what are some of the life occurrences that cause or predispose us to mental illness? Much mental disturbance results from poor parent–child relationships during the child's early years. Despite the current deemphasis of Freud in many psychological circles, he forced us to recognize the importance of early childhood in personality formation and its health or abnormality. The child's first social relationships are with whoever originally cares for it, usually the mother in our society. The relationship is one of total dependence of the infant on the mother. Numerous studies have shown how a cold, indifferent, punishing mother can cause enormous, even fatal, damage to the child. An overly protective mother, who either dominates or is highly indulgent, also damages the infant's personality formation.[10]

We have shown that private mental-health practitioners and family physicians remain the major source of mental therapy and counseling. It would be possible and natural for the family physician to recognize faulty parent–child relationships in his patients. Most parents, either those indifferent to or overly protective of their infants, are unable to recognize it themselves, and so are not likely to seek the assistance of a psychiatrist. The trained family physician, in the course of standard medical treatment, could identify unhappy parent–child relationships and seek help for the family. Unfortunately, few family physicians have adequate training to do so.

Many things can go wrong in the child's early years that lead to mental illness. Clearly, broken homes enormously increase tension and unhappiness for the child involved, although unhappy adults continuing to live together can be even worse. Overly rigid moral standards can produce severe guilt complexes, which are commonly involved in depression. Some patients have been known to experience conversion reaction by turning their guilt over masturbation into paralysis of the "offending" hand. On the other hand, children who are overly indulged and taught no values or concern for others often develop the personality disorders of drug addiction, alcoholism, and the like mentioned above.

[10] James C. Coleman, *Abnormal Psychology and Modern Life*, 2nd ed. (Glenview, Ill.: Scott, Foresman, 1956), pp. 108ff.

Excessive stress during adulthood can also produce mental illnesses and their physiological accompaniments. Highly traumatic or extremely stressful periods common to adulthood often lead to temporary or even permanent mental disorder. For example, everyone knows of people experiencing extreme anxiety and even depression because of divorce. One's own illness or impending death is obviously traumatic, as are these occurrences in the lives of a loved one. Consistent loss of significant interpersonal relationships often produce depression and even suicide. Emotional and sexual deprivation—not getting from life what we need—can cause aberrant behavior, though we are not always sure what is aberrant. We have noted that what society regards as mentally ill today it may soon regard as acceptable. In few cases of mental disease can we use the rather exacting diagnostic tests available in medicine generally.

A second, related problem pertains to issues about when the mental-health delivery system should intervene by providing treatment to a mentally disturbed person. Even if a person is acting strangely, do we have the right to force him into treatment or even place him in a mental institution?[11] Most states now make forced commitment to psychiatric hospitals very difficult to obtain, restrictions initiated partly as a result of relatives too anxious to rid themselves of the troublesome patient. How many people are experiencing major mental disturbance that no one around them is aware of? And of those we believe are emotionally disturbed, might not many get better of their own recuperative powers if we leave them alone? The limited curative successes of psychotherapy encourage the view that the mentally disturbed are best left alone or simply watched to avoid harm to themselves and others.

An additional barrier to successful delivery of mental-health services results from the low priority mental health is given and the fact that mental illness is a social taboo. Mental-health expenditures are an extremely small part of the total national health expenditure. This has traditionally meant that we do not have enough outpatient mental-health clinics. Even where those exist, many require substantial payments for their services, making them appropriate only to the middle-income and above. But the shame and fear surrounding mental illness persist despite some greater awareness, and this may well be the major stumbling block to effective mental-health services. One wonders how many sick and confused people are wandering around caught in the conflict between their own illness and needs for help and their fear of social ostracism.

Finally, it must be said that mental-health experts themselves usually admit that most forms of therapy achieve very limited success in the rehabilitation or cure of patients. This is particularly true with psychotics;

[11] For a recent discussion of this topic, see Salum A. Shah, Ph.D., "Dangerousness and Court Commitment of the Mentally Ill: Some Public Policy Consideration," *American Journal of Psychiatry*, May 1975, pp. 501ff.

and of course those with chronic brain damage are "incurable," although they can be helped significantly in their life adjustments.

Which of the many forms of therapy is used depends on the illness and the particular training and treatment philosophy of the therapist. Psychotherapy is a general term for treatment of mental illness that encompasses many specific approaches. One of the oldest forms of treatment is psychoanalysis, which is based largely on the principles of Freud. Psychoanalysis essentially uses a one-to-one relationship in which the patient unburdens himself through free expression and association of feelings and thoughts. It also makes much of the concept of the unconscious—the collection of painful fears, feelings, and experiences of which we are unaware but which have major significance for our behavior and mental condition.

Psychoanalysis is currently considered of limited usefulness in treating mental disturbance. It takes many months (even years) to conduct successfully and is an expensive undertaking. Its success is largely limited to certain forms of neurosis, and it is particularly unsuccessful with schizophrenia or manic-depression.[12]

It is increasingly common in psychotherapy to make use of drugs in treatment. Perhaps as much as twenty-five percent of all prescription drugs are given principally for their psychological effects, an importance which has led to the term "psychopharmacological" drugs. Some of the drugs—for example, lithium, used commonly in severe depression—are for the treatment of mental illness. Others, such as mild tranquilizers or sedatives (barbiturates), are used to limit the consequences of emotional or physical states that, if unchecked, might result in more severe mental disturbance.

A major tendency in treating mental illness is that of working outside the traditional therapist–patient relationship. "Social therapy," for example, attempts to treat mental illness as a community occurrence. This is essentially the same as "community therapy" and has been a major development in mental health since the 1950s. In this approach the focus is on those members of the community thought to be disposed toward mental illness—for example, mentally disturbed children. Here, again, the mental-health provider becomes both a social planner, seeking to develop the "healthiest" form of recreation or treatment for juvenile delinquents, and a public educator, attempting to give us all a better understanding of ourselves and of mental health and mental illness. Reactions to these social endeavors have not been entirely friendly, largely because of a public distrust of psychology.

Group therapy, also in vogue, is the treatment of many patients at the same time. The basic principle here is that patients will learn to inter-

[12] Roy K. Grinker, Sr., *Psychiatry in Broad Perspective* (New York: Behavioral Publications, 1975), p. 153.

act in an honest and healthy fashion with one another, not just with the therapist. In family therapy, the patient is treated in the belief that something in his family relationships needs correcting if he is to become permanently rehabilitated. "Milieu therapy" is like family therapy except that it considers needed changes in the patient's entire lifestyle. Finally, "hospital therapy" provides treatment during institutionalization. The most significant recent occurrence here is the growing use of part-time hospitalization for the patient's treatment. The patient may come to the institution for treatment during the day and go home at night.

RECENT THEMES AND ISSUES IN MENTAL HEALTH

We have already discussed several recent themes and issues in the field of mental health: outpatient versus inpatient care; efforts at moving therapy outside the therapist–patient relationship and into a focus on family life, community life, and other aspects of the patient's environment; attempts at defining mental health rather than focusing exclusively on mental illness; and the involvement of mental-health providers as agents of social change. Other themes and issues are also important for understanding the current situation and for determining what the future is likely to hold.

There is a growing debate over the morality and effectiveness of psychosurgery—the removal or destruction of parts of the brain as a method for altering a patient's behavior. The most infamous form of psychosurgery is the lobotomy, an incision into the frontal lobes of the brain that can significantly reduce anxiety and result in a calm emotional state. Between 1940 and the mid-1950s, some fifty thousand lobotomies were performed in the United States.[13] Critics of the lobotomy say it reduces patients to a "vegetablelike" state with little energy and emotion. Critics of psychosurgery say we know too little about which parts of the brain control what behavior and emotional patterns to be performing this kind of surgery. Others disagree, saying that it can offer hope in cases such as severe depression or manic behavior, in which other forms of treatment cannot help.

While psychosurgery and other methods of "physical" treatment, such as the use of electric shock, are declining in use, the currently popular therapy approach is behavior modification. Very simply, behavior modification uses rewards and punishments in a stick-and-carrot effort to change the unwanted behavior of patients. This approach is used particularly to treat character disorders, such as those common to habitual

[13] "New Ways to Heal Disturbed Minds: Where Will It All Lead?" U.S. News and World Report, February 16, 1976, p. 36.

criminals. The basic principle is that traumatic punishments and pleasing rewards should be used in a planned fashion to change behavior from the undesirable to the desirable. The concept of changing attitudes and feelings about the old and new behavior, emphasized in the psychotherapies, is deemphasized here. For example, alcoholics are punished through being shocked or subjected to painfully loud sounds while being shown bottles of liquor. In some cases the alcoholics develop so severe an aversion to drink that they become physically ill when they come into contact with it. The focus is not on counseling to change feelings and attitudes, but rather is on forced behavioral changes.

A somewhat less controversial theme in mental health is the developing interest in "ethnopsychiatry." This approach to mental health argues that traditional therapy models are deeply rooted in the cultures of Western Europe and are therefore inappropriate to peoples whose cultural foundations are from other parts of the world. The attempt to use standard therapies on ethnic minorities in the United States, this position states, is doomed to failure because these people are influenced by cultures other than those of the majority of Americans. The effort is to seek an understanding of mental health and mental illness in the context of the specific culture of which the patient is a part.[14] One product of this movement is a recent study comparing the attitudes and behavior toward death and bereavement of four ethnic groups in Los Angeles: Mexican-Americans, black Americans, Japanese-Americans, and white Americans.[15] This study demonstrated some differences in the frequency and intensity of death fears that can be of importance in the treatment of trauma resulting from the loss of a close relative.

Still another theme in mental-health research and theory is the relationship between emotional health, economic status, and occupation. The basic concepts are the relationships between mental well-being and social class and the influence of the work experience on mental health. Of course, there is also a relationship between social class and occupation, which gives the work experience an emotional significance beyond mere income. Some tentative conclusions have been reached: blue-collar workers and their families are less happy and well-adjusted than skilled workers; abject poverty leads to adverse mental consequences; and a valued and important work experience is a positive factor for mental health. Another aspect of the orientation toward mental health and working conditions is the interest in "organizational psychology" within business and even public management. Many university programs that train business-

---

[14] Antoinette A. Gattozzi, "Ethnopsychiatry," *Mental Health Reports—6*, Department of Health, Education, and Welfare, publication no. (HSM) 73–9139, 1973, pp. 150ff.
[15] Antoinette A. Gattozzi, "Death and Bereavement," *Mental Health Reports—6* Department of Health, Education, and Welfare, publication no. (HSM) 73–9139, 1973, pp. 48ff.

men, managers, and government officials now stress the importance of having employees who are "fulfilled." In other words, a contented worker performing tasks he feels are significant is the most highly motivated and the easiest to supervise. Relatedly, unhappy workers may become prone to accidents and illness.

Sociologists, psychologists, and even medical professionals have become especially fascinated with the psychological problems of death and bereavement. In the mental-health field specifically, the effort is toward minimizing the adverse emotional consequences of our death fears and finding the best adjustment to death's inevitability. These studies and theoretical developments, particularly those based on experiences of terminal patients, would seem particularly relevant for the medical profession and its continuous contact with the dying.[16]

Finally, two additional themes in the field of mental health are particularly significant for the rest of the health-care system. One is the recognition that mental illness is often related to particular life stages of the individual. Life stages are defined partly by the maturation and aging of the body and partly by the culture that influences when we are "adults" and when we are "old." The second theme is the growing belief that character and personality may well play a significant role even in those illnesses, such as cancer, that we have long regarded as essentially physiological.

Many of the specialties of the physician are based on the recognition that illnesses often relate to life stage. Pediatrics is medical care for the very young, geriatrics for the elderly. It should not be surprising, then, that mental illness is also related to age and life stage. As of 1970, according to one expert's estimate, there were a half-million psychotics or "borderline" psychotics under twenty years of age in the United States.[17] Suicide is among the five leading causes of death among adolescents in this country. Mental retardation and autism are emotional and mental disorders also common to the very young.

Life for those aged twenty years and older has its own particular threats to mental health. From about twenty-one years on, the individual is regarded as an adult, and pressures mount for marriage, career settlement, and education. Schizophrenia and depression, major psychotic illnesses, are common to this age group. This is also the time for ulcers.

In our society, at least, the lives of forty- and fifty-year-olds are often traumatic because they involve a recognition of the aging process. For men, it is often a fear of diminishing energies and a concern with lost opportunities. Many now believe that men during this period experience a process as severe as the woman's menopause. Many women in their

---

[16] Elisabeth Kübler-Ross, *On Death and Dying* (New York: MacMillan, 1969); Raymond A. Moody, Jr., *Life After Life* (Atlanta: Mockingbird Books, 1975).

[17] Martin, *Mental Illness and Mental Health*, p. 68.

forties and fifties also experience depression and emotional trauma due to aging and lost opportunities. Drinking among housewives of this age group is a particularly common social problem.

Being sixty years and older has its own threats of emotional disturbance. One must face retirement and the reality of impending death, since the average life expectancy in the United States is between seventy and eighty years. The great majority of patients in psychiatric hospitals are sixty years of age or older. The suicide rate among those sixty-five or older is the highest for any age group in our country. At this age, mental disturbance is commonly accompanied by physical deterioration.

The mental-health field makes a major contribution to America's health-care system by recognizing and investigating the interrelationships between age and life stages, on the one hand, and mental illness and mental health, on the other. Life is a total process, involving our personality, our bodies, those around us, and the values and emphases of the culture. This is extremely clear in the growing evidence of the pervasive connections between physical illness, personality characteristics, and stressful life situations.

We have discussed these connections in other sections of the book. Here we will only highlight some of the most recent research in the field.

> There are actually two kinds of evidence showing that one's thoughts and emotions have the ability to trigger somatic disease. One concerns stressful events, and their ability to trigger a welter of illnesses. The other concerns certain patterns of thoughts and emotions and their ability to trigger specific somatic diseases.[18]

Psychological stress is the label used for the unhappy emotions that usually accompany such life changes as being divorced, losing one's job, the death of a spouse, or such lesser stresses as the Christmas rush, changing residences, and minor violations of the law. There is evidence that these stress periods increase one's susceptibility to cancer, high blood pressure, alcoholism, gout, and arthritis.

The relationships between personality types or characteristics and particular illnesses are more controversial. Some researchers have argued that aggressiveness, time-urgency, and competitiveness are characteristics making the individual prone to a heart attack. Others have concluded that cancer victims are most often low-geared people, seldom given to outbursts of emotion, who have experienced frequent feelings of isolation and unhappiness from early childhood.

[18] Joan Arehart-Treichel, "The Mind and Body Link," *Science News*, Vol. 108 (December 20, 1975), pp. 394–95. See also, "The Case: Did Watergate Make Him Sick?" *Newsweek*, November 11, 1974, pp. 28–29, and "Backaches and Personality: A Test Can Save a Useless Operation," *Psychology Today*, May 1974, pp. 27–28. For a critical view of the theories of personality and their relationships to cancer, see, Mary G. Marcus, "Cancer and Character," *Psychology Today*, June 1976, pp. 52ff.

While relationships between personality characteristics and certain illnesses, such as rheumatoid arthritis, asthma, and ulcers are easily demonstrated, one suspects that other connections between personalities and major physical illnesses also exist and will someday be proven. Stress is at least a predisposing factor in many illnesses, and a precipitating cause in others. Much more research, jointly involving physicians and mental-health experts, must be done. Maximum healthfulness for Americans can only result when we integrate our knowledge of body and mind.

SUGGESTED READINGS

KESEY, KEN, *One Flew Over the Cuckoo's Nest* (New York: Signet, 1962). A novel that provides insight into the life of mental institutions, and reflects on the tyranny of the organization in dealing with eccentricity.

LAMOTT, KENNETH, "What to do When Stress Signs Say You're Killing Yourself," *Today's Health*, Vol. 53 (January 1975), pp. 30–34. A discussion of the symptoms and health implications of excessive work.

MAY, PHILIP R. A. and JEROME COHEN, "Development Operations in Mental Health Delivery Systems: An Urgent Need," *American Journal of Public Health*, Vol. 65, no. 2 (February 1975), pp. 156–59. A proposal for the development of a new mental-health engineer in care facilities to have personal responsibility for sustained patient care.

MILLER, DOROTHY H., "Worlds That Fail." In Anselm Strauss, ed., *Where Medicine Fails* (Chicago: Aldine, 1970), pp. 85–97. An essay on the sense of isolation, worthlessness, bitterness, and depression for institutionalized patients.

MUSTO, DAVID F., "Whatever Happened to Community Mental Health?," *Public Interest*, no. 39 (Spring 1975), pp. 53–79. Examines the results of a Canadian Maritime Province study that concluded that only seventeen percent of its population were "probably well."

"New Ways to Heal Disturbed Minds: Where Will It All Lead?," *U.S. News and World Report*, Vol. 80, no. 7 (February 16, 1976), pp. 33–40. A review of innovations in the treatment process of mental patients.

PAPPWORTH, M. H., *Human Guinea Pigs: Experimentation on Man* (London: Routledge & Kegan Paul, 1967). A commentary on the ethics of experiments with the mentally ill.

POPE, SAXTON, "The Containment of Mental Illness." In John D. Porterfield, ed., *Community Health: Its Needs and Resources* (New York: Basic, 1974), pp. 79–90. A discussion of the incapacity of most institutions and individuals to deal sympathetically with the mentally ill.

ROSEN, HAROLD, "The Impact of the Psychiatric Intensive Care Unit on Patients and Staff," *American Journal of Psychiatry*, Vol. 132, no. 5 (May 1975), pp. 549–51. A commentary on stress from patients undergoing intensive psychiatric care.

ROSENFELD, ALBERT, *The Second Genesis: The Coming Control of Life* (Englewood Cliffs, N.J.: Prentice-Hall, 1969). Presents ethical issues of the manipulation and control of human behavior.

SCHEFF, T. J., "Medical Dominance: Psychoactive Drugs and Mental Health Policy," *American Behavioral Scientist*, Vol. 19, no. 3 (January/February 1976), pp. 299–317. A description of national trends of the mental-health system and the importance of psychoactive drugs in treatment.

SELYE, HANS, *The Stress of Life* (New York: McGraw-Hill, 1956). A comprehensive view of the affects of stress and hypertension on one's health.

SHAH, SALEEM A., "Dangerous and Civil Commitment of the Mentally Ill: Some Public Policy Considerations," *American Journal of Psychiatry,* Vol. 132, no. 5 (May 1975), pp. 501–5. A discussion of the risks of commitment to the patient, related to the fear of potential danger of the mental patient to himself and others.

WALES, HEATHCOTE W., "The Rise, the Fall, and the Resurrection of the Medical Model," *The Georgetown Law Journal,* Vol. 63, no. 87 (1974), pp. 87–105. An examination of the definition of sanity.

10
INSTITUTIONAL CARE:
HOSPITALS

Just as the physician is at the center directing the flow of services for those needing medical care, so is the hospital the central institutional structure, virtually the hub of medical services. Our discussion to this point has centered on the human dimension of illness. We will now consider its institutional stage. We begin with a brief review of the evolution of the hospital, noting its changing function from serving as a poorhouse to its present distinguished status as a service institution. We outline briefly the statistical dimensions of the hospital "industry," identifying the size of the various components and their purposes, with side attention to extended-care facilities and nursing homes. A subsequent section revisits the cost issues of hospitalization, focusing on the significance of third-party payments for hospital services. This is a conspicuous and unique feature of the American "system"—a feature regarded by many serious students of the health market as the most important cause of our cost problem. In the ensuing chapter, we will probe some of the administrative and organizational problems besetting hospital services.

THE CHANGING FUNCTIONS OF HOSPITALS:
AN HISTORICAL VIEW

In earlier cultures, especially, the curative abilities of society's "medicine men" were derived from priestly medicine and incantations to the Gods or spirits for favored treatment. During the Middle Ages, barber surgeons emerged to treat the peasant class, while a professional group, formally designated as physicians, emerged to serve the well-to-do. Even then, jurisdictional feuds developed between the two specialties, largely reflecting the efforts of surgeons to distinguish themselves from their barber counterparts.

Advances in physiology and the discovery of the circulation of the blood by William Harvey (1578–1657) provide the foundation for modern medical care. Even so, physicians continued into the late nineteenth century in their search for a universal law of healing, based on speculations that are quaint by contemporary standards. There were, of course, no medical laboratories, no microscopes, no controlled experiments, and few hospitals.

During the Middle Ages, hospitals emerged initially as shelters for the poor, the sick, the orphans, and others wandering aimlessly throughout the countryside seeking sanctuary. Their growth reflected urbanization, and only later did doctors realize that such shelters were an appropriate laboratory for study:

> Thousands of new immigrants moved into the city from the countryside, where they soon fell victim to typhoid fever, tuberculosis, or other illnesses endemic in the unsanitary cities. Since the new arrivals had no families or friends who were willing to take care of them, they ended up in hospitals, and these rapidly grew in number. To a research-minded physician the overcrowded hospitals offered unprecedented material for clinic observation—and for autopsies.[1]

In some countries, such as Scotland, universities developed adjunct relationships with hospitals, so that medical students would have access to the ebb and flow of humans seeking sanctuary and medical care. In England, however, universities shunned such contact with the poorhouses. We find here the origins of the contemporary problem: university graduates tended to serve only the prosperous, with the impoverished masses losing the benefits of their care. Throughout much of the seventeenth and eighteenth centuries, and even into the nineteenth, most hospitals were more like shelters than places where people could expect to be cured of illness.

There is interesting speculation on the motives for herding the indigent into poorhouses. On the one hand there were the altruistic (often with religious inspiration) seeking to provide care for the infirm and the wandering transients. On the other hand, the need was felt to isolate those infected with contagious disease, such as lepers, those possessed with the devil (as revealed by deranged behavior), and so on. For many, in fact, the visit to such "hospitals" was the last stop on the way to the grave.

Hospitals, then, first housed the homeless and later gave medical attention to the poor who had become ill. This mixture of poverty and altruism set the stage for the evolution of the modern hospital, as an institution where the very best of scientific care could be expected.

[1] Bonnie Bullough and Vern Bullough, "A Brief History of Medical Practice." In Eliot Freidson and Judith Lorber (eds.), *Medical Men and Their Work* (Chicago: Aldine, 1972), p. 95.

There are many colorful accounts of the quality of care provided. In the premodern period, medical attention was afforded the poor on a charitable basis. The more wealthy secured attention in "homes." But in either station, the care by contemporary standards was rather chilling.

> Patients often were maimed or killed by the infection and shock result-ing from successful surgery. Nothing need be said of the unsuccessful. . . . The early hospital tended to become very crowded. Patients were accepted only when their complaints had reached crisis proportions. The indifferent medical care available—and the overcrowded conditions and all that they implied concerning cross infection and overworked staff—did not allow for a good prognosis for the average patient: Mortality rates of 25 percent of all admissions were not uncommon. For maternity cases, the figure was closer to 50 percent; and few mothers and new-born babies left the hospital without a disease or defect acquired while in the hospital's care.[2]

With the absence of contemporary technique and of knowledge about germ theory, there seemed little that these institutions could do to stem the tide of misery they faced. At the time of Louis Pasteur (1822–95), who discovered through the use of the microscope that each disease had its own microorganism, some forty-five percent of amputation patients were dying of gangrene. Through the work of Joseph Lister (1827–1912), the Glasgow physician, techniques were advanced for sterilizing during the operating procedure, with phenomenal benefits. Surgical mortality rates dropped from eighty percent to six percent.[3] With a sweeping revo-lution in the understanding of body functions, surgeons were willing to undertake operations never before thought practical. There was less at-tention to grand, speculative theories of the single cause of all morbidity, as attention now shifted to a disease-centered approach to the treatment of illness.

Early America was regarded as the "colonial outpost" of Europe's medical sophistication. During the colonial period, services were likely to be provided by ship's surgeons who had acquired skills (at best) as apprentices. The early practitioners performed all types of services, in-cluding surgery, mixing drugs, pulling teeth, and treating cows, horses and pet dogs.[4] Indeed, on the eve of the revolution, the Virginian William Byrd wrote: "America was a place free from those three great scourges of mankind—Priests, Lawyers, and Physicians." Life expectancy was about thirty-five years, with half the population dying before their tenth birth-day.

[2] Raymon D. Garrett, *Hospitals: A Systems Approach* (Philadelphia: Auerbach, 1973), p. 5.
[3] Ibid., p. 6.
[4] Bullough and Bullough, "A Brief History of Medical Practice," p. 97.

Scurvy, scrofula and scabies were common among the poor. Bathing was rare: one Quaker lady noted in her diary in 1799 that she withstood a shower bath "better than I expected, not having been wet all over at once for 28 years past." Body lice were omnipresent, as was the disease they carried—typhus fever. Frequent births and poor obstetrics accounted for the high mortality in mothers; the death rate among black women served by midwives was lower than among the whites served by physicians. Mental illness was seen as the work of the devil; the village idiot was either derided or tolerated, while the more violent were shackled and jailed.[5]

At the time of the revolution, 2.5 million people were served by 3,500 medical practitioners, with fewer than 200 of these holding degrees from medical schools. Medical techniques were not sophisticated:

Purging, emetics, and bloodletting were common remedies; surgery consisted of "cutting for stone" and amputations. With no anaesthesia, the best surgeons were the ones who could cut, hack and saw most rapidly, aided by the strongest assistants to hold the patient down. . . . Boston physicians were prescribing "Leaden Bullets," to be swallowed for "that miserable Distemper which they called the Twisting of the Guts."[6]

Emulation of the British hospital system began with the establishment of the Pennsylvania Hospital in 1751, the New York Hospital in 1771 and the Massachusetts General in 1811. The devastating consequences of infectious diseases encouraged growing public concern over quarantine measures and sanitary engineering. In the nineteenth century, we saw the introduction of vaccination for smallpox, the development of the stethoscope, the clinical thermometer, hypodermic syringes, the use of ether as an anaesthetic agent, and the rapid growth of the science of bacteriology, demonstrating the microbial origins of many diseases. In the early part of the twentieth century, advances were made in understanding the chemistry of the blood, and the use of x-ray machines allowed the visualization of organic systems.

From a passive receptacle for the sick, it [the hospital] became a house of hope and an active diagnostic and curative institution for all classes. The use of blood transfusions hastened the transformation.[7]

We noted early in chapter 3 the commercial character of medical services through much of the nineteenth century. A frontier spirit of entrepreneurship dominated. If the workingman could not secure credit, the free banking movement allowed individuals to start their own banks and print their own currency as needed. In keeping with the spirit of the

[5] John H. Knowles, "The Struggle to Stay Healthy," *Time*, August 9, 1976, p. 60.
[6] Ibid.
[7] Ibid., p. 61.

times, if an individual had difficulty gaining admission to medical schools, he might start his own.

> Anyone could claim to be a doctor and even establish a medical school. More than 400 medical schools were founded in the nineteenth century. Few had any connection with institutions of higher learning or even any recognized educational standards. Instead, they were proprietary institutions, run on students' fees, and designed to show a profit; the more students, the more profit. Few of them required a high school degree, let alone any college work, for admission; and the student, regardless of qualification, usually graduated at the end of two or three years without any real practical experience.[8]

There was a discernible shift, with the rapidly advancing research in microbiology, to adjudge that affliction was not simply the punishment for the self-indulgent. The notion that medical intervention involved trespassing on "divine territory" lost much of its force, when it was appreciated that morbidity was not God's punishment for those possessed by evil spirits, but reflected, instead, possession by microscopic organisms. A popular conviction spread that disease, at last, could be controlled. Such hope at the turn of the century encouraged populist notions that the government was an appropriate agency to advance the cause of national health. In 1916, Meyer London introduced a House Joint Resolution calling for a federal commission to draft a health-insurance bill. Woodrow Wilson, in his first inaugural address the next year, served notice that the federal government ought to safeguard the nation's health.[9]

Efforts to establish a national health system were deflected by the rising surge of conservatism after World War I. But advances in hospital care would be secured from other sources.

With the turn of the century, hospital construction became a favored form of philanthropy with private donors, including (among many others) Hopkins, Vanderbilt, Whitney, and Rockefeller. While many European countries, particularly Germany, had pursued programs of socialized medicine with state-funding for hospital construction, this country became dependent on community sources of support—and dependent, too, on fee-for-services from its patients.

It is startling to realize how early the broadening of access to medical care was accepted in European countries, considering the on-going debate about the "untested" adventures of a national insurance system in this country today. Free medical care for German workers was provided by the state in 1883, with those benefits later expanded to include sickness insurance for workers' families. Austria followed in 1888, Sweden in 1891,

[8] Bullough and Bullough, "A Brief History of Medical Practice," p. 97.
[9] Charleton B. Chapman and John M. Talmadge, "Historical and Political Background of Federal Health Care Legislation," *Law and Contemporary Problems*, Vol. 35, no. 2 (Spring 1970), p. 340.

Denmark in 1892, Belgium in 1894, and Switzerland in 1912. In the United States the early form of federal intervention reflected concern over the yellow-fever epidemic of 1878, starting in New Orleans and rapidly moving up the Mississippi River Valley. With the death of 30,000 Congress supported a bill to create a National Board of Health with supervisory quarantine authority. The law, passed in 1879, was allowed to expire after its four-year authority as it confronted strong states'-rights opposition. Throughout the latter part of the nineteenth century, *The New York Times* carried regular accounts of the cholera deaths sweeping many passenger ships traveling from Europe and the West Coast. Even so, proposals for a nationally sponsored quarantine law were viewed as part of federalist tyranny.

> Some papers hit the states'-rights issue head on. *The Chicago Tribune,* for example, wryly commented, "The cholera will make this country much sicker than an infraction of the Jeffersonian ideas will." *The Hartford Post* twitted the antifederalist holdouts with the following: "The gentlemen of Texas and Louisiana propose if they die of cholera to be able to thank the Almighty that they caught it in a constitutional way, strictly Jeffersonian, and with regard for states' rights."

In the debate over the 1892 quarantine legislation, Congressman Oates of Alabama explained: "It is desirable to keep out an invasion of cholera, and also of anarchists and communists. . . ."[10]

Between the founding of the distinguished Johns Hopkins medical school in 1893 (simulating the German model of scholarship) and that of the University of Chicago medical school in the 1920s, hospitals emerged as centers of the medical expertise. The research focus of medicine placed a premium on the sterilized setting for medical care. The populace began to lose its fear of hospital treatment, and the physician increasingly developed a dependence on its technology and the comfort of collaboration with specialists. Nineteen-ten, according to one source, was a watershed year: by that time the medical sector was probably doing, on balance, more good than harm. In a succinct essay, Chapman and Talmadge describe the transformation.

> In the nineteenth century, relatively few of the nation's citizens had access to hospitals and specialists. Laboratory tests were virtually unknown; the x-ray was discovered by Roentgen in 1896 but came into general medical use only after World War I; the electrocardiograph dates from 1912 but was not in general use until after 1930. By the mid-1930s utilization of hospitals, which were formerly turned to only in case of terminal illness or major surgery (if at all), was increasing rapidly. Medical diagnosis and treatment had gone far beyond the stethoscope and epsom salts stage. The general practitioner's black bag no

---

[10] Ibid., pp. 337–39.

longer contained all that patients needed and were beginning to demand.[11]

By way of recapitulation and integration, the scientific revolution following the discoveries of microbiology led, in turn, to the Flexner Report, accounting for a dramatic change in focus of medical education. This led, in turn, to the organizational or institutional "revolution," with the increased dependence of the physician on elaborate medical technology. The remarkable improvements in successfully diagnosing and treating patients were costly. Medical treatment had shifted from the home to the hospital, an institution that was both dazzling and formidable. As John H. Knowles explains:

> With less time spent with patients . . . complaints about the dehumanizing of medical care were increasingly heard. Doctors moved their offices close to the hospital and its technology. By the 1950s the house call had virtually vanished as doctor and patient met in the emergency wards and clinics of urban teaching hospitals or in offices next door.[12]

Almost every aspect of care reflects this organizational transformation. Childbirth and surgery have moved out of the family residence and into hospitals. Nursing homes now provide maintenance care for one million of our aged, a function still performed by the family in many other societies.[13] In recent decades there has been a substantial growth in the number of persons choosing to enter medical institutions rather than hire nurses to care for them at home. As one writer explains:

> During the first half of the present century, the hospital changed from a place where poor people died to a place where most of us are born, are subjected to elaborate checkups, undergo surgery, are treated for certain diseases, and eventually may die.[14]

With the growth of affluence, we now seek the "best" of medical care. And the view is now widely accepted that such care can be secured only in a hospital setting because of its sophisticated hardware and specialist teams. Furthermore, we have been educated to believe that the home could hardly provide the aseptic conditions so important to childbirth and surgery. The increased coverage of health insurance has further encouraged hospital use. There is evidence that physicians and patients often contrive to have care delivered through hospitalization rather than on a clinical or outpatient basis, for insurance coverage is more liberal when delivered there than in the physician's office. Professional organiza-

---

[11] Ibid., p. 343.

[12] Knowles, "The Struggle to Stay Healthy," p. 61.

[13] "Getting Old in Kids' Country," *Newsweek*, November 11, 1974. An additional one million of our sick are in hospitals.

[14] Carol Taylor, *In Horizontal Orbit* (New York: Holt, Rinehart and Winston, 1970), p. 16.

tions such as the American Hospital Association reinforce the aura of legitimacy surrounding these institutions. The federal government, too, has encouraged institutional care by paying for hospital bills for the aged and medically indigent and by financing hospital construction.

The historical perspective encourages one to marvel at the transitions from barbaric to "civilized" care. In a reflective essay that encourages some humility about the present state of the art, Howard H. Hiatt writes:

> Nancy Mitford may have been indulging in literary license when she predicted that "in another two hundred and fifty years, present-day doctors may seem to our descendants as barbarous as Fagon and his colleagues seem to us. . . . In those days, terrifying in black robes and bonnets, they bled the patient; now terrifying in white robes and masks, they pump blood into him." Wholesale bloodletting disappeared from our "therapeutic" kit long ago, but within my own professional lifetime, I recall seeing patients "treated" for multiple sclerosis by having blood pumped into them until they were polycythemic.[15]

However, contemporary problems abound. The present crisis in medical care includes uncontrolled expenditures that will inevitably dictate setting in place an allocative mechanism for services. In this context, thoughtful questions are being raised about the risks of excesses in hospitalization, medication, and surgery and about the inundation of the system by the worried well. Herbert Ratner explains:

> The modern hospital is a highly misused institution. Many people with hospital insurance have been paying their premiums for years and because they are dying to "get their money back," they are willing to go to the hospital for all kinds of minor things. This, in turn, drives the cost of hospital insurance up, and that makes the person all the more determined to use the hospital. Anywhere from 20 to 40 percent of our hospital beds are needlessly occupied. Studies show that it doesn't seem to make much difference how many hospital beds are put up in this country, they will always be used. . . . the number of people in hospital beds always rises to equal the number of beds available.[16]

Entwined with the issue of overuse is the determination of a rationing mechanism to control access to hospitals. We are confronted with pressures to expand hospital service to the large poverty groups that often surround medical centers in metropolitan areas. Hospitals themselves become the battleground between forces intent on experimentation and research and those concerned about patient care for individuals with "ordinary" afflictions. In one popular account, Fred Anderson charges:

[15] "Protecting the Medical Commons: Who Is Responsible?" *The New England Journal of Medicine,* Vol. 293, no. 5 (July 31, 1975), p. 236.
[16] Herbert Ratner, "Medicine," an interview with Donald McDonald, *Child and Family,* Vol. 11, no. 2 (1972), p. 102.

The second Establishment, hostile to the first, is based in urban hospitals. It is research and technology oriented, often salaried, and provides the world's best surgery and treatment for complex illnesses. The result is that, though this is the best country in the world in which to have a serious illness, it is one of the worst countries in the world in which to have a non-serious illness. . . . At the same time, we have outstanding open heart surgery, plastic surgery, surgical organ transplantation and diagnostic skills. It is a paradox which makes it possible for a patient to read in the waiting room literature of America's latest triumph of medical technology, while failing to receive quick, effective and inexpensive treatment for a sore throat.[17]

Anderson blames the medical schools, where the values and attitudes about worthwhile medical care are implanted. "The schools and their hospitals turn out excellent clinicians, scientifically imaginative researchers, who appear more concerned with a patient's electrolytes than with his humdrum good health." How do we determine the appropriate "mix" of technological resources with medical talent, as one makes sober assessments of local population needs? Just what are hospitals expected to accomplish?

THE STRUCTURE OF HOSPITAL FACILITIES TODAY

There is great diversity within and between the groups of institutions known as hospitals, extended-care facilities, and nursing homes. Like all components of the health-care delivery system, their consumers are people experiencing ill health or seeking to avoid it. Two basic characteristics, however, set them apart from other delivery components. First, hospitals are comparatively large organizations served by large staffs, heavy capital investments, and large administrative structures. This contrasts with the fact that eighty-one percent of all physicians providing direct patient care are practicing by themselves or with partnerships.[18] Our health needs are served by thousands of solo practitioners and small groups of physicians. But hospitals are large and growing in size. Today, about forty-five percent of all hospitals in this country have one hundred or more beds. It is estimated that by 1980 forty percent of all hospital beds will be in institutions with over five hundred beds. While hospitals are continuing to grow in size, however, physician-service units are not.

Health-care institutions are also distinctive because of the nature of

---

[17] "The Growing Pains of Medical Care," *The New Republic*, January 17, 1970, p. 17.
[18] American Medical Association testimony to the Subcommittee on Public Health and Environment, Committee on Interstate and Foreign Commerce, U.S. House of Representatives, "Hospital Cost Controls," p. 128, Serial No. 93-60.

their relationships to the patients. About sixty percent of all hospital patients are inpatients despite efforts to encourage outpatient services. Often outpatient services are provided through the hospital's emergency facilities. Thus, a majority of the patients receiving hospital services, and almost all of those receiving services from nursing homes and extended-care facilities, are residing, at least temporarily, in these institutions. Many are suffering from serious disease or, as in the case of nursing homes and extended-care facilities (ECFs), prolonged and even permanent illnesses.

Another slice of data revealing hospital services analyzes the distribution of hospital *beds* by hospital function. This is perhaps a more precise measurement of intended service than the number of hospital facilities taken alone.

First, we should note again the remarkable growth in the number of hospital beds serving the American public. In 1948, at the time the Hill-Burton program became operational, there were 3.4 beds per 1,000 population. The hospital-construction program was designed to minimize the serious disparities of hospital access. In the mid-1940s, some states had as few as 2 beds per 1,000 population. In three decades of construction (costing over $12 billion) the federal government absorbed 30 percent of building costs. By 1973, the ratio of short-term general hospital beds had increased to 4.3.

Shifts in public policy and medical technology indicate an interesting shift in the direction of services. From 1946 to 1973, long-term general facilities were reduced by one-half, from 0.6 per 1,000 to 0.3 per 1,000. There was an even sharper decline in bed ratios for tuberculosis hospitals, from 0.5 in 1946 to 0.05 in 1973. Another sharp decline was recorded for psychiatric care, from 4.1 to 2.0 per 1,000. When we add the decline of these long-term specialty facilities to the growth of short-term general facilities, we find an overall reduction of bed facilities, from 8.6 in 1946 to 6.6 in 1973. If we move from the nonfederal to federal hospitals, we find a similar decline, from 1.7 in 1946 to 0.7 in 1973.

The expansion of short-term facilities has been associated with a rapid increase of special-service facilities, including units that provide open-heart surgery. Radioisotope and renal-dialysis units have also proliferated.

There are other single-purpose agencies, as well. We have 217,000 beds for the mentally retarded, 49,000 beds for orphans and dependent children, 60,000 beds for the emotionally disturbed, 33,000 beds for alcoholics and drug addicts, 24,000 for the deaf and blind, and 5,000 for the physically handicapped.[19]

Let us look at the "ownership" of beds, as opposed to the sponsorship of hospitals. In 1973 we had 1,449,062 beds, of which the government

[19] Ibid., p. 133.

owned 696,259 (139,000 federal and 557,000 state), or close to half of the total. Nonprofit organizations owned 672,219 beds (193,000 church-owned and 479,000 "other"), and proprietary (profitmaking) groups provided only 81,000 beds. We see, then, that government remains the largest single sponsor of bed facilities in the United States. When we consider this, along with the substantial government funding of nonproprietary services, we must acknowledge government's substantial influence in developing health-care facilities.

Nursing homes, initially residential institutions providing nursing and personal-care services, have increased rapidly during the past quarter-century. Mose Ellis aptly describes the range of nursing-home care:

> Nursing home patients present a wide spectrum of illnesses and needs, often within one institution. Included in the category of nursing home patients have been the chronically ill, the self-care resident, the terminal patient, the potentially rehabilitative patient, the senile, and other classifications of long-term cases.
>
> The nursing home industry is as multi-faced as the patient load it serves. Nursing homes which are physician-oriented and offer medical services by skilled medical personnel are correctly classified as "Medical facilities"; others are little more than the final "home" for long-term geriatric cases. Most fall somewhere in between, and are not easily classified.[20]

Recent developments have had a major impact on the nursing-home industry. The result has been an increased connection between these institutions and the other components of the health-care delivery system. First, we have witnessed an enormous increase in the costs of short-term hospitalization and the growing suspicion that some patients are hospitalized unnecessarily. The growing proportion of our elderly population, who often require what is coldly called "maintenance care," has also increased the importance of the long-term institutions. Medicare helped remove the financial barrier to the use of these facilities by many aged citizens. On January 1, 1967, Medicare made millions of senior citizens eligible for posthospital, inpatient, long-term medical care. The principle is that after the patient passes the acute stage of his illness, or if the illness is chronic rather than acute, he should be transferred to a less expensive facility with convalescent and medical services. In an attempt to guarantee the quality of services in long-term institutions, Congress created the Extended Care Facility through Public Law 89-97. The congressional objective was to provide medical and convalescence service

---

[20] Mose Ellis, "The Extended Care Facility and the Medical Society—An Overview," *The Extended Care Facility, A Handbook for the Medical Society* (Chicago: American Medical Association, 1967), pp. 5–13.

for Medicare recipients through ECFs at less expense than in short-term general hospitals.[21] Government was now paying the medical bills. It was also hoped that nursing homes would upgrade services to meet ECF standards for certification in an effort to attract Medicare patients and dollars. Many nursing homes, and some hospitals and other institutions, did become certified as ECFs. By the end of March 1967, approximately three thousand nursing homes, or one-third of all nursing-home beds, had been certified. At that time, eight hundred hospitals and other institutions formed the remainder of ECF certifications.

Nursing-home bed facilities have more than doubled between 1963 and 1973, from 569,000 to 1,328,000. For 49 percent of their residents, Medicaid became the primary source of payment by 1973–74. Public assistance absorbed another 10 percent of costs, and the individual and his family resources absorbed 37 percent.[22]

The increased number and proportion of our elderly, the fact that many have only a small income or savings at retirement, and the unwillingness of many young families to house older family members, led to Medicare, generally, and to the use of long-term medical institutions as a type of retirement home, specifically. As we noted in chapter 8, Medicare has had enormous consequences for both long- and short-term institutions. It has helped insulate the aged from the costs of being hospitalized and of longer stays. As a result, even where beds are relatively scarce, the amount of hospital care received by the aged is not reduced as sharply as for other age groups, and thus they take a larger share of existing beds.[23]

There are several ways to classify the hospital structure. One approach is to classify institutions according to the length of patient stay per admission. Short-term general hospitals provide a broad range of services to patients staying an average of thirty days or less. When the hospital's services are specialized to emphasize the treatment of particular illnesses, they are sometimes referred to as short-term specific.[24] Of the approximately 7,500 institutions represented by the American Hospital Association, between 5,700 and 5,800 are nonfederal, short-term hospitals providing general or specialized services.

[21] Ibid., pp. 9ff.

[22] Health: United States, 1975, DHEW Publication No. (HRA) 76-1232, GPO, 1976, p. 85.

[23] Benefit-Cost Analysis of Federal Programs, A Compendium of Papers submitted to the Subcommittee on Priorities and Economy in Government, of the Joint Economic Committee, U.S. Congress. See, Martin S. Feldstein, "Econometric Analysis of the Medicare Program," January 2, 1973, pp. 182–99.

[24] American Hospital Association testimony to the Subcommittee on Public Health and Environment, Committee on Interstate and Foreign Commerce, U.S. House of Representatives, "Hospital Cost Control," pp. 32ff., Serial No. 93–60.

A second classification is based on the nature of ownership or controlling agencies. There are 420 federal hospitals, 750 proprietary hospitals, 1,000 church-owned hospitals, 1,700 owned by state and local governments, and 3,900 voluntary hospitals. Proprietary hospitals are "for-profit" institutions, often owned by physicians. They form a small percentage of the nation's bed availability, but tend to be a source of both interest and controversy.[25] Privately owned voluntary hospitals are non-profit institutions containing about 560,000 beds, or about 49 percent of the nation's total.[26]

A third way of classifying health-care institutions is on the basis of the type of treatment or service offered. We have already mentioned short-term general hospitals; others include: long-term institutions providing personal maintenance and a relatively small amount of medical care (ECFs, nursing homes); convalescent hospitals, which frequently focus on paralysis; psychiatric institutions concerned with both physical and mental disabilities; and tuberculosis and other specialized treatment institutions. The nation has 85 convalescent hospitals and 820 special hospitals.

Psychiatric, convalescent, and special hospitals are distinct because they treat patients with particular illnesses or health problems. Physicians refer patients to these institutions because they are thought to have the trained personnel and facilities to manage particular illnesses more effectively than general hospitals. The relationship between short-term general hospitals and long-term institutions, on the other hand, has more to do with the amount and frequency of medical services. General hospitals provide intensive medical services, while nursing homes and extended-care facilities provide fewer services over a longer period of time. While the two million inpatients in health-care institutions are currently about evenly divided between short-term and long-term facilities, it is hoped that savings can be realized by increased use of nursing homes and ECFs.

Institutions involved in health-care delivery are big business. We have noted the growth in the average size of hospitals and the recent rapid expansion in nursing-home and extended-care facilities. In 1972, short-term hospitals alone had 1.6 million full-time employees and treated 31 million patients during the year. There were 2.7 million employees in all types of these institutions.[27] On a daily basis they served an average

[25] Critics of profitmaking proprietary hospitals say that owner-physicians are tempted to have their patients use the hospital facilities needlessly in order to maximize income. A few observers believe that the profit motive can eliminate waste and increase cost effectiveness in hospitals. For the latter argument, see, Charles W. Baird, "On Profits and Hospitals," *Journal of Economic Issues*, Vol. 5, no. 1 (March 1971).

[26] Garrett, *Hospitals: A Systems Approach*, p. 8.

[27] Sidney H. Croog and Donna F. VerSteeg, "The Hospital as a Social System." In Howard E. Freeman, Sol Levine, and Leo G. Reeder, *Handbook of Medical Sociology*, 2nd ed. (Englewood Cliffs, N.J.: Prentice-Hall, 1972), pp. 275–76.

of 663,000 inpatients and 445,000 outpatients. The daily cost of operating the short-term hospitals was over $70 million.[28]

The significance of the hospital-industry's growth is seen in the fact that hospital plant assets in 1950 were $7,483 per daily census (or assets required per unit of output). That figure had increased to $33,814 in 1972. In the latter year, total plant assets of community hospitals (non-federal, short-term) were $22.5 billion, an increase of 800 percent over 1950 values. In 1950 there were 110.5 admissions and 900.5 patient days per 1,000 civilian resident population. The growth in facility use has been remarkable: in 1972 there were 149.1 admissions per 1,000 population.[29]

THE HOSPITAL COST PROBLEM REVISITED

In chapter 3, our summary of system trends briefly outlined the sources of cost pressure that have proved so perplexing and distressing. Here we will refine and elaborate on elements contributing to these unusual cost advances.

There are multiple pressures converging on hospitals to account for their soaring costs. Among the more important is the rapid growth of third-party payments, now accounting for some ninety-two percent of reimbursements for hospital and related expenses. The government has undertaken an investigation of the role physicians play in Blue Cross and Blue Shield programs, reflecting a concern that their presence on policy boards encourages a somewhat casual attitude about the increase of "prevailing" charges for hospital-related medical services. The government is not an innocent bystander in all of this, for its tax programs have encouraged the spread of private health insurance. The consumer is an actor, too, in his eagerness to secure reimbursements (in the form of expensive services) for his investments in health insurance.

A second bundle of forces is the dedication of hospital, physician, and patient to quality care. In the absence of defined budget constraints, there is no discernible limit to the kinds of medical technology providers seek. It has been difficult to establish societal standards for appropriate numbers of hospital beds and appropriate backup medical-technology systems. The desire to secure the very best is a conspicuous feature of the medical fraternity, with its preoccupation with cures, not costs. That desire is exceeded only by the emergency-care patient, seeking to avoid certain death by medical intervention.

[28] American Hospital Association testimony to the Subcommittee on Public Health and Environment, Committee on Interstate and Foreign Commerce, U.S. House of Representatives, "Hospital Cost Controls," pp. 32ff., Serial No. 93-60.
[29] *Hospital Statistics, 1972*, American Hospital Association, 1973.

Related to this category of forces is the rapid increase in hospital facilities, reflecting the inordinate pressure of each small community to have facilities. As we have noted throughout, hospital beds beget patients, and patients raise costs. Ironically, if the total capacity is not fully used, costs may increase anyway. Reimbursements made on behalf of patients must cover the overhead costs of idle beds.

A fourth factor is the shift in emphasis toward long-term care for the chronically ill. This shift has been associated with the trend to institutionalized rather than home care.

There are the more obvious cost factors. Undoubtedly, those supplying materials for medical services have been quick to exploit the upsurge of demand, with "downstream" price or cost effects that hospitals have been forced to absorb. These supplies include everything from syringes to syrup medications to mops. Related to the cost of materials are the increases in labor costs. These have two components: the increase in the rate of pay, engendered in part by higher minimum-wage laws and threats of unionization, and the substantial increase in the worker–patient ratio.

A sixth factor is the redesigned billing process, largely encouraged by the government's reimbursement schedules and the realization that providers can maximize revenues by increasing services. In the absence of crisp definitions of quality care, we are left with the awkward task of identifying which services are essential to patient care.

Finally, there is concern about cost pressures that reflect the heavy representation of nonprofit institutions in our delivery system. Paradoxically, the "nonprofit" designation is considered the source of difficulty, for in the absence of a clear maximizing goal (such as profit or net return), which would give explicit considerations to costs, community hospitals may be launching expansion programs unjustified in terms of community benefit–cost ratios. Hospitals have been dubbed as institutions with "uncertain" goals. But the speculation grows that hospitals maximize "activities." Such activity might reflect an interest in revenue maximization, the construction of hospital beds or floor space, the maximization of a full range of services, the maximum deployment of modern medical technologies, the maximum expansion of staff, and so on. All of these are facets of volume or size: statistically, as we have noted, there has been a discernible increase in the bed size of the "average" hospital, and there is ample evidence of expanded employment and technology. Defining the excesses of such expansion confronts us again with the perplexing definition of optimal quality care. Lacking community-based standards, hospitals have tended to "go for broke" in an effort to establish their prominence in the health-care field. That option will remain feasible if there are external subsidies for construction and extended reimbursement plans involving government and other third-party payers for patient care.

Let us review the logic for the cost pressures caused by third-party payments. We identified the considerable detail of this feature of our health system in chapter 3, and need not reproduce those data here. On the average, the consumer/patient pays only eight cents on the dollar for hospital services, and even with spiraling costs, this must appear as a bargain. No matter that premium costs are ultimately absorbed by the employer, the employee, or the taxpayer. Ted Frech and Paul Ginsburg make explicit use of the fully insured patient who is insensitive to "feedback" costs on his premium through his full use of insured medical care. They note that prices under such arrangements have "explosive tendencies."

> If the insurer pays 100 percent, the insured bears none of the cost of services (remember, we are ignoring the minor feedback through higher premiums or taxes for all consumers), and the price of services will be irrelevant to him. In this full-coverage case, while the quantity of service demanded by the consumer is clear (an amount where marginal utility of service in the form of medical care is zero), the supply and demand analysis of a market does not apply, for a competitive supply curve does not exist. Since the price charged the *insurer* by the medical care provider will not affect the quantity demanded by the *consumer*, the incentive is to charge a very high price to the insurer. The seller finds no limit to the demand price of consumers. The market pricing mechanism is eliminated by full-coverage benefits. Medical prices under such a program will have explosive tendencies. As the objectives of national health insurance would not be accomplished, full-cost benefits would not likely continue, unless accompanied by price regulation. . . .[30]

Although physicians may be sensitive to the financial resources of patients in prescribing a treatment regimen, there is evidence that hospital usage is directly related to whether the patient—or an insurance company—pays the bill. The inference is clearly established that physicians, just as patients, are reassured when an impersonal corporate structure—with seemingly endless resources—is obligated to pay the bill. Kong-Kyun Ro examined the hospital-stay patterns of nine thousand patients served by twenty-two short-term general hospitals, and found that patients who paid directly for their services had the shortest stays and the smallest bills. Patient visits to hospitals supported by the government were confronted with the longest visits and the largest bills. Individuals covered by insurance had intermediate length of stays, with intermediate-sized bills.[31] There is evidence, too, that the cost of hospitalization is directly correlated to the per capita income in the state in which the hos-

[30] H. E. Frech, III, and Paul B. Ginsburg, "Imposed Health Insurance in Monopolistic Markets: A Theoretical Analysis," *Economic Inquiry*, Vol. 13 (March 1975), p. 57.

[31] Kong-Kyun Ro, "Patient Characteristics, Hospital Characteristics and Hospital Use." In Victor R. Fuchs (ed.), *Essays in the Economics of Health and Medical Care* (New York: National Bureau of Economic Research, 1972).

pital is located, again giving credence to the argument that the rate structure is sensitive to consumer ability to pay.

In all of this, we hypothesize the individual's enthusiasm for hospitalization because of his illusion that this is close to being costless. If the individual calculates that he will "come out ahead" by disdaining the opportunity for hospital care in order to avoid burdening either the government or his insurer (realizing that he must eventually absorb those costs in tax payments or increased premiums), he may well lose more than he gains. So long as he alone abstains, the insurance principle of spreading or sharing costs works against him. All of this assumes, of course, that there are positive benefits, psychic or physiological, derived from hospitalization.

It is not impossible, for example, that a modest number of consumers may view hospitalization, not so much as medical intervention, but as a means of retreating temporarily from the pressures of everyday life, somewhat analogous to a motel or hotel visit. Hospital "care" is then seen more directly as a consumer good than as an investment designed to deal with a medical problem. Indeed, a few hospitals have identified consumer interests in this form of service. A short-term escape from problems through hospitalization in VIP facilities might be somewhat more expensive than American Plan vacation retreats at an area lodge, but the inhibitions of cost lose much of their force if an insurance company pays ninety-two percent of your hotel bill. The corporate executive may not be alone in making such calculations: the "ordinary" taxpayer can readily conclude about the rationality (in terms of *his* cost) of making full use of public services provided by his own tax dollars. Again, the bargain of such service is reflected by the fact that there has been very little increase in out-of-pocket medical costs to the consumer. With all other services increasing, often at two-digit annual rates, medical services may well appear as the one last bargain available to the consumer. As Martin S. Feldstein notes:

> In real terms the net cost to the patient of hospital care has hardly changed in 20 years. It is not surprising, therefore, that consumer demand has encouraged and supported the rapid growth of advanced and expensive hospital services.[32]

Feldstein denies that the price pressure for hospital care reflects the lag of supply to demand shifts. It reflects, rather, an increase in more expensive or exotic supplies and services for which the consuming public is quite willing to pay so long as it is "covered" by third-party payments.

[32] Martin S. Feldstein, "The Medical Economy," *Scientific American*, Vol. 229 (September 1973), p. 155. See also "Research on the Demand for Health Services," *Milbank Memorial Fund Quarterly*, 1973; and "The Rising Prices of Physicians' Services," *The Review of Economics and Statistics*, Vol. 52, no. 2 (May 1970).

"Because the net out-of-pocket cost appears so modest, at least in the short run, the patient is willing to buy more expensive care than he would if he were not insured."

> Unfortunately the production of high cost hospital care is a self-reinforcing process: the risk of very expensive hospital care stimulates patients to prepay hospital bills through relatively comprehensive insurance, while the growth of such insurance tends to make hospital care more expensive. In this way our current method of financing hospital care denies consumers the opportunity to register effectively their preference between higher-cost and lower-cost hospital care.[33]

Concerns about inundation of the system and about the "moral hazard" of indiscriminate use of hospital services emerge, then, not only when government pays the bill, but also when private insurance is available. The stereotyped view of the indigent ill "plundering" society's resources by swarming our medical facilities has its counterpart in the application of the private-insurance principle. A Social Security study explains:

> Insurance is bought to avoid the risk of unexpected expenditure, but because it provides a reduction in price at the time that the hospital care is purchased, it has the concomitant effect of artificially increasing the demand for such care and its price. In fiscal year 1950, patients paid about a third of their hospital bill directly. By 1973, this proportion was reduced to one-tenth, with government paying the largest share at 53 percent, private health insurance paying 36 percent, and philanthropy making up the remaining 11 percent.[34]

The patient may, for quite rational reasons, believe he deserves the very best medical treatment. His insurance premiums represent a "sunk" cost, and quality treatment represents the only possible return. He may believe his employer bears the costs of those premiums. And if he is reminded that extravagant use of sophisticated service can only raise insurance rates in the future, he has two ready responses: he gains more as a consumer of medical care today than he loses as a premium payer tomorrow.

The fringe costs of medical protection are substantial. Of the cost of a 1976 automobile, an average of $117 goes to meet the payroll costs of auto workers' health insurance. The question of just who, in the final analysis, pays for such a payroll tax is beyond the scope of this discussion, but several parties are involved, including (as we note above) consumers, production workers who lose wage increases, and the production workers not hired as a consequence of heavy labor costs. The employer is not

[33] Feldstein, "The Medical Economy," p. 155.
[34] Barbara S. Cooper, Nancy L. Worthington, and Paula A. Piro, "National Health Expenditures, 1929–1973," *Social Security Bulletin*, Vol. 37 (February 1974), pp. 13–14.

alone in absorbing these costs. Yet the popular myth persists that fringe benefits are costless "add-on" benefits for the employee to the extent these are paid for by the employer. And in terms of tax deductions for medical expenses, it is much more economical for the employer to charge one hundred percent of these operating costs as a business expense than for the production worker to declare premium charges in his personal tax returns. Again, the government "pays."

It has been estimated that in 1970 personal income-tax deductions provided taxpayers with a $600 million subsidy in the purchase of health insurance. Another $1.3 billion was deducted for out-of-pocket medical expenses. The premiums paid by employers are also deductible, a subsidy of $2.5 billion. The total is around $4.4 billion. Bridger M. Mitchell and Ronald J. Vogel have observed:

> . . . the federal government directly spent $2.9 billion on medical services for the poor through the Medicaid program the same year. Thus, the effect of federal policy has been to "spend" more health care dollars on middle and upper-income taxpayers than on the poor.[35]

The advantages of participating in group health plans provided by employers is obvious. In 1970, a sample survey indicated that of the total premiums for private health insurance of $17.2 billion, employers paid an estimated $9.8 billion.

> By participating in a group plan, they [the employees] gain access to substantial economies of scale in insurance underwriting and are generally able to obtain coverage at an 8 to 10 percent loading cost for moderate sized firms, versus loading costs of 50 to 100 percent for individual policies. During World War II and again during the most recent period of inflationary controls, wage stabilization efforts have stimulated increases in nonwage forms of income. Finally, federal tax policy, which exempts *all* premiums paid by employers from corporate payroll and personal income taxation, is more attractive than the partial deductibility of personally paid premiums.[36]

Related to the reimbursement mechanisms now in place is the charge that hospitals have little incentive to control costs or even ration access to services. They have been issued a blank check by the government and the Blues, and if the "going rate" becomes the standard for reasonable charges, then this rate displays its exponential growth. Hospital administrators vehemently protest this characterization, contending first that they are the victims rather than the villains in the cost-inflation

---

[35] Bridger M. Mitchell and Ronald J. Vogel, "Health and Taxes: An Assessment of the Medical Deduction," *Southern Economic Journal*, Vol. 4, no. 4 (April 1975), p. 660.
[36] Ibid., pp. 664–65.

issue. They are confronted with spiraling costs in securing materials and services and should not be faulted for shifting such cost burdens to the consumers of services. Second, the physician determines what services should be provided, not the hospital.

In their testimony to a congressional committee, the American Hospital Association explained:

> . . . The AHA, like all responsible hospital administrators and physicians, agrees that patients who can properly be treated as outpatients should not be treated as inpatients, and that inpatients should receive only that degree of care which their medical condition requires. . . .
>
> Hospitals do *not* determine intensity of treatment. . . . Hospital administrators cannot admit or discharge patients; they cannot prevent treatment which doctors consider necessary. Indeed, under the bylaws of a hospital, decisions about medical treatment are reserved *exclusively* for the medical staff.[37]

Defenders of short-term general hospitals also believe that charges of wastefulness and inefficiency in organization are overdone. These observers claim that any large organization will experience some duplication and inefficiency but that those costs are more than offset by the economic benefits of large organizational size. They also believe that emphasizing the use of long-term institutions is based on the belief that cost savings will automatically accrue, but this, in fact, may not be the case. Interestingly enough, at least one economist believes that for Medicare, "The net effect of the extended care facilities is to *raise* cost per hospital episode."[38] As for increasing use of outpatient facilities, hospital supporters note that this development is already well underway.[39] Hospital administrators stress that increased total expenditures for institutional care are at least partly a reflection of growing use of their services, which in turn is largely a result of governmental action through the Medicare and Medicaid programs.

Hospital administrators also emphasize that quality care is inherently expensive. There are no conspicuous economies of scale realized in the expansion of medical services, and if our current national purpose is to make quality health care available to all, we must simply pay the fee. These defenses notwithstanding, heavy public investments in the extension of hospital facilities and public subsidies to encourage the flow of additional medical personnel have not produced the counterinflation bias one would reasonably anticipate in the market. One cannot avoid specu-

[37] American Hospital Association testimony to the Subcommittee on Public Health and Environment, Committee on Interstate and Foreign Commerce, U.S. House of Representatives, "Hospital Cost Controls," p. 93, Serial No. 93-60.
[38] Feldstein, "The Medical Economy," p. 184. Italics added.
[39] *Hospital Statistics, 1972*, The American Hospital Association, 1973.

lating that the "blank check" syndrome has softened hospital resistance to higher costs. In a market where charges of extravagance may be difficult to authenticate, the sense of prosperity and activity characterizes most facilities. It is difficult to obscure the impact of a $130-billion revenue flow.

With reimbursement assured for at least ninety-two percent of hospital patients, the prospect of a diminished revenue flow because of "bad debts" is diminished. When the ill are presented to a hospital facility, it is less and less necessary to calibrate a treatment regimen in terms of "constrained" patient resources. On the face of it, investments in care can now reflect the nature of the affliction without reference to the economic limits of the patient's resources. With reimbursements assured, the physician could ideally dispense with unnecessary care for the wealthy while concentrating on the "real" medical problems of his patients. In the technical jargon of the economist, the physician can be "income neutral" in defining appropriate measures of care.

Stuart H. Altman, HEW deputy assistant secretary for health planning (identified as the government's "industry watchdog"), reflected the puzzlement of economists in accounting for hospitals' increasing costs. He noted that about fifty percent of the cost increase was attributed to additional expenditures:

> The problem we have and the problem everyone has is to differentiate in that 50 percent how much of it was due to the fact that this industry has been a cost-plus industry, where someone sits behind them with essentially a blank check, providing funds for new equipment. Now, it is a very difficult thing to decide how much of that increase was marginal at best in terms of improved medical care. We have a feeling, and so do most experts, that there is a significant amount of so-called fat.[40]

PATIENT PERSPECTIVES ON THE QUALITY OF HOSPITAL CARE

Not all pressures for changing the health-care delivery institutions are economic. Many are attitudinal and political. Hospitals are often considered highly self-contained and isolated organizations, which go about their business with little concern for or relevance to the health-care system, and for the community that surrounds them. This "cocoon mentality"

---

[40] "Medical Policies and Costs," Hearings before the Subcommittee on Consumer Economics of the Joint Economic Committee, 93rd Cong., 1st Session, May 15 and 16, 1973, pp. 116–17.

is most dramatic when instances of administrative red tape or insurance requirements deny critically ill persons the care they urgently need.[41]

The majority of a patient's interpersonal contacts in hospitals are with physicians and nurses. The charge is often made that these hospital personnel are insensitive to the attitudes, feelings, and fears of patients from minority groups. The following are excerpts from a study of the delivery and reception (or nonreception) of health services to Mexican-Americans in the Rio Grande Valley:

> The family usually is reluctant to relinquish its responsibility for sick members and frequently resists hospitalization. The impersonal environment of a hospital or mental institution seems cold and unpleasant to the Mexican-American, who values the affective interpersonal relations of his family environment. Hospital schedules and unfamiliar food are distasteful to the Mexican-American patient. Finally, the hospital is feared as "a place where people go to die."[42]

Unfortunately this morbid view of hospitals is too frequently accurate. Testimony by a physician from a grossly understaffed Indian Health Service Hospital illustrates this tragic condition:

> We average about one needless death about every six weeks to two months. Either a mistake or lack of personnel or lack of equipment, or a combination of these are the causes for the deaths.
>
> Case in point. A 40-year-old woman with tuberculosis—pulmonary tuberculosis—which usually doesn't kill people. This lady died because she drowned in her own secretions because no one could get into her throat to suck the secretions out often enough to keep her from drowning.
>
> Another case in point. A little infant, four months old, in the hospital for a week for salmonella, extremely ill when she comes in, hard working physicians and nurses make her better. She responds nicely to therapy. She's about ready to go home, but she's in a back room now because she's not acutely ill. There are plenty of other children that are acutely ill and have to be placed in the hall or in the front rooms. The patient is seen at four o'clock doing well, fed. Next rounds are made at

[41] A clear statement of the need for this type of evaluation is contained in the testimony of Dr. Patrick O'Donoghue, Associate Director, Health Services Research Center, Institute for Interdisciplinary Studies, American Rehabilitation Foundation, "Health Maintenance Organizations," Hearings before the Subcommittee on Public Health and Environment, Committee on Interstate and Foreign Commerce, U.S. House of Representatives, Serial No. 92-91, April 1972, pp. 1203ff.

[42] William Madsen, "Society and Health in the Lower Rio Grande Valley." In John H. Burma (ed.), *Mexican-Americans in the United States* (New York: Harper and Row, 1972), p. 329.

eight o'clock, patient found dead in her crib. The patient did not even die from the disease for which she came in. Had she been at home she probably would have lived through the whole thing. But because she was here, supposedly in a hospital, which supposedly has sufficient people to see her and take care of her, she gets poorer care than she would have at home. She dies of unknown causes.[43]

These incidents help to explain the growing aggressiveness facing health-services consumers and what they consider an intolerable lack of concern for patient welfare. As we noted at the outset, the early history of our hospitals encouraged this lack of concern; they were places where health care was provided to passing strangers or the very poor. However, as hospitals became the center for much of the health care we all receive, consumers became more critical of the inadequate or inconsiderate delivery of services. Some hospitals have also been recently rebuked for providing special "red carpet" services to the wealthy.[44]

Short-term general hospitals are particularly susceptible to the charge that they organize their services, purchase expensive medical equipment (which can cost hundreds of thousands of dollars), and expand facilities with little attention to how these elements fit into the health-care needs of their community. The fact that the nation has a surplus of hospital beds, but a scarcity of inpatient facilities in many rural and low-income areas, is tragically ironic. And as noted above, institutions with an excess bed capacity pass the fixed costs of those facilities to patients who do receive care. Thus, "over-bedding," as it is usually called, results in the inflation of hospital costs.

Nursing homes, too, are constantly criticized for the quality of care they provide. This reputation derives in part from the fact that they tend to have a large number of geriatric patients, who need a wider range of services. They are vulnerable to "horror stories" about mistreatment of resident patients. Because most are profitmaking institutions, there are prevalent anxieties that cost-cutting reduces access to needed care. At least one economist believes that nursing homes, now the fastest-growing component in expenditures for medical services, should be organized as public utilities, "not only for the protection of the consumer, but also . . . to bring the nursing home into the main-stream of medical care and coordinate its operation with that of local hospitals and other health-care facilities."[45]

[43] Testimony of an anonymous physician, "Indian Health Care," Hearings before the Permanent Subcommittee on Investigations of the Committee on Government Operations, United States Senate, (Washington, D.C.: GPO, September 16, 1974).

[44] Taylor, *In Horizontal Orbit*, pp. 20ff.

[45] Leahmae McCoy, "The Nursing Home as a Public Utility," *Journal of Economic Issues*, Vol. 5, no. 1 (March 1971), pp. 67–68.

SUGGESTED READINGS

BAIRD, CHARLES W., "On Profits and Hospitals," *Journal of Economic Issues,* Vol. 5, no. 1 (March 1971), pp. 57–66. A review of charges of inefficiency in not-for-profit hospitals.

BRIAN, EARL E., "Government Control of Hospital Utilization," *The New England Journal of Medicine,* Vol. 286, no. 35 (June 22, 1972), pp. 1340–44. Brian traces the influence of government in moderating hospitalization.

ETZIONI, AMITAI and PAMELA DOTY, "Profit in Not-for-Profit Corporations: The Examples of Health Care," *Political Science Quarterly,* Vol. 91, no. 3 (Fall 1976). An incisive treatment of the nonprofit structure of hospitals and the cost problems that evolve from this form of organization.

FELDSTEIN, MARTIN, "Hospital Cost Inflation: A Study of Nonprofit Price Dynamics," *American Economic Review,* Vol. 60, no. 5 (December 1971), pp. 853–72. A detailed account of the cost pressures confronting hospitals.

GRANFIELD, MICHAEL E., "Resource Allocation Within Hospitals: An Unambiguous Analytic Test of the A-J Hypothesis," *Applied Economics,* Vol. 7, no. 4 (December 1975), pp. 241–49. An introduction to the Averch-Johnson Hypothesis of hospital management.

JOSEPH, HYMAN, "On Economic Theories of Hospital Behavior," *Journal of Economics and Business,* Vol. 27, no. 1 (Fall 1974), pp. 69–74. An introduction to the issue of reprivitation of medical services.

KNOWLES, JOHN H., "The Hospital," *Scientific American,* Vol. 229, no. 3 (September 1973), pp. 128–37. A survey on the development of hospitals.

LEVESON, IRVING and ELIZABETH RODGERS, "Hospital Cost Inflation and Physician Payment," *The American Journal of Economics and Sociology,* Vol. 35, no. 2 (April 1976), pp. 161–74. A discussion of the high costs of operation faced by hospitals.

MUSHLIN, ALVIN I. and FRANCIS A. APPEL, "Extramedical Factors in the Decision to Hospitalize Medical Patients," *American Journal of Public Health,* Vol. 66, no. 2 (February 1976), pp. 170–72. Examines hospital use, including a consideration of what elements are considered in hospitalizing a patient.

O'CONNOR, ROBIN, "American Hospitals: The First 200 Years," *Journal of the American Hospital Association,* Vol. 50, no. 1, (January 1, 1976), pp. 62–72. A review of the evolution of the hospital.

PHILLIPS, DONALD F., "American Hospitals: A Look Ahead," *Journal of the American Hospital Association,* Vol. 50, no. 1 (January 1, 1976), pp. 73–81. A commentary on the future prospects for hospitals.

Quality Assurance of Medical Care (Symposium by Regional Medical Programs Service of St. Louis, Missouri, January 23–24, 1973. Published by the Health Services and Mental Health Administration, U.S. Department of Health, Education and Welfare, February 1973). A monograph containing practical information on evaluation techniques and standards for patient care.

Technology and Health Care Systems in the 1980's (Washington, D.C.: GPO, DHEW, Health Services and Mental Health Administration, National Center for Health Services Research and Development, DHEW publication [HSM] 73–3016). A presentation of papers by national authorities on medical technology.

11

HOSPITALIZATION
AND THE ADEQUACY
OF MEDICAL CARE

This chapter reviews the larger issue of the hospital and our quest to provide quality care for all. We will identify the limits of society's resources and the problems of defining priorities. We will review testimony on the "technological imperative" of physicians—their instinct to provide the very best care possible. A focal point will be the decision-making process within the hospital, particularly the administrator's task of mediating interests of the physician, the patient, the board, the government, and the community.

THE MEDICAL "COMMONS" AND THE PROBLEM OF DEFINING "APPROPRIATE" CARE

We cannot, of course, isolate the central role of the hospital from the roles played by those who deploy medical resources. The hospital remains an instrument of service, but it is an instrument directed by several hands. Reflection on the role of hospitals must include analysis of those who control the policies.

As emphasized throughout, one of the central concerns of all parties is that medical-care programs are now absorbing an inordinate amount and share of our resources. In the absence of any evidence of restraint, control mechanisms will have to be instituted. In 1968, Garrett Hardin wrote an essay entitled "The Tragedy of the Commons," which has been one of the most widely discussed and republished articles in recent years.[1] The hypothesis of this provocative treatise is simple: society's resources could be likened to the common pasture shared by cattle; the use of the

[1] *Science*, Vol. 162 (1968), pp. 1243–1348.

community's relatively free resource posed no problem so long as the demands on the village green were moderate. But with any sharp increase in the demands on the common, there was risk of overgrazing: while previously the welfare of society was advanced through use of the village commons, there is now the risk that we will destroy the mutual interests of the individual and the community. The prospect is not simply that we have moved to a zero-sum game, in which the advantage of one is simply offset by the proportionate disadvantage of the other. The prospect is that we may be destroying finite resources, with irreparable injury confronting present and future generations. "Ruin," concluded Hardin, "is the destination toward which all men rush, each pursuing his own best interest in a society that believes in the freedom of the commons. Freedom in a common brings ruin to all."

In chapter 10, we reviewed the problem of our excessive demands upon our so-called free resources for medical care. If the paradigm of the common has relevance to the medical field—as some medical authorities believe—we must also be concerned with the unique position of the providers of care.

In allocating health resources, four questions are often posed: What measures do we have to identify the effectiveness of various treatment procedures? Is there some risk that we may, in fact, be exaggerating the benefits of medical intervention, or "overtreating" patients? Are we making excessive use of surgery? And to what extent are we rationalizing technologies, including hospital facilities themselves, in order to reduce costs? Let us briefly review these issues.

Howard H. Hiatt, M.D., reviews the issue of "raids" on the medical commons and identifies several medical practices that are now considered to have no value or an undetermined value:

> One could cite a substantial number of procedures that were at one time practiced rather widely in this country, many of them within relatively recent years, but that have now been virtually abandoned. Such a list might include gastric freezing for peptic ulcer, colectomy for epilepsy, bilateral hypogastric-artery ligation for pelvic hemorrhage, renal-capsule stripping for acute renal failure, sympathectomy for asthma, internal-mammary-artery ligation for coronary-artery disease, the "button" operation for ascites, adrenalectomy for essential hypertension, complete dental extraction for a variety of complaints thought to be the result of focal sepsis, lobotomy for many mental disorders, and writing for aortic aneurysm.

Hiatt points out that most such practices fell into disuse, not because improved techniques were discovered, but only because they were found to be without value.

No careful pilot studies were undertaken to evaluate the.
they were introduced. As a result, even though some merite
tion on an experimental basis, they remained on the medical ⟩
much too long, at costs that went beyond those of the econo⟩
sources inappropriately used.[2]

Hiatt identifies the possible extravagance in resorting to hospitals' intensive-care units, now a well-established medical facility, to deal with
acute illnesses. One study involved patients suffering from pulmonary
edema. Griner compared those admitted to an intensive-care unit of a
university hospital with those admitted to the hospital's general medical
floor. The study indicated no difference in mortality and an insignificant
increase in the length of stay for patients in the intensive-care unit.
(Charges for one day of care at the general medical services of one Boston teaching hospital in 1975 averaged $250; the charges per day for the
intensive-care unit exceeded $400.)[3]

Another area of concern is the practice of tonsillectomies. Some
pediatricians have concluded that over 90 percent of the one million such
operations per year are probably unnecessary. If this habitual exercise
could be confined to only the required cases, the annual cost of $400 mil-
lion could be reduced to $40 million. The conservative estimates of deaths
expected from general anesthesia alone might be cut from 70 to 7.[4]

Questions are also raised about the cost effectiveness of hospital
coronary-care units: there is evidence of cost increases, but only ambiguous evidence of their effectiveness. Hiatt further questions whether
the recent decline in deaths from carcinoma of the uterine cervix can be
attributed to examinations.

> . . . this cause and effect connection has by no means been conclu-
> sively demonstrated. Since the death rate began falling some years be-
> fore there was widespread use of the examination, and, further, since
> the rate of decline has been much the same in different areas, irrespec-
> tive of the proportion of women screened, serious questions must be
> raised concerning the role of the procedure.[5]

As an even more exaggerated example, some 38,000 coronary artery
bypass graft operations were conducted in 1973, at a cost exceeding $400
million. About 400 hospitals have bypass teams. One advocate of the
operation indicated that the United States should prepare to do 80,000

[2] Howard H. Hiatt, M.D., "Protecting the Medical Commons: Who Is Responsible?"
The New England Journal of Medicine, Vol. 293, no. 5 (July 31, 1975), pp. 236–37.
[3] P. F. Griner, "Treatment of Acute Pulmonary Edema: Conventional or Intensive
Care?" *Annals of Internal Medicine*, Vol. 77 (1972), pp. 501–6.
[4] Hiatt, "Protecting the Medical Commons," p. 237.
[5] Ibid., p. 237.

coronary arteriograms a day. If this recommendation were implemented, radiologic costs alone would exceed $10 billion a year. The cost of surgery would exceed $100 billion annually.

In fairness to the medical academy, the testing procedures required to authenticate new medical techniques are imperfect, and they require longitudinal measurement of patient progress and isolating genetic and environmental influences. But the thrust of the Hiatt study is that members of the medical fraternity grow comfortable with existing procedures but do not become adequately aware of their unknown potential for either cure or damage.

Certainly the public must accept partial responsibility for this state of affairs, for it is obvious that the typical American is action-oriented and expects the attending physician to "do something" as a visible demonstration of his technical virtuosity and his concern for the patient's welfare. Herbert Ratner makes a compelling point:

> It is really ironic that the doctor who tells the mother that her sick child does *not* need an operation only gets paid his small house-call fee. For this he frequently has to spend an inordinate amount of time reassuring the anxious mother, parrying subsequent telephone calls and then, stimulated by the mother's anxieties, he may end up spending a restless night wondering whether, perhaps, his diagnosis was wrong. On the other hand, the doctor who proceeds under the principle that it is better to remove nine normal appendices than have one rupture (a bad medical principle) lays his magic hand on the abdomen and rushes the child to the hospital for a "life-saving" appendectomy. For this he gets a substantial surgical fee for a short period of cutting and sewing, a good night's sleep, and is looked upon as a savior. In other words, rescuing a reluctant patient from an unnecessary operation results in much pressure—consumer pressure, so to speak—and a small fee; whereas, performing an operation, even when it is unnecessary, makes one a hero and the recipient of an heroic fee.[6]

The American has also been caricatured as flabby, neurotic, suicidal; as suffering from overnutrition, undernutrition, malnutrition; and as an amateur chemist, a calorie counter, an apothecary juggler, and a vitamin and food faddist, seeking the right combination of pills to set a mood and reshape the body. He is also immersed in the "diseases of civilization," while nurturing the illusion that good health is a commodity that can be purchased at will.

Related to the extravagances of intervention is the failure to appreciate the remarkable restorative capacities of the human body. It is unusually resilient and responds with marvelous ingenuity to abuse. Lewis Thomas makes the point in a colorful fashion:

[6] Herbert Ratner: "Medicine," *Child and Family*, Vol. 11, no. 1 (1972), pp. 7–8.

The human organs' surest tendency is toward stability and balance. It is a distortion, with something profoundly disloyal about it, to picture the human being as a teetering, fallible contraption, always on the verge of flapping to pieces.

As Thomas explains, there ought to be acknowledgment—even celebration—that most of us enjoy good health most of the time. He adds:

The great secret, known to internists and learned early in marriage by internists' wives, but still hidden from the general public, is that most things get better by themselves. Most things, in fact, are better by morning.[7]

Even so, we believe we can improve on nature. The hospital system emerges as a sort of gigantic spa, "offering, like the labels on European mineral water bottles, preventives for everything from weak kidneys to moroseness."[8]

Although this portrait reflects some measure of literary license, it does raise the more profound problem of how greatly do we actually prize our good health? Medical economist Victor Fuchs suggests that we seek good health only to the extent that such measures do not intrude on the pleasurable aspect of our lifestyles. Fuchs explains:

It requires only a casual study of human behavior to reveal the fallacy of their proposition. Every day in manifold ways people make choices that affect health and it is clear that they frequently place a higher value on satisfying other wants; e.g., smoking, overeating, careless driving, failure to take medicine.[9]

We identify "more" with "better," affluence with prestige, and consumption with pleasure. But not all consumption maintains good health. Joseph H. Newhouse and others summarize the case for the limits of medical intervention:

During the past 15 to 20 years there has been little increase in life expectancy in the United States, and there is no reason to believe that increased resources spent on health will alter this situation appreciably. Social factors responsible for premature death—such as poverty, smoking, alcoholism and automobile accidents—are little affected by the availability of health services. Similarly, the major biologic determinants of life expectancy—such as cardiovascular disease and cancer—are not dramatically influenced by current forms of therapy. Provision of additional health care is therefore not likely to influence mortality statistics

[7] Lewis Thomas, "Notes of a Biology-Watcher," *The New England Journal of Medicine*, Vol. 287, no. 15 (October 12, 1972), p. 762.
[8] Ibid., p. 761.
[9] Victor R. Fuchs, "Health Care and the United States Economic System: An Essay in Abnormal Physiology." In John B. McKinley (ed.), *Economic Aspects of Health Care* (New York: Prodist, 1973).

more than slightly unless research advances lead to new therapies affecting several of the major causes of death.[10]

Nor is there convincing evidence that multiphasic screening and annual physical examinations have any pronounced effect on life expectancy.[11]

If individuals are not willing to accept responsibility for their own health, to what extent then are hospital resources obligated to care for problems created by personal excesses? In 1975, 75,000 American males died of lung cancer, more than the total number of victims of the three next commonest forms of cancer; this in spite of extensive advances in cancer surgery, radiotherapy, chemotherapy, and so on. It is estimated that 90 percent of all cancer in this country is a result of environmental factors, with cigarette smoking much implicated.

By way of summary, we make the case that some conventional treatments—including surgery—are unnecessary and add considerably to hospital cost inflation, to say nothing of the human costs. We have placed some blame on the public for its impulse to depreciate the body's self-corrective capacities and for insisting that the physician perform some magic to effect recovery. We have also emphasized that many of the much-heralded new techniques for dealing with chronic illness, such as cancer, have had only negligible benefits to date. Although an advancing society must invest in research and development, including experimentation in the medical field, we tend to forget how some of these costs impinge upon the "medical commons." Establishing priorities for the use of limited funds will require an enlightened collaboration between the government, consumer groups, patients, physicians, and hospital staff. For although the system continues to face unabated claims for attention to medical problems, we must emphasize what seems most ironic of all—that the solution to most medical problems cannot be secured by hospital technology.

THE TECHNOLOGICAL IMPERATIVE

We have continually identified the effort of medical teams to do their very best. This requires not only being attentive to patient needs, but also building a medical facility that allows the most skilled diagnosis and treatment. Some critics view this impulse to disregard costs in the quest for the best as analogous to the "Veblen effect," a form of ostenta-

[10] Joseph P. Newhouse, Charles E. Phelps, and William B. Schwartz, "Policy Options and the Impact of National Health Insurance," *The New England Journal of Medicine*, Vol. 290, no. 24 (June 13, 1974), p. 1352.

[11] B. Bates and J. A. Yellin, "The Yield of Multiphasic Screening," *Journal of the American Medical Association*, Vol. 222 (1972), pp. 74–78.

tious consumption. Here, again, it is difficult to fault medical teams for seeking the most reliable diagnostic equipment, but the critics point out that the costs of much medical technology is spiraling.

The imperative to go "first class" in the treatment regimen builds medical costs. There is, in all of this, something unique to the medical sector. The physician not only does the best with what he has, he also seeks the best. Victor Fuchs contracts such performance with automobile manufacture:

> Automobile makers do not, and are not expected to, produce the best car that engineering skills permit. They are expected to weigh potential improvement against potential cost. If they do not, they will soon be out of business. Moreover, the improvements must be those so perceived by the consumer—which may be very different from those perceived by the engineer.[12]

The impulse toward a single, best procedure is not uniformly true for all fields of medicine. For example, a dentist typically has several treatment options in dealing with an abscessed tooth. He may propose a restoration, with penicillin injections to reduce infection; he may propose root-canal work; or he may propose simply to extract the tooth. If the tooth is extracted, he may propose a temporary bridge, a permanent bridge, or none at all; and his decision undoubtedly reflects his judgment of the patient's ability to pay and his "taste" for restorative work. It is not coincidental that well over ninety percent of dental services are paid for by the patient. This undoubtedly encourages consultation with the patient to review alternative cost–benefit ratios that best coincide with the consumer's perceptions.[13] Such conferral is not always practiced by the physician, possibly reflecting the professional persuasion that he, not the patient, knows what is best. The physician may fear alarming the patient by elaborating on the possible pitfalls of alternatives, even though legal obligations of informed consent press him to that position. Fuchs again reminds us of the physician's unique position in influencing the treatment process:

> . . . a large part of the demand for medical care is determined by the physician. It is the physician who suggests hospitalization, . . . prescribes drugs, . . . orders tests and x-ray examinations, . . . calls in a consultant. . . . Thus, the physician, in addition to being a supplier of medical care, is also the consumer's chief advisor on how much medical care to purchase.[14]

[12] For discussion, see Victor Fuchs, "The Growing Demand for Medical Care." In Fuchs (ed.), *Essays in the Economics of Health and Medical Care* (New York: National Bureau of Economic Research, 1972), p. 66.
[13] Ibid., p. 66.
[14] Ibid., p. 65.

Economists studying the sources of inflationary pressure have noted the "enriched" volume of activities provided by the hospital. Feldstein feels that hospital-cost inflation is not fully explained by increased public demand for services: ". . . a complex of factors has led hospitals to alter their product in ways and to a degree which actually exceeds public desires."[15]

Related to this is the development of expensive "halfway" technologies, the supportive machines that sustain life, but offer no cure for the affliction. We might fully understand the origin of an affliction, yet realize there is no potential for restoring the organ or for repairing it through medication or surgery. We substitute, instead, an artificial support system designed to compensate for, rather than cure, the disease process.

We return to the earlier conjecture that health, or even longevity itself, is not substantially influenced by the investments hospitals undertake. Edward J. Burger, Jr., M.D., of the National Science Foundation offers confirming testimony for this hypothesis:

> What stands out . . . is that, having achieved control of much of bacterial infectious disease in this country, we are now faced with a series of major contributors to mortality which include diseases about which we have insufficient scientific understanding to permit truly effective prevention and therapy. Chronic degenerative diseases and myocardial infarction are obvious examples. . . . we have an additional set of contributors to mortality (such as cigarettes and the combination of alcohol and driving) which, although intervention is technically possible, are outside the classical agenda of medical problems. In the first group, our professional energies are science-limited. The solution to the second group of problems awaits some more definite social decisions.[16]

The ethical issue of the "prudence" of intensive medical care involves, not only complex problems of measuring costs, but also the more vexing task of defining benefits, particularly when benefit calculations are broadened to include estimates of the individual's "net worth" to society. Most physicians would undoubtedly prefer their current professional practice and would advocate improved supportive techniques, whatever their cost. Issues of costs are problems that should worry the hospital administrator or its board, not the medical fraternity.

[15] M. S. Feldstein, *The Rising Cost of Hospital Care* (Washington, D.C.: Information Resources Press), 1971.

[16] Edward J. Burger, Jr., M.D., "The Nation's Health and Expenditures for Health: Thoughts on National Policy," *Journal of Medical Education*, Vol. 49, no. 10 (October 1974), p. 932.

WHAT ARE HOSPITALS MAXIMIZING?

One of the ironic products of the concern over soaring hospital costs is the realization that profitmaking institutions often perform better than their nonprofit counterparts. This has led to considerable analysis by economists, attempting to identify the logic for the improved efficiency and cost performance of private, profitmaking institutions.

One obvious defense is that the profitmaking institutions do much more "skimming." They are much more selective in the patients and/or afflictions treated and are attracted to "profitable" service-intensive, short-term patient care. This leaves to public and community institutions the responsibilities for high-cost, low-benefit treatment regimens.

But economists have been intrigued by the ambiguity of hospital goals, particularly in a nonprofit setting. In the economic analysis of a business firm, any firm foregoing profits to produce to the point where average price of the product or service is equal to average cost will be charging a lower price. Thus, the consumer benefits. But there is anxiety that, in the hospital sector, the patient is not the exclusive beneficiary in this institution dedicated to patient welfare. Why the paradox?

A private-sector service firm, operating for profit, makes price and output decisions to reflect both cost and demand variables. The price it is able to charge will reflect the number of service units in relative proximity to the market, the extent to which the service product is specialized, the ease of entry of competing units into the market, and so on. The varieties of market settings facing hospitals are obvious. Many hospital administrators, more recently confronted with intensified competition because of the proliferation of hospital units, have acquired an interest in marketing techniques—indeed, in the full array of business-administration skills for both cost control and productivity improvement.

The nonprofit hospitals—units usually identified as voluntary institutions—are not typically owned by the government, nor are they in most respects accountable to it. They are quasi-public, serving the public through a board that includes community representatives. If these hospitals eschewed all interest in a "net" return for their activities—for most enjoy the status of nonprofit institutions—they would provide more services at a lower price than their profitmaking competitors. Such theory notwithstanding, there are frequent charges of extravagance in the use of resources, reflecting the uncertain accountability of these institutions. And one "extravagance" involves the allegation identified above: a bias toward quality.

The implications of this can be represented in graphic form. In

Figure 11-1 we represent the equivalent of an isoquant for a hospital. The isoquant represents alternative combinations of quantity and quality of service the hospital can provide, each combination providing a constant total of service. The mix of inputs that can be read from different positions on each isoquant represents the minimum of resources necessary to

Figure 11-1

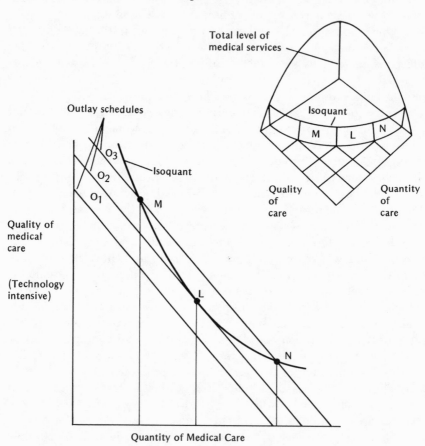

effect a cure. (In reality we have a family of such isoquants reflecting different levels of investment necessary to secure remedies for different illnesses. The more serious the medical problem, the greater both the quantitative and qualitative investments necessary to serve the patient.) In the upper lefthand reaches of the isoquant, we have a service regimen that is quality intensive. This requires specialists and sophisticated medical hardware.[17] As we follow the isoquant down to the right, we identify a mix of services that may be more time-intensive than service-intensive. Such a mix will require the services of a general practitioner and a larger array of paramedical personnel, perhaps with more reliance on medication and the natural restorative qualities of the body.

We compare the isoquant with the income levels, specifying the consumer's purchase of medical service. We represent the outlay schedules of three patients with equivalent medical problems, but with varying incomes. The different impulses of these individuals to spend money for medical care reflects not only their "taste" or preference for such care, but also the discomfort of the illness and, of course, their income. The greater the intensity of desire for treatment and the greater the income, the further from the origin is the outlay schedule. That schedule depicts all ranges of quality and quantity available to each patient as constrained by his income and expenditure decision.

We now introduce the physician, who frequently must determine the appropriate resource mix for treatment. If we are concerned with the consumer having the outlay schedule O_2, the patient is assured recovery by purchasing quality and quantity in combination L. But if the patient has more income, as seen in outlay schedule O_3, the physician may opt for the resource mix M. At combination M, we have a higher quality of service and a smaller quantity. But why would the physician spend more time in patient care than is required? Nonprofit voluntary hospitals operate much like a producer cooperative. The nonprofit status of the producer cooperative does not preclude, of course, the maximization of benefits for those who serve the cooperative. Indeed, the cooperative is often created to maximize the net advantage of its members. As Ryland Taylor explains:

> The voluntary hospitals presently escape some of the discipline of market forces only because the physicians, by limiting their numbers and imposing sanctions on competition, have escaped these same forces themselves. Increasing the levels of competition in medicine is not an easy task. Physicians traditionally argue that an increase in the supply of doctors will cause the quality of medical care to deteriorate.[18]

In Taylor's view, the risk of going overboard on quality care might be reduced if the payment rewards to the physician are linked to considerations of cost—benefit ratios to the patient, hospital, and society. Such considerations are, of necessity, introduced with a group-health

---

[17] This analysis draws heavily on the lucid discussion by Ryland A. Taylor, "Principles of the Economic Behavior of Hospitals," *Nebraska Journal of Economics*, Vol. 11 (Spring 1972), pp. 45–53.
[18] Ibid., p. 53.

plan, particularly those with fixed fee-prepayment arrangements. With the revenue flow fixed by the number of subscribers and typically invariant to the flow of services provided, and with physicians calibrated to "net" returns generated by the system, the economic incentives for the quality bias and proliferation of services would lose some of their force. Participating hospitals and physician teams would be concerned with an "optimal" quantity-quality mix of services, mindful of maintaining consumer–patient satisfaction with the system, along with considerations of providing a net return. With its nonprofit orientation, the system tends to work as a producer cooperative; and the physician's reward is based upon the hospital system's prompt attention to his prescription of a high-quality, service-intensive regimen. His capacity to secure a high income is, in part, a function of the efficient response of the hospital staff, his access to contemporary technology, and the volume of activity this support system makes possible. There may be no clear market constraints discouraging a cost-plus pricing, particularly when physician referrals of patients to the hospital are largely influenced by the supportive position of its facilities, rather than by price differentials of for-profit, nonprofit and prepaid group medical systems.

The above narrative draws our attention to yet another concern of the community hospitals. A key to the patient-referral system is the physician's satisfaction with services provided. With the increase in bed facilities and the general excess capacity throughout the system, it is clear that the physicians affiliated with a hospital wield enormous influence in determining hospital policy. In one account, the hospital staff introduced cost-benefit analysis in urging the closing down of its maternity ward. The hospital physicians protested, explaining that maternity care remained an element in their portfolio of consumer services. The hospital responded to the protests by adding a wing and investing in more facilities for maternity care. If the patient is dependent on physician judgment in securing health, the hospital is even more dependent on physician description in determining to which hospital he will refer patients.

When we look at the hospital administrator as a separate force, with goals that can be distinguished from those of the patient, physician, and community, one senses a strong bias toward size. There are analogies to the sales maximization of the corporate executive, with his relative autonomy from the "scattered" influence of its many shareholders. Administrative personnel, in the private sector, may establish target profit rates and then maximize sales subject to that constraint. Or they may establish management-by-objectives, with moving targets year by year that encompass such elements as market-penetration rates, production volume, sales volume, and the like. Analogies can be made to the hospital, where there appears to be a reflex for increasing bed capacity, increasing staff, increasing technology, increasing physician appointments, and the like.

With third-party payment, federal subsidies for construction, and a pro-liferation of federal, state, local, and community agencies concerned with quality care, the stage is set for an expansionist mood. The rationale for such expansion may be rooted in nothing more complicated than the quest for authority and prestige that accompany the management of a large and expanding, rather than a small and stable hospital unit.

If the community hospital decides to use its surplus revenues for capital expansion—as many private corporations would do—the criticism can be made that the capital market is not allowed its influence in deter-mining the relative profitability of alternative investment prospects. By drawing on internal funds, the issue of returns is bypassed, except as con-sideration may be given to this by the hospital board itself.

Medical economist Rashi Fein supports the view that hospitals have ambiguous, perhaps nonmonetary, maximizing goals:

> A hospital . . . can hardly be considered competitive. It exists as a not-for-profit institution whose behavior patterns are guided by various ac-tors who are trying to maximize a number of nonmonetary performance characteristics, whose accounting systems are constructs that, in part, reflect the characteristics of payors and third parties in particular, whose incentives to economy and efficiency in the light of payment mecha-nisms are often weak. The physician, too, is motivated by goals other than maximization of profit or of income. It is, for example, sometimes suggested that the concept of target income is important in understand-ing physician-price behavior.[19]

In some cases, the charges of extravagance are not confined to over-investment in technology and facility, but are also related to the overin-dulgence of VIP patients and the administrative staff. It is difficult to establish the quantitative significance of individual "case studies" of alleged abuse of hospital revenues. But the *New Republic* picks up on the investigatory reporting of Ronald Kessler of the *Washington Post*. The newspaper study focused on the finances of the Washington Hospital Center, again a nonprofit, "charitable" institution in the District of Co-lumbia. Average patient charge in the hospital was $170 daily. In this 1972 analysis, the *Post* found that 10 of the 38 hospital trustees had en-gaged in conflict-of-interest transactions with the hospital. The hospital had a VIP suite served by a gourmet chef. Such facilities involved a loss of $21,000 a year to the hospital. The *Post* alleged inflated staff salaries: the assistant administrator received a salary of $39,000. The administra-tor received $55,366, along with free use of a Ford LTD and $16,000 for the college education of his children. The chief anesthesiologist made about $200,000 a year because the contract gave him a percentage of

---

[19] Rashi Fein, "Some Health Policy Issues: One Economist's View," *Public Health Reports,* Vol. 90, no. 5 (Sept./Oct. 1975), p. 389.

profits from his department. Men with similar positions, the *Post* noted, sometimes earned between $300,000 and $500,000 a year.[20]

Another criticism, perhaps reflecting not so much an absence of considerations of net return as an absence of complete accounting systems, is the appearance of "whimsical" pricing for various services. Some of the fees charged have little connection to actual costs of operation; these fees may reflect intuitive judgments about what services are necessary and about the opportunities for reimbursement or the patient's ability to pay. In one account:

> Some of the unprofitable departments—for example, the emergency room—are carried at a loss as a public service. The intensive-care nursing units, surgery, and clinics also do not cover the costs. Traditionally, a few departments like medical-surgery nursing, laboratories, pharmacies, and x-ray are expected to carry other departments. Hospital markups of 1,000 percent on antibiotics and pain killers are not uncommon; x-ray fees and radiologists' salaries are astronomical. Clearly, this type of pricing assumes that the user of lab facilities has a greater ability to pay than the user of emergency facilities (often the same person). Is this pricing really a "public service," or is it charging the most for those things customers are least informed about?[21]

HOSPITALS: HOW MANY ARE ENOUGH?

The scramble to shift to state and regional areas the responsibility for planning and the efforts to determine actual needs has not yet halted the pressure of local citizenry for additional hospital facilities. The logic for such pressure is not difficult to understand. Access to first-class medical facilities, preferably with stand-by excess capacity, is one of the prized "amenities" of any community. It is considered as important to the welfare of the family as the quality of schools, the cleanliness of the air, the level of property taxes, and the like. Because of the peculiarity of the commodity of medical services—avoiding the "bad" of affliction rather than purchasing a "good"—the satisfaction of stand-by facilities in close proximity might be likened to the construction of a flood-control facility. The risk factor of a flood may be somewhat lower than that of a heart attack, but in either event, one can sleep better knowing that emergency facilities are at hand. But how do we identify the benefit-cost ratios to assign to such investment when, more often than not, the citizen enjoying

[20] "Prospects for Health Insurance," *The New Republic*, Vol. 168 (February 3, 1973), pp. 17–18.
[21] Alan Reynolds, "The High Cost of Health," *National Review*, Vol. 25, no. 25 (July 20, 1973), p. 784.

the protection is not the same one who pays the taxes to secure them? Just as the insurance principle sharpens the individual's enthusiasm for extravagant medical care, so does the existence of a grant program in Washington encourage local enterprise to secure these funds.

Closing down a major city hospital because of an eroding population and revenue base creates much more political havoc than closing down a university or—to use the classic analogy—changing the location of a cemetery. The authority given to local HSAs to guide and control hospital construction has yet to be fully tested, both in principle and in practice.

THE POLITICS OF ECONOMY AND THE RHETORIC OF PROTEST

We are now confronted by disenchantment with organizations of all forms and by taxpayer revolts against government at all levels. The public has developed a sharpened interest in the performance of the medical sector, not an unreasonable preoccupation for individuals who work, on an average, more than one month a year to support the health-service industry. The political "sensitivity" to the issue of extravagance will become more explicit. A few instances of protest are provided below. Although these criticisms appear shrill, one-sided, and unfair, they help identify the thrust and scale of protest.

Let us note some congressional views. Senator Ralph W. Yarborough charged: "Our health care system . . . is in shambles. We have allowed our marketplace view of economics to govern our handling of our people's health needs.[22] Yarborough charged that of the $63 billion spent for health care in 1969, about $14 billion was sheer waste. Part of that waste was attributed to private insurers, who took over $1.7 billion as their cost of doing business. "Not only does this figure represent an enormously unnecessary bureaucratic or administrative expense and not only does it provide skimpy coverage for most Americans, but it also encourages hospital overuse. . . ."[23] He estimated an annual savings of $575 million in construction costs if we diverted attention to ambulatory care and extended-care facilities rather than hospitals. If hospitals were in full operation seven days a week, he estimated that the average stay could be reduced by half a day and another $700 million saved. Coordinated and consolidated use of maternity and pediatric services would save another $250 million annually. Ambulatory testing for patients before hospital

[22] *National Health Insurance,* Hearings before the Committee on Labor and Public Welfare, U.S. Senate, 91st Congress, 2nd Session on S-4323, September 23, 1970. Part I, p. 2.
[23] Ibid., p. 2.

surgery could save 118 hospital days per 100 patients, for a savings of $300 million annually. Another $1.8 billion could be saved by preventing excessive use of hospitals. Dr. John Bunker of the Stanford Medical School has estimated that surgery could be reduced by some 25 percent, reducing the number of operations by nearly 4 million a year. This would lower national hospital-bed requirements by 26 million days, for another savings of $1.6 billion. He further contended that $3.6 billion of the $12 billion spent for private physician services could be saved if group practices were substituted for private practices.

> . . . If we could initiate 2,000 group-practice programs in the next five years and staff them each with 20 physicians, along with other members of the health team, they could serve 60 million people. That would require 40,000 physicians out of a total of a quarter of a million. The same number of solo physicians, however, could only meet the needs of 30 million people.[24]

Note the testimony provided by John D. Young, HEW Assistant Secretary/Comptroller. A target for federal budget cuts in 1970 was the twenty-year-old program supported by the Hill-Burton Act, which provides funds to construct new hospitals and modernize existing facilities. Young explains:

> It is clear we have too many hospital beds. We have an estimated 25 percent vacancy rate in hospitals, and that raises the costs of medical care. So we recommend no more funds for Hill-Burton, and now Congress has put back some $200 million. Money that is no longer needed.
>
> Now, the department would argue that in certain areas, such as central cities, hospitals are in poor shape and funds ought to be diverted to them. Some of the Hill-Burton money should go for that, but we cannot do that without congressional approval. So what Congress will do, since a lot of people recognize the problem in central cities, is both: They'll keep the Hill-Burton plan and then start a new program at a higher level.

Caspar Weinberger alluded to what Theodore White had called the "Iron Triangle" of fierce resistance to budget reduction:

> The special-interest groups who feel they are benefited directly, the civil service groups who administer these programs and don't want to lose their jobs, and the staffs of the congressional committees who don't want to lose their jurisdictions combine together to create very strong support for existing programs. We don't have a countervailing force.[25]

When confronted with these charges, Walter Mondale replied:

[24] Ibid., p. 3.
[25] Quotations from "With Good Intentions," *Forbes*, Vol. 114 (October 15, 1974), pp. 28–29.

I reject their arguments on Hill-Burton. They keep hanging onto those figures, saying there are too many beds. We say, "Where?" "What kind of beds?" "Are they adequate?" They don't want to talk about that. They don't look at the number of hospital units that are run down and useless, that need modernization. We revised the program five years ago to specify that the money only go to facilities in areas where there's a demonstrable need. They're just wrong.[26]

The United Auto Workers' president, Leonard Woodcock, has also testified about the shameful inadequacies of treatment, considering the very large investments and sophisticated medical technology now in hand. His union's negotiated health-care plans cover some 1.7 million members and retirees. But these plans protect only for episodes of illness treated through hospitals or other institutional services. "We estimate our negotiated health insurance programs presently cover no more than about 50 percent of our members' health costs." The union protested a 50-percent increase of 1970 premiums, and it was calculated that less than 20 percent of the increased premiums provided for new benefits: inflation had absorbed the major part of the increase. When protests were made, the Michigan Blue Cross and Blue Shield mounted an educational campaign to encourage participating members to see doctors and use hospitals less often. Woodcock replied:

> This is a ludicrous remedy to the fundamental problem of the frightening inflation of medical service costs. It goes counter to sound notions of early diagnosis and treatment. It overlooks the fundamental fact that only physicians prescribe treatment and order hospitalization.[27]

Woodcock complains of the myth that the consumer is sovereign in the area of health care. He frequently lacks the opportunity to confer in any detail with physicians about the complexities and traps of the misguided medical marketplace.

There is concern, too, about the quality of existing care. The National Advisory Commission on Health Manpower (1967) studied 15 representative reports on health-care quality. It found the following disconcerting evidence:

1. The Public Health Service National Center for Communicable Diseases makes use of medical laboratory facilities. Twenty-five percent of reported laboratory results on known samples were erroneous.

2. An evaluation of all major female pelvic surgery performed during a 6-month period in a community hospital revealed that, in the opinion of expert consultants, 70 percent of the operations that resulted in castration or sterilization were unjustified.

[26] Ibid., p. 36.
[27] *National Health Insurance*, Hearings, pp. 228–29.

3. The medical records of a random sample of 430 patients admitted to 98 hospitals in New York City during May 1962 were reviewed by expert clinicians. In their opinion, only 57 percent of all patients and only 31 percent of the general medical cases received "optimal" care.[28]

An *American Legion Magazine* article offers the following testimony of disenchantment:

> Anyone who has had to wait three months to see a specialist, anyone who has waited two hours in a doctor's office *after* he got his appointment, anyone who's struggled to pay a medical bill which he thought was covered because he had insurance *knows* that something is wrong.

> No one doubts that we have good medicine and fine doctors. But who wants to keep reading about miracle heart transplants when the business of affording regular shots for the kids seems more and more of a miracle?[29]

To the dedicated health-care providers—and their numbers are legion—the shrill quality of this protest is a source of exasperation and frustration. For every anecdote or statistic reporting abuse, they would cite ten that attest to the professional integrity and inordinate care displayed by medical teams, including hospital administrators. In their view, a popular revolt against establishments, including the hospital structure—traditionally placed on the high ground of professionalism and service—would guarantee tragic losses of quality care for the public.

SUGGESTED READINGS

GORMAN, MIKE, "The Impact of National Health Insurance Delivery on Health Care," *American Journal of Public Health,* Vol. 61, no. 5 (May 1971), pp. 962–71. Perhaps no set of issues clarifies society's involvement in the health-care system as fully as those of national health insurance. Gorman looks at the quality and effectiveness of health-services delivery under an NHI program.

"Health Care Delivery in Rural Areas," from *Health Care Crisis in America,* Hearings before the Subcommittee on Health of the Committee on Labor and Public Welfare, United States Senate, April 7, 1971, pp. 1–7. Discusses health care for rural Americans, for whom services are generally considered insufficient.

KESSEL, REUBEN A., "The A.M.A. and the Supply of Physicians," *Law and Contemporary Problems,* Vol. 25 (Spring 1970), pp. 267–83. A discussion of

---

[28] Evidence cited by Fred Anderson, "The Growing Pains of Medical Care," *The New Republic,* January 17, 1970, p. 16.

[29] Roul Tunley, "Medical Care at Less Cost Is Possible," *The American Legion Magazine,* August 1970, p. 8.

the limited supply of physicians, the resultant costs of health care, and the consequences for efforts at self-diagnosis and treatment by patients.

KILPATRICK, JAMES, "The Hospital and the Bureaucrats," *Nation's Business*, May 1975, p. 11. A discussion of how some doctors and hospitals place patients into hospitals for economic gain rather than for medical reasons, and a review of governmental efforts to stop these practices.

MECHANIC, DAVID, "Ideology, Medical Technology, and Health Care Organization in Modern Nations," *American Journal of Public Health*, Vol. 65, no. 3 (March 1975), pp. 241–47. Mechanic takes a cross-cultural view of medical care's "peripheral effect on health," and discusses the growth and elaboration of medical technology and the related increase in expectations for effective medical care in modern nations.

RAPP, MICHAEL, "Federally Imposed Self-Regulation of Medical Practice: A Critique of the Professional Standards Review Organization," *George Washington Law Review*, Vol. 42, no. 4 (May 1974), pp. 822–49. An excellent discussion of the problems of overuse of medical services and of how PSROs are attacking this problem.

SCOTT, CHARLES D., "Health Care Delivery and Advanced Technology," *Science*, Vol. 180 (June 29, 1973), pp. 1339–42. Stresses the importance of technology in health care, and values the contribution of those developing technology.

SUCZEK, BARBARA, "America: In Sickness and In Health," *Society*, September/October 1973. Discusses some of the emotional, financial, and societal aspects of a major American illness, chronic kidney failure.

THOMAS, LEWIS, "Notes of a Biology-Watcher," *The New England Journal of Medicine*, Vol. 287, no. 15 (October 12, 1972), pp. 761–62. Thomas criticizes the then-new concept of HMOs, from a perspective of our major illnesses as "blind accidents that we have no idea how to prevent."

PART THREE

Current Directions of System Change

12
THE SEARCH FOR PERFORMANCE STANDARDS IN HEALTH CARE

The socialist and playwright George Bernard Shaw fully explained economic theory in his satirical attacks on capitalism and physicians. He complained bitterly of the unjust distribution of output in a private-enterprise economy in which consumer sovereignty or personal income alone determined command of resources:

> A New York lady, having a nature of exquisite sensibility, orders an elegant rosewood and silver coffin, upholstered in pink satin, for her dead dog. It is made: Meanwhile, a live child is prowling barefooted and hunger-stunted in the frozen gutter outside.

George Stigler, a contemporary price theorist, offers a counter parable:

> Dr. John Upright, the young physician, devoted every energy of his being to the curing of the illnesses of his patients. No hours were too long, no demand on his skill or sympathies too great, if a man or child could be helped. He received 2,000 pounds net each year, until he died at the age of 41 from overwork. Dr. Henry Leisure, on the contrary, insisted that even patients with broken legs be brought to his office only on Tuesdays, Thursdays and Fridays between 12:30 and 3:30 p.m. He preferred to take three patients simultaneously, so he could advise while playing bridge (at which he cheated). He received 2,000 pounds net each year, until he retired at the age of 84.[1]

In one of his most famous plays, *The Doctor's Dilemma* (produced in 1906) Shaw charged that "until the medical profession becomes a body of men trained and paid by the country to keep the country in health, it will remain what it is at present: conspiracy to exploit popular credulity and human suffering." Again, he emphasized that supply and demand, not

[1] George Stigler, *The Theory of Price* (New York: Macmillan, 1952), p. 17. The quotation from Shaw is found in *Fabian Essays* (London: Allen & Unwin, 1948), p. 24.

professional ethics or science, held sway. "However scientific a treatment may be, it cannot hold its place in the market, if there is no demand for it; nor can the grossest quackery be kept off the market if there is a demand for it."

When Shaw was writing his satirical essays of social protest, the world population was less than half its present size. A high proportion of children died before they were a year old because of starvation, malaria, diphtheria, cholera, and tuberculosis. Today we still face a *Doctor's Dilemma*, even though our issues are somewhat modified. How do we allocate resources in the health-care field if we abandon reliance on consumer sovereignty? If we do not use the pricing mechanism—and we must not if we assert that health is a right and not a privilege—how are we to ration health services? How do we define "need"? Although biomedical research has produced miracles in extending life expectancies and although we have cultivated the illusion that medical intervention has the ready potential for transforming the quality of human life, economists remind us we are far from the "edge of abundance." These questions are the focal point for the discussion in this chapter.[2]

THE LIMITS OF THE PRICING MECHANISM

Our claims for health-care services are not uniformly distributed, simply because income in our society is not equally distributed. Thus, in the absence of subsidies, people's capacities to command attention to their health problems vary considerably. We have noted that the poor have many more physical and mental ailments and until recently had very limited access to quality medical care. It is a moral imperative in our society that human needs for medical attention should not be denied because of humble socioeconomic status. In brief, the pricing mechanism should no longer serve as the rationing mechanism.

As emphasized previously, the pricing mechanism has been faulted for encouraging geographic misallocations of medical skills. Perhaps it is unfair to blame all such misallocation on this mechanism, for certainly physicians are attracted to those areas where fashionable amenities of life and cultural activities are present. Many people doubt that subsidies can encourage a physician to undertake general family practice in thinly populated areas. Similarly, the occupational distortions, with the concen-

[2] For discussion of current ethical issues in health care see, Lord Zuckerman, "The Doctor's Dilemma: The Right to Health. Choices and Priorities in Research and Development in the Biomedical Field." In Robert M. Kunz and Hans Fehr (eds.), *The Challenge of Life*, Roche Anniversary Symposium Basel, Switzerland, August 31 to September 3, 1971 (Basel and Stuttgart: Birkhäuser Verlag, 1972).

trations in field specialties, may well reflect definitions of accomplishment or status that transcend the pricing mechanism. Pride in a special craft may provide sufficient psychic rewards to offset the attraction of subsidized income for family-practice specialties. These dimensions of misallocation of resources may well reflect cultural rather than economic considerations.

Once we surrender the role of the pricing mechanism—and that is our present posture—we must find other criteria for allocation of scarce resources. So far there has been very little serious discussion of alternative criteria. It is essential to the design of any modified process to specify just what needs are to be served. If consumer income is to have less influence on how resources are allocated, can we simply turn to the health-service providers for a solution? As Feldstein asks: "Should not health be allocated to maximize the level of health of the nation instead of the satisfaction which consumers derive as they use health services?"[3] But how are we to define "maximum levels of health"? If consumer satisfaction is not to be a controlling element in resource use, are we left with only the professional's discretion in dishing out lavish (or niggardly) helpings of health-care services without reference to the appetites of consumers or even the limits of public resources? Again, "if individual preferences are not to be counted, what are the benefits and costs to be weighed?"[4]

The search for purpose in the health-care field may appear tedious simply because good health at first glance is an obvious goal. This, however, is hardly the case. In brief, we have not yet specified the components of the production function of maintaining good health. And the definitional issue of what we want to produce must be resolved before we can rationally plan an appropriate production function.

Countries with nationalized health programs have been forced to provide explicit definitions of the degrees of urgency in gaining access, although a major mechanism (typically unintended) is the queuing process, or what economists have dubbed the "time cost" in waiting for attention. Related to this is a sorting mechanism, through which health professionals must define degrees of urgency of treatment. It is simple enough to define emergency care in terms of preventing immediate death. But once death is not an immediate threat, the screening mechanism may not be explicit. Today, in truth, we are confronted with a series of *ad hoc* decisions, which largely reflect the intuition and values of the physician and related health-care providers.

Our federal government—and the American public—must now deal with these vexing issues. The federal government has hoped to dampen

[3] M. S. Feldstein, "Economic Analysis, Operational Research and the National Health Service," *Oxford Economic Papers,* Vol. 15 (March 1963), pp. 19–31.
[4] A. J. Culyer, "The Nature of the Commodity 'Health Care' and Its Efficient Allocation," *Oxford Economic Papers,* Vol. 23, no. 2 (July 1971), pp. 189–211.

the arbitrary authority of professional judgment by encouraging review by PSROs or by peers. In time, it hopes to prevent the potential abuse of peer reviews by encouraging a majority of nonprovider presence in the Health Systems planning boards. It is hoped that consumer representation will permit a more balanced view of medical needs, with patient interests appropriately blended with technical opinion. It is further hoped that norms of performance can be established nationally, with deviation from such norms serving as benchmarks for investigation and review. Also, Congress has allocated funds for the study of quality standards for health-care services. All these expedients are subject to serious criticism. Peer review, it is charged, is like sending the foxes to care for the chickens. Consumer review is like sending the novice to rate the technician. And the use of national standards involves an implicit admission that the care the "average" patient receives is somehow an appropriate norm for national care.

Obviously, the issue of resource use has not been resolved by shifting authority from the economic market to the administrative or political process. For here we have equally serious questions about the definition of society's interests, including the complex problem of defining benefits to recipients of care relative to the cost of those paying the bill.

DEFINITION OF OUTPUT

The economist conceptualizes the maximization of community health by drawing a community-welfare function. The ideal distribution of resources is represented as Pareto optimality. Pareto efficient conditions exist when the adjustment of resource use improves the satisfactions of some without diminishing the welfare of others. If we could explicitly define the community-welfare function and statistically specify its determinants, we would then be able to identify the mix of services that maximize societal welfare. In a more practical sense, however, an individual's perception of what will improve his personal welfare may not, in fact, coincide with the hypothetical welfare construct of architects of national health programs. There is always the risk that such planners will take a nirvana approach to health-care systems, offering the ideal without reconciling dreams with reality.

Let us briefly sample some of the views of what constitutes good health and of what is required to maintain it. Obviously, good health requires both preventive and remediation activities, for we seek a robust body, lively spirits, and programs that reduce crippling diseases to an absolute minimum. We seek medical-rehabilitation services that are dignified, through institutions that are sensitive and humane. The World Health Organization has concluded: "Health is a state of complete physical, mental and social well-being, and not merely the absence of diseases and infirmity."[5] Sigerist writes that "Health is . . . not simply the absence of disease: It is something positive, a joyful attitude toward life, and a cheerful acceptance of the responsibilities that life puts on the individual."[6] Wylie explains that "Health is the perfect, continuing adjustment of an organism to its environment. Conversely, disease would be an imperfect continuing adjustment."[7] Hoyman concludes that "Health is optimal personal fitness for full, fruitful, creative living."[8] Romano writes: "Health consists of the capacity of the organism to maintain a balance in which it may be reasonably free of undue pain, discomfort, disability or limitation of action, including social capacity."[9] And H. L. Blum offers the following: "Health consists of (1) the capacity of the organism to maintain a balance appropriate to its age and social needs in which it is reasonably free of gross dissatisfaction, discomfort, disease or disability; and, (2) to behave in ways which promote the survival of the species as well as the self-fulfillment or enjoyment of the individual."[10]

These definitions are remarkable in their attention to psychic and social variables, including the individual's capacity to operate effectively in his environment. A healthy individual is one who can avoid pain, but more positively has a joyous attitude toward life's challenges and the ability to adjust to their rhythm. These psychological variables are somewhat removed from the "curative" approach of much of contemporary treatment. And they involve qualities that are often difficult to quantify. There is some distance between society's search for the euphoric quality of "feeling good" and the physician's pronouncement that the patient can be sent home from the hospital. But Seth B. Goldsmith reminds us:

> Just as the inability to clearly define the objectives of any program or organization leads to the operational difficulty of measuring advancement toward diffuse goals, so our inability to define health leads to the obvious problem of not being able to measure health status. This diffi-

[5] World Health Organization: *The First Ten Years of the World Health Organization,* (Geneva: WHO, 1958), p. 459.

[6] H. H. Sigerist, *Medicine and Human Welfare* (New Haven: Yale University Press, 1941), p. 100.

[7] C. M. Wylie, "The Definition and Measurement of Health and Disease," *Public Health Reports,* Vol. 85 (February 1970), p. 103.

[8] H. S. Hoyman, "Our Modern Concept of Health," Paper presented to the American Public Health Association, Detroit, November 16, 1961, p. 1.

[9] J. Romano, "Basic Orientation and Education of the Medical Student," *Journal of the American Medical Association,* Vol. 143 (June 3, 1950), pp. 409–12.

[10] H. L. Blum, "A Working Definition of Health for Planners: Merging Concepts." University of California School of Public Health, Berkeley, 1971, pp. 1–22. Mimeographed.

culty of conceptualizing health is perhaps the major constraint on the development and usefulness of health indicators.[11]

One of the most intriguing issues in the evaluation process is to give reasonable attention to the external variables that influence health. As noted earlier, health officials have been quick to emphasize that disability and mortality often reflect careless and extravagant lifestyles and that the major killers, such as cancer and heart failure, are not subject to known techniques of disease control. If our well-being is sensitive to variables outside of the health-care system, it is not always reasonable to evaluate the effectiveness of our health-care system in terms of treatment.[12]

MEASUREMENT ALTERNATIVES

Good health is inextricably caught up in the web of societal relationships, including the economic, social, and medical. Measures of health must include capacities to "cope." The individual's acquiescence to cultural norms are assumed reasonable parameters of health.

The evaluation of medical effectiveness requires—both for logic and fairness—considerations of all intervening variables. First, there are internal biological realities of interdependence. The effectiveness of surgery to remove (or replace) an organ may well depend on the vitality of related support systems. Thus, the ratings on effectiveness of such surgery must, of necessity, take account of the entire biological structure. A profile of individual health is frequently taken into account in much of the medical care now provided.

Much more elusive are the external environmental conditions, including the quality of life surrounding the afflicted patient. The range of external influences has been described graphically by Victor Fuchs and can be seen in Figure 12-1. We start with the inputs to the medical industry: labor, technology, capital, and materials. Health services provide outputs, such as hospital facilities for those seeking a retreat from worldly pressures. Such consumer-good outputs are not intended to restore health, but provide a sanctuary. Similarly, the industry provides considerable evidence to insurance companies and others about the nature of injuries, evidence used to determine reasonable reimbursements for accidents and the like. Similarly, there is a considerable volume of diagnostic work, in

11 Seth B. Goldsmith, "The Status of Health Status Indicators," *Health Services Reports,* Vol. 187, no. 3 (March 1972), p. 213.
12 Eric Helt and James Pelikan, "Quality: Medical Care's Answer to Madison Avenue,"*American Journal of Public Health,* Vol. 65 (1975), pp. 284–90. "If the provider has no control over housing or nutrition he cannot be held responsible for health outcomes."

Figure 12-1 A Schematic View of the Economics of Health

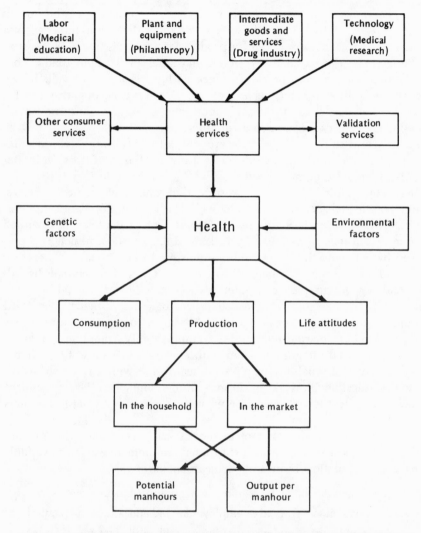

From Victor R. Fuchs, "The Contribution of Health Services to the American Economy," in Victor R. Fuchs, ed., *Essays in the Economics of Health and Medical Care* (New York: National Bureau of Economic Research, 1972), p. 23.

which the "worried well" are reassured about their health. These may not normally be included in service indices for they do not involve any major treatment process. The health of the individual served by the industry is influenced by both his genetic functioning and his environmental conditions. The latter may help explain why the individual suffers the affliction in the first place and may well help predict the pace of his recovery.

Achieving good health can lead to consumption, intended for immediate pleasures, or investment activities involving the production of goods or the generation of income. In either capacity, the qualities of the human agent are tested by use, and in some cases suffer deterioration because of such activity. The major outlet for productive activity is the market sector, although one can reasonably contend that much of the individual's "consumption" of the good life takes place within the home as well. In the economic sphere, the outputs are reflected by improved opportunities for labor-force participation; these opportunities, in turn, increased with improved chances for labor-force productivity.

Several study projects are searching out the full range of variables leading to (or eroding) health. One study by the Northeast Ohio Regional Medical Program postulates that age-adjusted death rates be predicted by hospital discharge statistics, the volume of medical services, and genetic and socioeconomic factors.[13] The Human Population Laboratory of the California State Health Department in Berkeley has studied three dimensions of health: physical, mental, and social. Each is measured by a twenty-three page self-administered questionnaire. There are thirty-three specific complaints involving five types of functional disability and eleven symptoms associated with chronic illness. Mental health is measured by a set of questions on psychological well-being. The third segment, dealing with social health, is designed to map four dimensions of social health: marital relationships, employability, community involvement, and social integration. Goldsmith contends that these tests offer a high measure of reliability of physical health, but with a research instrument of questionable validity. In an oblique comment: "The instrument does an excellent job of measuring what it measures, but what it measures is in doubt."[14]

Conceptually, measures of medical service have taken three forms. The first gives attention to the institutional and human resources available to serve a population. Indices of such care include:

1. physician availability, by region and major professional activity
2. registered nurses by field of employment and educational preparation
3. registered nurses employed for public-health work, by type of agency
4. registered and practical nurses in practice, estimated number and the rate per 100,000 population
5. nonfederal hospital beds by type of hospital

[13] Northeast Ohio Regional Medical Program, Part II: Health Related Data. Section IV: *Hospital Discharge Study*, Cleveland, 1968, p. 25.
[14] Goldsmith, "The Status of Health Status Indicators," p. 217. For further studies, see National Center for Health Statistics, *An Index of Health: Mathematical Models* PHS Publication No. 1000, Series 2, No. 5 (Washington, D.C.: GPO, 1965).

The rapid increase in both the capital costs and human-support services represents an inventory of capacity and skill. Frequently the case is made that the existence of such a resource is a reliable indication of the delivery of services. For example, the argument is advanced that the increase in the number of supporting personnel in hospitals for each day of patient care is an appropriate index of the improved quality of such care. Nevertheless, the existence of such resources requires their effective deployment.

A second measure of service involves activity analysis. Here attention is shifted from the inventory of resources to their use. This is an important step to reality. Indices for such use include:

1. hospital admissions per 100,000 population

2. nonfederal bed-use rates by type of hospital

3. annual physician visits per person, by age and sex

Activity counts are flawed because one cannot always assume that all activity is for productive purposes. Government agencies have been known to simulate activity, to participate in the well-known "numbers game" in order to build an impressive statistical base for more generous funding.

The third category measures output. This is the most important index and, for that reason, all the more controversial. Most attention has centered on mortality statistics because of the simplicity of distinguishing life from death. When one moves to morbidity data, one is immediately confronted with serious qualitative issues. How do we measure varying degrees of sickness, varying intensities of morbidity? How does one differentiate, in turn, the economic, psychic, and social penalties attached to varying degrees or varying classifications of illness? The issue becomes more critical as we realize that individual perceptions of self-affliction vary considerably with socioeconomic status.

As we attempt to remedy affliction and disease, we see an interaction not only of internal and external realities but also of mental and physiological considerations. Elinson, for example, has suggested that appropriate targets for evaluation should include the five "Ds": death, disease, disability, discomfort, and dissatisfaction. A sixth element, "social disruption" has also been considered an appropriate issue for attention.[15] Looking at the more positive side of the same coin, Donabedian, in his classic study, specifies outcome as "recovery, the restoration of function and survival." In further studies, he identifies eleven categories of health outcomes and two categories of satisfaction. He has stressed, too, that the evaluation of the treatment process must consider all three categories

[15] As noted by Barbara Starfield, "Measurement of Outcome: A Proposed Scheme," *Milbank Memorial Fund Quarterly*, Winter 1974, p. 40.

listed above: structure, process, and outcomes. Outcome evaluation must be linked to inputs, and a fair treatment of input measures must consider the available technological and human resources.[16]

Increasingly, it is appreciated that consumer attitudes, including health knowledge, are determinants of health. It is difficult to identify statistically the value of these attitudes, particularly since they may interact in an obscure fashion with the prevention, treatment, and recovery process. This draws our attention once again to the depressing evidence of the consumer's indifference to his personal health.

PERSONAL PERCEPTIONS OF HEALTH AND LIFESTYLES

To what extent can we legitimize public intervention to advance the health of citizens who display little interest in self-care? It is a popular view that preventive care offers the most rewarding of all payoffs; yet the evidence of improved health is mixed, but largely disappointing. (The most frequent customers for preventive care are white married female college graduates enjoying moderate to high incomes.)

There are several explanations for lack of interest in preventive care. First, the individual may fear that prescriptions for good health might require a radical alteration of lifestyle: pressure to cut down on eating, recreational activities, socializing habits, and so on. Second, he may have a genuine fear of what might be uncovered. Even his speculation may set in motion an emotional reflex in which the individual prefers innocence to diagnosis. A third sociological variable is the individual's speculation that health is controlled or determined by external reality, with minimal influence of medical intervention. A scenario is set, in which fatalism plays a considerable role. Probing one's health may only anticipate, rather than deter discomforting sequences surrounding the tragedy of life and the inevitability of death. A fourth reason is the cultural criticisms of those who seek medical attention. There is some social stigma attached to preoccupation with bodily processes. Finally, individuals may be reluctant to invest the $100 to $200 required for a thorough physical examination.[17]

The capacity of the system to ensure or "produce" health requires at least some measure of consumer cooperation or support. The key to eco-

[16] A. Donabedian, "Evaluating the Quality of Medical Care," *Milbank Memorial Fund Quarterly,* Vol. 44, Part 2 (1966), pp. 166–207. "Promoting Quality Through Evaluating the Process of Patient Care," *Medical Care,* Vol. 6 (1968), pp. 181–202. "A Guide to Medical Care Administration: Vol. II: Medical Care Appraisal: Quality and Utilization," The American Public Health Association, 1969.

[17] Several of these observations are provided by Nola J. Pender, "A Conceptual Model for Preventive Health Behavior," *Journal of Public Health,* Vol. 2, no. 6 (June 1975), pp. 385–90.

nomic health is not access, but an attitude of personal concern about lifestyle and consumption patterns.

The Canadian government, in an experimental project involving 1,500 persons, asked each to identify features of their lifestyle, including smoking, drinking, exercising, driving practices ("Do you wear seat belts?"), physical status (including blood pressure, weight, blood cholesterol, presence or absence of high health risks reflected in recent screenings), and the personal and family health history regarding specified diseases. With such information in hand, a computer program was used to identify the "health-age" of the responding individual. Making use of probability tables (including causes of death for each age-specific respondent), the researchers compared the respondent's actual age to his "appraised" age. The printout also provided suggestions that would lead to what has been called a "compliance age."

Take, as an example, Mr. Moderate. His actual age is 45 years. Because he is a nonsmoker, because he drinks only moderately and undertakes moderate exercise, his "compliance age" is only 40.8 years. The 12 most frequent causes of death are checked against his lifestyle. If he fails to follow prescriptions for health proposed by the computer, he is given an "appraised age" of 41.1 years.

In contrast, Mr. Indulgent is also 45 years of age, but has a sedentary job and smokes and drinks heavily. He is also overweight. He has an appraised age of 53.2. If he follows the computer prescription, his compliance age would be 42.7. This is possible if he reduces his weight by 14 percent, cuts out smoking, reduces his alcohol consumption, uses a seat belt, and has an annual medical checkup. By the laws of probability he could extend his life expectancy by 10.5 years.

This program has been used by about thirty private physicians in Canada, as well as by some occupational health groups, to give patients a statistical profile. The purpose is to motivate individuals to change potentially harmful lifestyles and encourage regular medical checkups.[18]

A University of Chicago research team studied differing perceptions of symptoms of illness. It classified three groups. One group was described as symptom-insensitive. These were individuals who failed to secure medical attention for symptoms that physicians regarded as serious. A second group was symptom-sensitive in that they and their physicians agreed the symptoms warranted attention. A third group was symptom-hypersensitive and sought medical care for symptoms that physicians considered trivial. The researchers elicited independent professional judgments of the medical significance of complaints in order to fashion a normative standard for the appropriate response to symptoms. In this project, twenty-two symptoms were identified, including weight loss, in-

18 Louise Rickenbacker, "Preventive Medicine: Helping People to Help Themselves," *The Labour Gazette,* January 1975, pp. 57–58.

digestion, sore throat, "pains in the gut," and so on. The presence of these symptoms was spread over five age categories, and physicians were asked to identify those symptoms that warranted consultation. By checking the actual use or nonuse of medical consultation against physician opinion of whether such contact is warranted, it was possible to construct indices of claims for services that exceeded and fell short of norms established by the physician group.

The study showed that mature adults between thirty-five and sixty-five went to see a doctor less often than they should have. Nonwhites also see a doctor less often than was warranted by medical opinion. Persons living on farms in rural areas are much less likely to see a doctor about symptoms of illness than are persons living in cities (or persons in rural areas not living on a farm). Persons below the poverty level are not likely to see a physician for symptoms medical opinion indicates require attention. People who have no doctor as a regular source of care also fall into the group neglecting medical attention.[19] The physician's definition of the need for medical care suggests far more attention than a majority of our society considers necessary.

There is an awkward contradiction between public pronouncements that we can never invest too much in health care, and the disinclination of many to make even modest investments in personal hygiene. Victor Fuchs has noted:

> . . . surveys have shown that many people do not brush their teeth regularly, even when they believe that brushing would significantly reduce tooth decay and gum trouble. Smokers who acknowledge the harmful effects of smoking refuse to stop, and a group of executives whose obesity was called to their attention by their physicians took no action to correct a condition which is acknowledged to be injurious to health.

> . . . one of the problems that should be squarely faced in framing a social policy for health services is that people differ in the relative value that they place on health. . . .

> A study of low-income Negroes in Chicago revealed very little awareness that a significant decline in infant mortality had actually occurred. This suggests that changes in life attitudes, if they are related to changes in health levels, probably occur only after a lag.[20]

If the collective society perceives its obligation to provide minimal health care for all, to what extent can that society tolerate the ignorance and indifference of individuals to sources of good health already available

[19] D. Garth Taylor, Lu Ann Aday, and Ronald Anderson, "Social Indicators of Access to Medical Care," *The Journal of Health and Social Behavior,* Vol. 16, no. 1 (March 1975), pp. 39–49.
[20] Victor R. Fuchs (ed.), *Essays in the Economics of Health and Medical Care* (New York: National Bureau of Economic Research, 1972), pp. 30–31.

to them? More specifically, does society have an open-ended obligation to offer lung surgery to individuals who refuse to terminate a heavy smoking habit? Is it obligated to offer heart transplants for individuals who refuse to lose weight? Does it have unlimited obligations to provide kidney machines for individuals who refuse to surrender a habit of heavy drinking? Does it have unlimited obligations to render emergency operative treatment to those with a lifetime history of reckless driving? Does it have obligations to provide complete dental care, including oral surgery, for individuals who refuse to brush their teeth?

It is difficult, of course, to untangle ignorance and indifference from the other environmental features that encourage a cultural apathy. An individual with little prospect for improving himself economically may resign himself to a fatalistic posture. The dissipation of hope may well lead to a decay of spirit, which in turn leads to poor care of the body.

LONGITUDINAL ANALYSIS AND POSTTREATMENT EVALUATIONS

Related to this issue of preventive and multiphasic screening is the proposition that the health industry must fully embrace longitudinal responsibilities for individuals following curative treatment. In an appropriate analogy, John Williamson explains:

> To determine the effectiveness of the maintenance of a 707 jet aeroplane, we should not go into the shop, close all of the windows and doors, take an inventory of the maintenance equipment, the tools, the qualifications of our mechanics, the processes utilized in repairing the 707, the check-off sheets used, and what-not, and never look outside to see if the plane flies.[21]

In this "outside" monitoring of the patient, we are confronted with myriad variables that influence recovery. The task is to determine and sift out elements that are the significant impediments to recovery.

Williamson acknowledged the serious limits of internal care, limits that often come to light only after the patient has left the treatment center:

> In one clinic, . . . we found that diagnostic outcome indicated that 70 percent of patients with urinary tract infections were not being diagnosed by the physicians.

[21] Hearings, *Health Maintenance Organizations,* Subcommittee on Public Health and Environment of the Committee on Interstate and Foreign Commerce, House of Rep., 92nd Congress, 2nd Session, on HR 5615 and HR 11728, 1972, p. 1221.

We studied this in detail and found it was due mainly to physician failure to heed laboratory test results. Quality achievement activity eventually resulted in a policy of screening all admissions for those infections, reducing the missed diagnoses considerably.

In another hospital we found that patients were dying in the CCU [coronary care unit] at a rate almost double the expectations set by the criteria. We found the cause to be the misuse of fluids and electrolytes, and the crucial drug Leidocaine. Education helped these physicians improve and the death rate was reduced by half.

In another hospital, we found patients discharged from coronary care units were not back to work one year later, at a much higher rate than we anticipated. We found that nearly half of these patients had not had a coronary to begin with. They had been brought into the coronary care unit originally on suspicion of a coronary, but it was ruled out. But the patient went back home, thinking he had heart trouble, and did not go back to his regular life activity as found a year later by routine evaluation. Follow-up is being considered as a policy in this hospital.

Fourthly, patients in . . . a leading prestigious university hospital had the same symptoms on follow-up four months after discharge from a hospital that they had when they came in. It was identified that the cause was the university staff, when they found there was no organic lesion, discharged patients without treatment and without follow-up.[22]

Such testimony reflects a surprising lapse in the treatment process, detected only after the patient had left hospital and physician care.

ECONOMIC MEASURES OF HEALTH INVESTMENTS

There are perplexing contrasts in both morbidity and mortality rates internationally. The Swedes, often cited for their high suicide rate, moroseness, and penchant for drinking, have a mortality rate (not age specific) for males forty-five to fifty-four of only fifty-two, close to half the rate for the American index of one hundred. Each culture seems to produce its own peculiar "mix" of problems, as indicated in our earlier treatment of these international data.

Increasingly, economic criteria have been introduced into discussions of health care, particularly in the search for performance and output standards. Some studies reveal surprising results. One, for example, contends that much more damage to health is realized by contaminants in our air than can be offset by our heavy investments in health. This leaves us with the conclusion that a more prudent investment in reducing such contaminants might be better than construction of additional hospitals or

22 Ibid., pp. 1224–25.

the training of more physicians. Because we have increased health expenditures dramatically in the previous decade, and because there has been no marked decline in the death rate since the 1920s, questions are being raised about the economic sense of such extravagance. Because there is no correlation between income and health in cross-section surveys in the United States, the conviction grows that we have hit a ceiling in the production function of health care. We are, in effect, running into diminishing returns.

It has also been suggested that we have overestimated the advantage of wealth by assuming that high income begets good health. But the line of causation might just as likely be reversed. Certainly an individual who is in superb physical condition is more likely to be alert, energetic, and have a positive attitude about his job challenge. Where these qualities are rewarded in industry (as is often the case), the quality of health explains, rather than is explained by, income.[23]

The purpose of introducing economic criteria into the health-care field is to make use of benefit–cost payoff alternatives. To some, the uses of such criteria are vulgar in the sense that they treat investments in human health care as analogous to capital investments. The presumption is that we would be able to distinguish rational from irrational investment activity. The rational health-care investments would be made only if there were convincing proof that the payoff of remedies exceeds the cost; and in a more exacting sense, if the rates of return for health-care investments exceed alternative investments, such as capital growth or investments in education.

Behind such concern is the realization that the payoff must typically be represented as a discounted stream of income to be secured by a rehabilitated patient. What is his earnings potential with health care, compared with that realized without health care? Although there are obvious alternative payoffs, the economists are attracted to this bread-and-butter dimension.

We have access to tables that identify the present value of a lifetime stream of incomes for various age groups. The higher the interest rate used for such discounting, the lower the present value of the income stream. Median values of income can be calculated for each age group, and the value of the income path varying with age is itself discounted. For example, with a 7.2 percent discount rate applied, the discounted value of lifetime income for American males between the ages of 30 and 40 in 1960 was $70,515. By age 60, the discounted income stream had dropped to $29,853, and by age 70 was only $9,395. We see, then, that by economic criteria alone, it is much more rational to make investments for those in their prime working years of 30 to 40.

[23] Fuchs, *Essays in the Economics of Health and Medical Care*, p. 20.

Calculations of the benefit–cost ratio of medical services should consider the internal rate of return of such investment. This is the rate of return that will equalize or equate the time stream of treatment costs with the time stream of benefits. As noted above, it is necessary to identify the benefits of such treatment over a time frame. Such benefits can be identified in terms of avoiding more serious remedies requiring, say, the deterioration of untreated conditions. Benefits of treatment should take account of the extension of life expectancy, with a discounted stream of extended income reflecting probable earnings over a probable working career.

Treatment benefits should also consider improvements of productivity made possible by more regular attention to a job. These calculations are not always easy to make even though estimates of potential earnings are common considerations in settlements of liability claims in life-insurance cases. If the person receiving treatment is a housewife, whose contributions of service have not been monetized in terms of national income accounting, some estimate would have to be made of the value attributable to family support.

Even more vexing are cases of benefit measure for children. How does one measure the loss of life or the serious illness that causes crippling effects and lifetime damage? How does one measure malnutrition during infancy that causes irreversible brain damage? The payoff for adequate food must take into account the rewards of "normal" mental development (and its psychic benefits to those working and living with a normal individual). In yet another case, a successful inoculation campaign with a new miracle drug will have economic benefits: it can increase the total labor supply and the effectiveness or marginal productivity of labor.

In an illuminating study, Burton A. Weisbrod attempts to identify the cost–benefit ratios of medical research for poliomyelitis. Although his estimate of a return rate of twelve percent is built on a series of assumptions that many might challenge, Weisbrod points out some of the limits in the attention to economic criteria.

First, research to develop a vaccine for polio undoubtedly involves advances of medical intelligence, with spillover benefits to facilitate control of other diseases. It is difficult to impute a single beneficial output to massive team research on a wide range of issues. Second, there are external benefits of inoculation. The cost of one inoculation must, therefore, consider the reduced prospect of contagion and thus the reduced affliction of other individuals. In one sense, the more general the inoculation, the less the threat of infection to the individual who refused the discomfort or cost of such inoculation. This is analogous to the free-rider difficulty in welfare theory, or the famous "lighthouse" case, in which an individual shipper refused to absorb the pro rata costs of lighthouse construction while enjoying the benefits of its construction. Third, probabilities must be attached to affliction and even to the constancy of income stream with good health. In an uncertain economic environment, the estimates may be subject to considerable ranges of error. Fourth, net benefits of good health must consider not only the contributions of a healthy individual to the advance of the national product, but also his consumption of goods as well. In an accounting sense, the payoff of extending life expectancy should consider the "net" rather than gross advances to the national product. And finally, Weisbrod explains:

> Because of the narrowness of the operational measures of benefits used in this paper, including its abstraction from the pain and anguish accompanying disease, there is little doubt that the real value of the medically successful polio research—and the price that buyers would pay for the vaccinations—is greater than what is estimated in this paper. The "value" of reduced illness and increased longevity is, one might guess, greater than simply the effects on earnings.[24]

As we have noted, exclusive attention to economic criteria has distressing consequences. If we analyze the discounted stream of potential income by age group, clearly persons in their late twenties to forties are the best investment for health, for they have ahead of them a substantial income stream. The very young do not fare so well, because of additional support required until they reach working age. Similarly, the senior worker is a poor investment, for there is a limited time span in which to amortize the investment in productive activity. Indeed, an economist might also want to give attention to the burden of the elderly on the national product, expecting subsistence while currently contributing little to that product. Obviously, economists do not advocate closing down children's hospitals, nor do they repudiate humane and thoughtful medical services for the aged. But they would want to emphasize that these investment decisions reflect "noneconomic" values, including the respect for life, regardless of age and potential contributions to the gross national product.

Gorham has reminded us that the benefit–cost process does not, in fact, constitute a "prepackaged instant decision-maker intended to replace judgment, common sense, and compassion, or turn resource-allocation decisions over to computers." Or as former HEW secretary Gardiner made the point: "We are not dealing with pieces of hardware, but with human beings whose needs are obvious."[25]

[24] Burton A. Weisbrod, "Costs and Benefits of Medical Research: A Case Study of Poliomyelitis," *The Journal of Political Economy*, Vol. 79, no. 3 (May/June 1971), pp. 527–44.
[25] The Secretary's Letter, "The ABC's of PPBS [see below]," HEW, Vol. 1, no. 3 (July 1967).

It is important, however, to begin the task of quantification and, indeed, to identify the criteria necessary for evaluating the output of program planning. We must introduce principles that reflect the values of the community. In an era and in an area in which benefit–cost analysis is rare, there is little danger in excessive quantification or of too much calculation.

In October 1965, the Bureau of the Budget issued a directive requiring major government agencies to undertake a planning-programming-budgeting system (PPBS). Each department was asked to identify its objectives and weigh the benefits of pursuing those objectives with their costs. Budget requests would then be made on the basis of these calculations. The technique is similar to cost–benefit analysis. Ideally, if all programs performed benefit–cost analysis with the same measurement process, it should be possible for public officials to compare a payoff matrix of alternative public investments. In this ratio, the agency calculates the present value of all benefits and subtracts the discounted stream of costs. The resulting "net" return identifies the net advantage of the program. The task of optimizing public investments is thereby enormously simplified. The comparisons are only helpful, of course, if they include *all* costs and benefits. This is the rub: how does one measure the pain, grief, and disruption to family life caused by illness or accidents? How does one identify the payoff of a highway-safety campaign, of the nutrition module in the home economics class, of the brake-testing or anti-smog devices required by certain states? In brief, the major difficulty is the measurement of benefits which are often generational, often benefiting individuals unknown to the recipients of such care. As William Gorham explains, the major issue is intangible benefits which "are difficult, if not impossible to measure."[26] As Aaron Wildavsky has explained:

> If quantifiable economic costs and benefits are not everything, neither would a decision maker wish to ignore them entirely. The great advantage of cost benefit analysis when pursued with integrity, is that some implicit judgments are made explicit and subject to analysis.[27]

Similarly, Rashi Fein has cautioned against complete reliance on benefit–cost ratios. Nevertheless, "it should be sought—for even in the seeking we learn a lot, we think the problem through, we specify things more carefully. It is foolish to reject the attempts to measure and [instead] rely on vagueness."[28]

[26] As quoted by Dorothy P. Rice, "Measurement and Application of Illness Costs," *Public Health Reports,* Vol. 84, no. 2 (February 1969), p. 99.

[27] As quoted by J. Lyden and G. Miller, *Planning, Programming, Budgeting: A Systems Approach to Management* (Chicago: Markham, 1967), p. 387.

[28] R. Fein, *Problems of Assessing the Effectiveness of Child Health Services,* HEW, Occasional Papers, No. 1, Washington, D.C., May 5, 1967, p. 14.

We return to our original theme. How do we measure the value of medical outcomes if we have no price for the services provided and no crisp definition of market value provided by a competitive-pricing structure? If we are left to definitions of need rooted in psychological aspirations rather than effective demand (namely, money), we are confronted with the value identification of life itself. An individual's will and enthusiasm for survival may not be congruent with collective decisions. The inverse may also be true: his willingness to die because of the agony of terminal illness may not be supported by the collective decision of professionals within the medical establishment.

Because of the intense passion most of us have to preserve life, it is difficult to cast the issue of prudent investments within the context of benefit–cost analysis. Consequently, the mortality rate assumes an important position in popular measures of public health. But this can be a misleading or distorted measure of the health-care system. For example, heavy investments might be made in the treatment of mental diseases with no immediate or significant influence on the death rate.

It is probably unreasonable to leave to the physician alone the responsibility for the awesome question of optimal investments in health care. Most of us abhor the prospect of encouraging premature death by responding passively to the needs for care when these cannot be justified by the calculus or "break-even" analysis. In an emergency situation, is it reasonable to ask the physician to be mindful of our scarce economic resources and to limit medical care, whatever its humanitarian rationale, for that reason? Herbert E. L. Klarman properly describes the compulsion to provide full service:

> The clinician caring for his own patients is not expected to assume this posture [of rationing scarce goods] and should not. He must continue to act as if human life and health were invaluable. It is for society to introduce the constraints that make this objective unattainable, if only to diffuse the awful responsibility for decisions affecting life and death.[29]

It would indeed be frightening for patients, struck with critical illness and rushed to the operating room, to find treatment delayed while operating physicians huddle around a desk calculator, discounting the patient's estimated income stream with estimates of emergency-care costs in order to determine whether to proceed with the surgery. Obviously, if resources are available, it is unthinkable that service be denied. There are, however, hard choices that must be made, as the limits of our capacity to expand health services make clear.

[29] Herbert E. L. Klarman, "Present Status of Cost–Benefit Analysis in the Health Field," *The American Journal of Public Health*, Vol. 57, no. 11 (November 1967), p. 1952.

SUGGESTED READINGS

BELLOC, NEDRA B., LESTER BRESLOW, and JOSEPH R. HOCHSTIM, "Measurement of Physical Health in a General Population Survey," *American Journal of Epidemiology,* Vol. 93, no. 5 (1971), pp. 328–36. Identifies disability, chronic conditions, symptoms, and energy level of a sample population to determine how demographic characteristics influence social health.

BERKMAN, PAUL L., "Measurement of Mental Health in a General Population Survey," *American Journal of Epidemiology,* Vol. 94, no. 2 (1971), pp. 105–11. An eight-item index of psychological well-being to measure mental health.

CHILDS, ALFRED W., "The Functions of Medical Care," *Public Health Reports,* Vol. 90, no. 1 (January/February 1975), pp. 10–14. A catalogue of the range of services provided by the professional in medical markets.

ETZIONI, AMITAI, "Alternative Conceptions of Accountability: The Example of Health Administration," *Public Administration Review,* Vol. 35, no. 3 (May/June 1975), pp. 279–86. A commentary on the importance of individuals with presumed authority in determining the forms of medical care to be provided.

HIATT, HOWARD H., "Protecting the Medical Commons: Who is Responsible?," *The New England Journal of Medicine,* Vol. 293, no. 5 (July 31, 1975), pp. 235–41. An indictment of the casual way conventional treatment regimens are established, only to be uncovered later as harmful or useless.

HOCHSTIM, JOSEPH R., "Health and Ways of Living." In Irving I. Kessler and Morton L. Levin, eds., *Community as an Epidemiologic Laboratory* (Baltimore: Johns Hopkins, 1970), pp. 149–76. An analysis of community and its effect on social health.

HUNTLEY, ROBERT R., MARIAN OSTERWEIS, and JULIANNE HOWELL, "Assessing the Quality of Medical Care in Ambulatory Settings," *Journal of the American College Health Association,* Vol. 24, no. 3 (February 1976), pp. 146–49. A study of the quality of care afforded patients in an ambulatory setting, viewing patient perceptions, cost findings, and technical performance.

KASS, LEON R., "Regarding the End of Medicine and the Pursuit of Health," *Public Interest,* Vol. 40 (Summer 1975), pp. 11–43. A challenge to the traditional view that therapeutic expertise of providers can either restore or maintain health.

LINN, LAWRENCE S., "Factors Associated With Patient Evaluation of Health Care," *Milbank Memorial Fund Quarterly,* Vol. 54, no. 4 (Fall 1975), pp. 531–48. Considers the patient viewpoint in the analysis of the care he receives.

RENNE, KAREN S., "Measurement of Social Health in a General Population Survey," *Social Science Research,* Vol. 3, no. 2 (1974), pp. 25–44. A discussion of the research techniques involved in determining the basis for social health.

RICE, DOROTHY P., "Measurement and Application of Illness Costs," *Public*

Health Reports, Vol. 84, no. 2 (February 1969), pp. 95–101. A statistical treatment of the costs of morbidity and mortality.

RUTSTEIN, DAVID D., ET AL. "Measuring the Quality of Medical Care," *The New England Journal of Medicine,* Vol. 294, no. 11 (March 11, 1976), pp. 582–88. A proposal for a clinical method for output measurement.

STARFIELD, BARBARA, "Measurement of Outcome: A Proposed Scheme," *Milbank Memorial Fund Quarterly,* Vol. 53, no. 1 (Winter 1974), pp. 39–50. Examines the issue of what we should measure to determine the appropriate "outputs" of the health-care industry.

TAYLOR, D. GARTH, LU ANN ADAY, and RONALD ANDERSEN, "A Social Indicator of Access to Medical Care," *Journal of Health and Social Behavior,* Vol. 16, no. 1 (March 1975), pp. 39–49. A study of the consumers' perception of their need for care.

13

THE FEDERAL RESPONSE

The federal government—as all evidence on this point makes clear—has become fully immersed in providing health care. It has belatedly recognized that reimbursement provisions have set in motion rapid price and cost increases. There are four aspects to the federal government's response to this problem:

1. the devolution of a Health Systems Agency planning structure
2. the development of committees to review use and quality, identified as the Professional Standards Review Organization
3. support for the principle of prepaid group practice, commonly called the Health Maintenance Organization
4. the development of a national insurance system, with a combination of payroll and general tax measures designed to meet all major medical expenses of the public

In this chapter, we will be concerned with only two of these four programs: the HSAs and PSROs. In a nationalized system, we would presumably still have to deal with issues of allocating resource use and defining appropriate quality standards of care. If that activity is not anticipated before the fact, it will be realized of necessity after the fact, simply because resources allocated for health care would have defined budget limits. Although increases in funding might be anticipated year by year, the finite limits to resources in any one year would compel providers to make the hard choices regarding resource use. Both the HSA and the PSRO are realities, and the HMO is making advances in the face of unrealistic government demands upon their services. Although subsequent legislation may alter somewhat the form of the review procedures for planning and use, the issues discussed here are central to any health-care planning process.

MECHANICS OF THE PLANNING PROCESS

As we noted in our previous chapters, effective planning requires a definition of need and the specification of immediate targets; and these elements, in turn, must take account of the demographic features of the service area. Population characteristics relevant to health services include age and sex structure, socioeconomic status, occupational composition, ethnicity, and educational attainment. It is possible to project morbidity patterns for such populations and hence identify anticipated service levels for health care. Such projections are not likely to reflect fully the present normative judgments of appropriate care, but rather the historic standards of affliction and service. Definitions of need reflect the mixture of consumer expectations, professional judgment, and even access to service.

The supply side of the evaluation process requires an inventory of health services available to the area, along with logistic considerations of transportation access, the impediments of cost, and so on. The inventory includes both medical talent and technology. More complete profiles of the health scene will involve not only cross-section surveys of the existing resources available, along with a summary of present consumer needs, but also trend values over a span of time. This last can anticipate gaps between supply and demand in the near and distant future. As the disparities between capacity and needs are made explicit, one must identify priorities for treatment. There are, of course, alternative means to reach specified objectives. It is important to synthesize professional, technical, financial, and institutional judgments about the most effective treatment strategy, including preventive services, emergency medical service, ambulatory-care service, inpatient service, home health services, and so on. It is in the translation phase that the credibility of the plan meets its obvious test. Plans are not academic abstractions but practitioners' documents: resources should follow need. The purpose of planning is to facilitate that process. Statements abound on the purposes of planning. The American Association for Comprehensive Health Planning provides a position paper declaring:

> Barriers to quality of effective, acceptable, available and accessible care must be removed. They can and should be removed in part through cost containment efforts for facility and operational expenses and investments; but other efforts should be pursued.

> There are other ways of achieving cost containment beyond price/ capital controls which must be also pursued, such as providing ambulatory and home care in lieu of institutional care; budgetary incentives; or environmental-management programs which reduce illness or disability.

[Also, we should secure] better distribution and task responsibility, commensurate with revised credentialing among health workers.

Short-term gains should be invested in preventive programs, for long-term results.[1]

Another classification system of purposes measures effectiveness, efficiency, and equity. Effectiveness is (a) availability of health services where and when these are needed, (b) access to the most up-to-date medical technology and skills, and (c) continuity of care—the coordination and integration of health-center treatment with a recovery and rehabilitation program at home and in the job environment. Efficiency is the production of (a) health services with the lowest possible cost consistent with high quality, and of (b) a service mix most valued by the consumer. Equity is the distribution of services in a fair manner.[2]

The World Health Organization Expert Committee on Health Statistics has advanced analysis distinguishing efficiency, effectiveness, and efficacy. Efficacy represents the benefits to the individual of medical services as reflected by his own satisfaction with such care. Effectiveness, in contrast, represents the objective rather than the subjective reality: it is the outcome of treatment in relation to stated objectives. Efficiency relates the end results to the resource mix (commonly called "factors of production") necessary to provide the output. This input–output ratio represents dynamics: the flow of services provided by organizational arrangements and treatment procedures. The structure, in contrast, represents statics: the resource base available to serve the population.[3]

INTELLIGENCE AND INFORMATION SYSTEMS

The planning process described above, including the definition of desired outputs, will require the collection of information. Such medical information is the foundation for rational planning of resource use. Conceptually, the sequence of gathering and using information can be seen in Figure 13-1. We start with fact finding, and on the basis of the inventory of problems, we identify goals appropriate for treatment. Thus, by study of reality, we identify the "facts" and then determine problem areas. With activities ordered according to their appropriateness for analysis, we

---

[1] *National Health Policy and Health Resources Development.* Hearings before the Subcommittee on Public Health and Environment, House of Representatives, 93rd Congress, 2nd Session, March–May 1974, pp. 521–22.
[2] This classification system is proposed by Verne Gibbs, acting administrator of CHP in Washington, D.C. Ibid., pp. 608–9.
[3] Kerr L. White, "Health Care Arrangements in the United States: A.D., 1972," *Milbank Memorial Fund Quarterly,* Vol. 50, no. 4 (October 1972), p. 30.

Figure 13-1

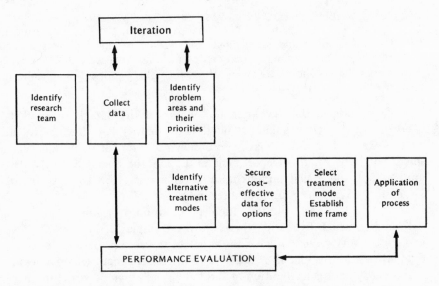

then identify alternative treatment possibilities. These are weighed according to cost effectiveness. The final stage is implementation. Later there is a feedback and evaluation of output.

In all of this, there are methodological risks. First, there is a genuine threat that the data-gathering system will dominate research activities, with the most vexing aspect in the flow process—establishing priorities—neglected. It is commonly felt that if we accumulate sufficient data, obvious solutions will be self-evident. This temptation is particularly serious because of the burdens of gathering data. Demoralization in filling out forms is even more likely if there is no well-defined way in which the information will be used. Those who are involved in the firing line of providing service may not, under the pressures of the workday, find time to participate in the planning process.

There are also the problems presented by aggressive computer salesmen who contract for sophisticated hardware without appreciation of the complexities and subtleties of the medical-care process. The engineer or systems analyst unfamiliar with health-care institutions may confuse matters further, by programming for a flow of materials of only tangential or trivial value to operating and planning decisions. More specifically, there may be an overemphasis on data gathering along with its coding and publication, and a lingering absence of intelligent data analysis. White makes the point with force:

> What is needed is a health intelligence service in the military usage of the term. Information needs to be tabulated, analyzed and arrayed so that it will illuminate problems, pose questions and assist in decision-

making. In the arena of social systems, particularly those as sensitive as health, contemporary values and political considerations are as important as quantitative inputs. Nevertheless it is not too much to expect that information and intelligence will elevate the level of empiricism and improve the climate for decision-making. At least politicians and administrators should be aware of the possible or probable implications of different courses of action.[4]

There are, in the developmental stages of the data base, obvious needs to bring various agencies together to identify key times series in health-care studies and to clarify terminology. Terms or definitions vary somewhat between the Department of Labor, the Social Security Administration, the Social and Rehabilitation Service, the Department of Defense, the Veterans' Administration and so on.

The evaluation of the individual program must be linked to "external" environments. In reality, there are three stages in the flow of services. In the first stage, we have the input to the service pattern—namely, the patient with his mix of medical disabilities. Treatment effectiveness is based partly on a consideration of the individual's genetic structure. Second, we identify activities provided by the health-service unit, including visits, activities, admissions, diagnoses, services, and other treatments. Finally, we identify the environmental and domestic influences that may well affect the recovery status, including access to a home environment of care, adequate nutrition, a regimen that follows medical prescriptions, and so on. The "outcomes" represented by effectiveness of treatment depend on the interaction of these three sets of explanatory variables. Such performance evaluation can be person-centered, with the data analysis following longitudinally the flow of services as their effectiveness is constrained by genetic and environmental influences. Or the evaluation might involve measures of activity or the number of services provided.

Behind these considerations of process is the issue of talent. White indicates that we need to produce a "new breed" of health-care administrator. These should be individuals

> who are prepared, not to preside over line-item budgets and individuals whose only accountability is for their "activities," but rather to use contemporary ideas and methods derived from industry, particularly service industries, to manage what are essentially social service systems. Whether this education is best conducted in schools of public health, medicine, business administration, public administration or industrial management is less important than that it be done creatively, intensively and rapidly. Vastly improved managerial expertise is a prerequisite for any meaningful improvement in our health care system at the operating and geographic levels.[5]

[4] White, "Health Care Arrangements in the United States," p. 29.
[5] Ibid., p. 33.

White does more than call for a new breed of managers. He seeks new patterns of competition, new standards for output evaluation, new forms of industry-wide cooperation, and new public regulation.

THE PLANNING PROCESS

Let us identify major options for improving the effectiveness of the health-care sector. We will offer brief sketches of six options, proposals suggesting that the health-care industry be democratized, atomized, moralized, equalized, supervised, and socialized.

DEMOCRATIZING HEALTH CARE

This policy option is a major feature of almost all reform programs, for it forces the planning agencies to give equal—if not greater—representation to consumer interests than to provider interests. Mandating such representation has political appeal and reflects the vogue of the new consumerism movement. As we noted earlier, the medical market is unique in its deviation from competitive norms. An unusual feature is the surrender of consumer sovereignty to physicians because of their ability to define "need." If the market for services is tight, if technical professional skills are in short supply, if the consumer is somewhat innocent about technical issues and alternatives in a treatment regimen, can we still not give the consumer sovereignty by placing representatives in key planning functions? As we will note later, this is accomplished by having consumer representatives compose fifty to sixty percent of all regional HSA planning boards, with a similar representation at the state's planning council. The PSRO movement provides for four consumer representatives "knowledgeable about health matters" to serve on the statewide PSRO review council.

There are several weaknesses in this structure. Here are some major concerns:

1. How does the consumer define his interests? He has usually only his own and other limited experience to support his counsel. If the market or medical professionals cannot assess consumer interests, how would one expect an appointed consumer to acquire such expertise?

2. How does the consumer secure technical information to deal with the issues of resource use in the health-care field? Obviously, a major effort will have to be made to identify benefit–cost ratios. Will the consumer have the time or ability to develop these insights? Is there not a risk that he will be intimidated by the pronouncements of the professional planner?

3. Consumer interest represents many publics: it is a tormenting responsibility for the representative of all needs to define the appropriate allocation of limited resources. While ideologically attractive and symbolically comforting for patients to realize that one of their own is on the planning council, there is many a slip between nominal representation and constructive influence.

These are distressing considerations. But we should not dismiss too quickly the potential for constructive influence. Consumers, with self-confidence and courage, can give fresh force to the grievances of patients and the perceptions of both the worried well and the worried sick. For it is in meeting the most obvious and fundamental of patient needs that the health-care industry has failed.

ATOMIZING THE HEALTH-CARE INDUSTRY

This option has appeal to many economists who emphasize the constructive potential of economic incentives and the mischief in the health-care sector created by licensure, restrictions of entry, prohibitions of advertising, the compact of silence in physician criticism of colleagues, the unique monopoly advantage of emergency-care facilities, third-party payments, and so on. This policy option requires federal review of Sherman Antitrust statutes to identify restrictions of trade by the American Medical Association. It would include prohibition of AMA control over entry standards to medical schools, the growth of public subsidies to increase the flow of graduates from medical schools, removal of many advertising restrictions, modified job structures with liberalized licensing standards, and the continued growth of outpatient hospital facilities. Generic drugs would be available to patients rather than the brand-name labels of the major pharmaceutical firms. Programs would also encourage the flow of foreign medical graduates and encourage new forms of group practice. Emphasis would be given to expanding consumer education about treatment options, compelling the industry to advertise its product in terms of both price and quality.

Although many of these elements appear a shocking threat to professionalism (and, to many, would certainly erode some of the standards for quality care), we should not overlook the capacity of competitive forces to improve services. With additional emphasis on education, the consumer would have a greater opportunity to discriminate intelligently in his purchase of medical services. It is not unthinkable that hospitals should be required to publish mortality rates by affliction, recovery rates for alternative forms of surgery, the credentials of physicians in terms of years of service and operating success, the rate structure for services, and so on. A medical ombudsman might be appointed to alert consumers of their rights to such information.

Just as the government wants to stop making retrospective reimbursement to health-care providers, so should patients have the privilege of prospective budgeting. They should have access to service-rate information, along with industry "norms" for both professional staff and hospital, and have some reasonable estimate of the characteristic additional charges. Although the consumer's impulse for discrimination is greatly reduced because of third-party payments, it is not impossible to identify the extent to which extravagant consumer demands for service ultimately affect premium costs for health care.

MORALIZING IN THE INDUSTRY

This policy option may seem the least attractive of all, for it involves jawboning and the admonition that providers exercise more restraint in pricing their services. One important aspect of the moralizing theme is exhorting individuals to live more moderate lives. If we identify the overeating, excessive drinking, and use of stimulants as irresponsible behavior, such preachment for "virtuous" behavior can do much to improve general health.

Undoubtedly, many providers would be scornful of any attempt to sensitize physicians, nurses, and others to the service aspects of medical care. Statements encouraging individuals to rededicate themselves—with less attention to pecuniary rewards and more to the psychic pleasure of service—are likely to be received with derisive laughter. The contemporary value structure emphasizes that the good wage represents the good life. The health-care sector has too long exploited, underpaid, and overworked employees. The mood now is to "catch up." Although the moral aspects of physician service are already covered by the Hippocratic Oath, many would be startled by pleas that they extend their services, while being less mindful to personal gain. Physicians now see themselves besieged by the proliferation of malpractice suits brought by hostile patients and unscrupulous attorneys.

It is tempting to dismiss "economics by admonition" out of hand as a rather naive appeal to morality. We lack ethical standards to buttress economic decisions on a price schedule. Few physicians are wandering listlessly through the corridors of their medical facilities, brooding about the excesses of their earnings or the burden of their service charges on hapless patients. Thus, the most promising prospect for this option lies in consumer education in health care, education that can properly center on the ethics of self-abuse and neglect.

EQUALIZING ECONOMIC FORCES

One of the most appealing policy options is to try to manipulate the structure so that interest groups are dealing with one another as equals. Again, this demands improving the bargaining power of consumers, educating them about medical-service options, increasing the alternative modes of health-care delivery, encouraging immigration of foreign medical graduates, and lowering the barriers of access for occupational groups. The strategy is not to atomize the industry, but to create equality of influence.

Its most conspicuous form is the HSA structure, with consumers influencing resource use, and the positive encouragement of the HMO and other group structures for the practice of medicine. The proposition of patient choice enjoys sanction by both the AMA and government. Competition, in this modified form, would have a restrictive influence on prices and cost adjustments, while serving as a spur for improved efficiency in the industry. The "equalizing" tendency does not decry the role of the profit motive, as might be true in moralizing strategies. Profits encourage effective services. The market structure is reinvigorated. This posture draws on the theory of countervailing power popularized by Galbraith. In a more formal sense in economic theory, we have a situation of bilateral monopoly in which geometric demonstrations can be made that equality of monopoly power may produce results that approximate the competitive market.

SUPERVISING THE INDUSTRY

This position treats the producers as equivalent to a public utility, with natural monopoly advantages. We cannot reasonably anticipate duplicate telephone systems, gas lines, postal services, sewer lines, or police protection. Some private-sector industries enjoy "natural" monopoly advantages. The public seeks to protect itself from the abuses of such market advantage by rate regulation. Public utilities are provided a "fair return" through rate adjustments for services. Commission hearings are conducted to examine cost patterns and to grant reasonable markups that assure the maintenance of the capital structure, improved technology, and adequate incentives for personnel to serve in the public utility. The analogies with medical service are persuasive. It is not surprising that the public-utility model serves frequently as the paradigm for health-care regulation.

The National Planning and Resources Development Act of 1974 backed away from previous administration proposals that states be required to regulate health-care providers receiving federal funds. There is considerable difference in flexibility and discretion between contracting for services at negotiated prices and operating within the rate controls of a utility. Apparently Congress felt that rate regulation would represent a precipitous step toward complete control of the industry.

The origin of the cost pressures in health care are fully illuminated in the following description by Paul M. Ellwood:

> . . . when you have a patient who is fully insured and undergoing some elaborate procedure in the hospital, all of the incentives are right for all parties concerned. Under those conditions, the patient, whose bills are very high, is satisfied because all of those bills are paid. The hospital is pleased because it gets to use all kinds of fancy equipment, and is being reimbursed on a cost-plus basis.

> The doctor, who is trained in medical school to do the most elaborate and technically demanding procedures, is gratified because he wins high praise from his peers when he does that sort of thing. The insurance company, which makes money by reinvesting premium income, not by keeping more money than it pays out for health care, also benefits. Thus, it is not surprising to find, as we found in a piece of recent research, that 64 percent of the dollars currently spent for health care in the United States are going for episodes that cost more than $1,000.[6]

Limits of the public-utility model. Is the utility model for rate control the appropriate remedy for the health field? Paul Ellwood, among many others, has many reservations. First, any control mechanism should create incentives for protective behavior among health-care providers. Rate regulations may not accomplish this; indeed they may increase the use of medical resources, encourage the overbuilding of hospitals, inhibit innovations, increase costs, and encourage even more regulation of the industry.

Let us consider the case of Sweden. Under its national insurance plan, each Swedish community decides how many beds it should have. Since the federal government meets construction costs, there is little reason for regional officials to resist the popular enthusiasm for ready access to hospital beds. By 1970, Sweden had from 6.2 to 10 beds per 1,000 population, (compared with 4.5 beds per 1,000 in the United States). The luxury of stand-by facilities would not be decried if it were not true that supply creates a further demand. There is nothing in rate regulation that necessarily discourages hospital construction.

But more significantly, if a definition of a "fair" rate of return is established, the utility can increase its returns by increasing its investments. Rate setting in the airline industry, for example, is based on operating costs, including costs of amortizing capital purchases. The more airplanes

---

[6] *National Health Policy,* pp. 797–98.

purchased, the larger the capital base to justify an upward rate adjustment. As Ellwood explains:

> . . . if incentives are structured wrong, by tying reimbursement to a hospital's investment in capital facilities, then you provide an incentive to create more capital facilities. In the case of airlines, this has led to a situation where one airline has two 747s that they have never flown with passengers, and where the airline's average load factor has dropped from approximately 70 percent of capacity in 1950 to 50 percent in 1970, primarily as a result of this peculiar set of incentives.[7]

There is also the risk that the regulatory agencies will discourage innovation, particularly cost-cutting innovation. This perverse consequence reflects the sympathies that develop quite naturally between the regulators and the regulated. Regulatory agencies often strive for stability and order, and they share the distress of industry representatives with major innovations that threaten the status quo.

> In the ICC, for instance, the introduction of "piggy-backing" came about only after a prolonged delay because the agency thought this packaging practice would disrupt the competition between railroads and give trucking firms an unfair advantage over railroads.
>
> An even more bizarre example was the FCC's decision to approve the construction of an additional transatlantic submarine cable even though Comsat's communications satellite system had ample reserve capacity to accommodate traffic growth, and was demonstrably more economical than undersea cables. ICC's action seemed to be motivated by a desire to protect the existing producer against the economic threat of an advanced technological system, and by the agency's reluctance to deal forthrightly with the issue of "sunk costs." . . . The history of regulatory law is replete with such examples, and the health industry surely is not exempt from their probable occurrence.[8]

A further risk is that regulated rates may in fact produce much higher costs for medical care than might otherwise be available. The airfare for the unregulated Pacific Southwest Airways between Los Angeles and San Francisco is $16.50, compared with the cost of $32 to travel the same distance from Washington to Boston on a regulated line. It has been estimated that consumers are paying as much as $4 to $5 billion annually to "cover" unnecessary extravagances of regulated services.

The economist is also concerned that the rate structure may not have the effect of equalizing demand and supply. If, in contrast to the previous example, the rate is kept at a low level, the stimulated demand may create a queuing problem. This raises once again the issue of priority of resource use, the vexing task of determining who is to have access to hos-

---

[7] Ibid., p. 799.
[8] Ibid., p. 800.

pital beds and doctors' services. If the rate structure does not (in contrast to the arguments above) provide for adequate returns to the industry, delays in expansion will compound the problem. As price theorists never tire of emphasizing, one cannot legislate "solutions" to the problem of human need simply by legislating lower prices. Often these expedients only increase the number of patients clamoring for services, while diminishing any economic rationale to extend supply.

Economists are also inclined to identify the "tarbaby" effect of regulation: it is difficult to contain the web of regulation, once initial rate structures have restricted supply. For with restrictions on supply, the pressures of demand are compounded, setting in motion further pressures to regulate rates. Thus, initial efforts to control hospital rates might well lead to control of physician services, which may lead to programs to control the costs of hospital purchases, and so on:

> If we go one step further and start controlling which hospital staffs doctors can be on, in effect, you create physician monopolies. That brings us back to the beginning of the regulatory cycle again, and would ultimately lead to controls over the fees doctors are permitted to charge, or (as one Canadian province has done) the imposition of ceilings on physician incomes. Incidentally, where this scenario has unfolded almost completely, the rate of medical inflation is even more rapid than in the United States.[9]

It may seem fanciful to build analogies between commercial airline service and medical services, but there is evidence of resistance to innovations in the health-care field too. One state's planning agency rejected the construction of an outpatient surgical center because it appeared to threaten a revenue flow to an existing inpatient surgical center. The proposed center would have reduced surgical costs by one-half. Probably HMOs have been resisted because they might reduce the flow of patients to hospitals. Physicians with established practice might also oppose them, for their patients could be attracted to a more economical service plan.

SOCIALIZING THE INDUSTRY

This policy option can take many forms; but in the extreme case, it means government ownership of the capital and support systems for medical services, with medical personnel working, in effect, for the state. In most forms, coverage is extensive, even though modest copayments at point of entry to the system are designed to discourage the "worried well" from clogging the system. The rationing system for services involves formal definitions of priorities of care, with emergency needs securing im-

9 Ibid., p. 801.

mediate attention. Services are not available, then, on a "first-come, first-served" basis. The extensive waiting time required for noncritical afflictions is a major criticism of the system. Physicians complain of inadequate pay scales, and patients complain of delayed access and, on occasion, impersonal service. We have ample case studies of ventures of this sort in Great Britain, Canada, and most European countries. Health-care legislation proposed by Senator Edward Kennedy also involved a comprehensive system. Paradoxically, evaluations are often lyrical in their praise or devastating in their criticism. Estimated costs in the United States run to $100 billion, and critics have charged that such a price tag is wildly extravagant, considering pressures for attention to other social problems. Advocates point out, however, that the estimate is less than our current expenditures on health-care services: socializing health-care delivery need not involve additional expenditures, but simply a better distribution of existing resources.

LEGISLATION FOR HEALTH SYSTEMS AGENCIES

The federal government has acknowledged that much of existing legislation in the health-care field has fostered a somewhat fragmentary approach to the problem of planning. Such legislation included CHP (Comprehensive Health Planning), RMP (Regional Medical Programs), Hill-Burton experimental health services delivery systems (EHSDS), and area health-education activities funded by RMP. Legislative authority for many of these programs expired in June 1974, setting the stage for reform.

HSA legislation permits the representation of five major components to the health-care system: consumers, providers, third-party payers, health-education institutions, and the government. Its underlying philosophy is to maintain a private health-care system, with strength and vitality assured by additional competition. Competition is to take the form of enlarging alternative delivery systems, including attention to ambulatory care, preventive medicine, environmental health, and so on. A further assumption of the HSA structure is that definitions of priority needs are best formulated by the system itself or, more specifically, by the five elements that constitute the system. Top-down planning, would thus give way to the obligation of localities to define priorities of need and appropriate resource use. A further feature acknowledges that although there are many interests at the local level, these can best be compromised and integrated through a single planning agency. The planning function would be adequately supported with federal funds, and the integration of regional plans within the state would be achieved through state authority. But it was anticipated that state regulatory bodies would rely heavily on local planning bodies for advice in deploying resources for the state.

Each HSA is not required to develop a comprehensive plan to meet the health needs of residents in its geographic area or problem area. It is mandated that priority be given to meet acute shortages caused by maldistribution of health-care services and wherever possible to redeploy such services from surplus to deficient areas.

In all of this, it is clear that the federal government has attempted to remove planning responsibilities from Washington, D.C., with the reasonable admission that the federal structure does not have the capacity to reorganize services to satisfy the full range of consumer and provider interests throughout the country. There is pressure, in addition, to simplify the advisement process. HSA legislation provides for the establishment of a fifteen-member council to advise the Secretary of HEW on national health policy. Federal Health Administrator Frank Carlucci described the embarrassing abundance of committees:

> We have some 368 advisory committees in HEW to the point that some of our people spend most of their time attending or staffing advisory committee meetings. I . . . found that there are approximately 2,800 individuals that serve on these advisory committees. . . . Frankly, if you get too many advisory committees, nobody pays any attention to the product. We eliminated some 90 committees in the past year. We need to eliminate more. As you eliminate them and get them down to where they are manageable, the product of any one individual committee becomes meaningful.[10]

The efforts to secure legislation from both the House and Senate took the form of compromised bill Public Law 93-641, passed January 4, 1975. The preamble to the legislation acknowledged that the infusion of federal funds into the health-care system had contributed to the inflationary pressures. Further, the system had failed to produce either increases of adequate supply or a more appropriate distribution of health resources. Congress identified the following areas for HSA priority:

1. the provision of primary care for medically underserved populations, especially those located in rural or economically depressed areas
2. the development of multi-institutional systems for coordinating or consolidating institutional health services, including obstetric, pediatric, emergency-medical, intensive, and coronary care, and radiation-therapy services
3. the development of medical group practices, health-maintenance organizations (HMOs), and other organized systems for providing health care
4. the training and increased use of physician assistants, especially nurse clinicians

[10] Ibid., p. 400.

5. the development of multi-institutional arrangements for sharing support services

6. the promotion of activities to achieve needed improvement in the quality of health care, including needs identified by the review activities of PSROs

7. the development of institutions to provide various levels of care (intensive, acute, general, and extended) on a geographically integrated basis

8. the promotion of activities for the prevention of disease, including studies of nutritional and environmental factors affecting health and the provision of preventive health-care services

9. the development of a system for uniform cost accounting, simplified reimbursement, and reporting on service use, as well as improved management procedures for health-service institutions

10. the development of effective methods of educating the public about proper personal (including preventive) health-care methods and about effective use of available health services

These are, of course, sweeping mandates.

A fifteen-member health council was designated to advise the Secretary of HEW. Each HSA is expected to have between five and twenty-five members. The HSA has responsibility for establishing a health-systems plan and an annual implementation plan. The majority of an HSA's governing body must be health-care consumers, up to sixty percent of total membership. This majority will be representative of the social, economic, linguistic, and racial populations within the health-service area. The remaining members are providers, representing physicians, nurses, dentists, health-care institutions (e.g., hospitals and HMOs), health-care insurers, professional schools, and allied health professionals. At least one-third of the members must be health-care providers. Membership also includes publicly elected officials, other representatives, government agencies, and persons who reside in the nonmetropolitan areas of the health-service area.

Each HSA has been directed to:

1. improve the health of residents in the service area

2. increase the accessibility and acceptability, continuity and quality of health services

3. restrain cost increases of health-care services

4. prevent duplication of health resources in the service area

Each is obligated to draw up a health system plan (HSP), with a detailed statement of goals, through the use of public hearings. Further, each HSA will coordinate its activities with each PSRO and other appropriate agencies in the health-service area. Statewide Health Coordinating

Councils (SHCC) have also been formed to review each HSA's plans. It is made up, in part, of representatives from each of the state's HSA planning units, again with proportions of provider and consumer representation to avoid dominance of either.[11]

This legislation, with exquisite simplicity, has shifted the problem to local HSAs, with the mandate of improving access to and the effectiveness and quality of care, while inhibiting cost pressures. The obligations cover such a broad expanse of issues that it would be difficult to find any component of health care neglected. Such nobility of purpose requires, of course, remarkable leadership, highly skilled research personnel, and a new spirit of collaboration between agencies and institutions that so often have been adversaries in the scramble for resources.

POLITICAL CONCERNS IN HSA PLANNING

State and local governments have often been skeptical of the "new federalism," which includes revenue-sharing programs established by the federal government. Such programs demonstrate the impossibility of a federal capacity to identify local needs, to set priorities in administering to such needs, and to monitor the output of categorical grants. Even though the legislation was cast to advance local control, the legislation is undoubtedly the first step in a program of national health insurance, with this preliminary stage establishing a local and regional infrastructure.

Provisions of the 1974 legislation were designed to replace the network of technical personnel serving existing Regional Medical Programs (RMPs), with funds supporting the RMP structure terminated January 1, 1976. As the new planning functions evolved, the governor of each state was obligated to confer with elected representatives in all levels of state government. The opportunity for urban control of the planning function was minimal. Mel Bergheim, senior staff associate of the National League of Cities, contended that HEW really wanted to secure "a local outlet for the Federal pipeline, one that could be controlled. And since local elected officials are not easily controlled, HEW did not want them built into the system." He also alleged that HEW was "trying to create a vertical planning bureaucracy totally controlled by what HEW puts in at one end—money."[12]

[11] Legislative provisions can be found in National Health Planning and Resources Development Act of 1974, Public Law 93-641 (S. 2994). Text of Public Law, Statement on the Part of the Managers, and Summary of the Legislation prepared for the Subcommittee on Health of the Committee on Labor and Public Welfare, U.S. Senate, February 1975, GPO, Washington, 1975.

[12] Julie Bingham, "Health Care: Readying the System for Major Changes," *Nation's Cities*, March 1975, p. 10.

The key political issues center on the following questions. How is the planning unit to be designated geographically? How is the planning committee to be formed? What authority will the planning committee enjoy? And, finally, to whom should the committee, as Health Systems Agencies, report?

Each health service area is designed to serve a minimum population of 500,000 and does not ordinarily divide a Standard Metropolitan Statistical Area (SMSA) unless the governor has produced evidence that a boundary incorporating these areas would be unworkable. Consideration is also given to the "appropriateness" of each geographic planning unit, based on such factors as transportation patterns, political boundaries, economic trade areas, and the availability of data. Further, each planning unit contains health facilities to satisfy primary and secondary health needs, with at least one center providing highly specialized health services. The designation of areas is made by state governors in consultation with elected officials in the state's political subdivisions.

With the designation secured, the Secretary of HEW confers with the governor of each state to nominate the appropriate health system agencies. As noted above, the new HSAs are made up of a majority (but not more than sixty percent) of health-care consumers from the area, with the remaining members representing health-care providers. Membership of the governing body includes elected officials in the agency's health-service area.

There is some ambiguity about accountability. State planning agencies, called Statewide Health Coordinating Councils (SHCC), receive plans from the regional HSAs and coordinate these with statewide priorities. The state, through its governor, forwards these plans to Washington.

The authority given to HSAs is extensive. They review and approve—or disapprove—all proposed federal grants, federal formula grants spent by states within the area, contracts, loans, and loan guarantees under the Public Health Service Act, the Mental Retardation Facilities and Community Mental Health Centers Construction Act of 1963, and the Comprehensive Alcohol Abuse and Alcoholism Prevention Treatment and Rehabilitation Act of 1970. HSAs also assist state health planning and development agencies in judging the need for new health services, such as HMOs. Each year they recommend projects and priorities for modernizing construction and converting medical facilities.

There is obvious logic in the federal redistribution of decision-making authority: it gives the federal government an option for doing much less in a situation in which it doesn't know quite what to do. Practically, definitions of need can better be made at the regional level. Nonetheless, the difficulties of priorities and costs plague us, no matter at what level they are determined. The problems, in effect, are not resolved by regional decision making; they are simply scattered. The optimism reflects the contention of the classic liberal that a myriad of "small" decisions will lead to choices that are, more often than not, correct.

There is a characteristic anxiety of the "feds" about local decision. Because state and local governments are hungry (if not starved) for resources, there is much concern that the planning process may divert resources from their intended purpose and end up subsidizing inner-city welfare programs. There is concern, too, about the politicization of local activity: city·mayors, aldermen, councilmen, and county boards of supervisors are eager to find new sources of revenue to support their spending. One might reason that this political crossfire represents the very essence of establishing priorities, for in this situation local needs can be made explicit. But such political pragmatism may swamp principle: Washington, because of its distance from the scene, can often assume a philosophical posture about maintaining "principle" in the use of resources. Local officials, with their feet to the fire, are exposed to a scorching pressure from friends and foes alike.

There is concern, too, about the absence of well-trained planning experts. Each planning unit will have to develop and refine a data base from which statistical dimensions of need emerge. There is a built-in presumption that gaining such information will help resolve ideological issues:

> Developing a solid data base will help to offset the strange stranglehold which all too often is exercised over the planning process by misinformation, fear, ideology, and the tug of professional and institutional politics.[13]

Related to all such concerns is the realization that those with the most technical knowledge of how to deliver health services are also those under the most pressure for alternative uses of their time. Private physicians, hospital administrators, and health-agency heads do not have uncluttered agendas. They typically move from crisis to crisis, with little time for reflective discussion about the philosophy and purpose of overall efforts.

Health providers often view these newly emerging agencies with a mixture of hope and fear. The state political structure emerges as the gateway for the entry of federal funds, and the state itself is required to identify long-term plans integrated with explicit definitions of priority. Many providers see the entire planning structure simply as a maneuver by HEW officials to subvert rather than extend local control. Health personnel participating in the planning process may well resent the investment of time and energy this requires. But they also fear that their own interests are being compromised by the same planning process. They be-

---

[13] Avery M. Colt, "Elements of Comprehensive Health Planning," *American Journal of Public Health,* Vol. 60, no. 7 (July 1970), p. 1196.

come unwilling partners in a process of federal and state intervention and interference with their present practices. But if they fail to participate, they may suffer a loss of influence and authority—perhaps even money.

Does the mandate that the majority of each planning council be made up of consumers detract from "professional" decision making? Is it likely that representatives of the indigent, the elderly, and the ill have authority, skill, and a data base to articulate the perceived needs of their constituencies? How can adequate representation be secured for the myriad interest groups?

These planning exercises will undoubtedly require a redeployment of economic resources. Inevitably, of course, some will believe they have been outmaneuvered by coalitions of adversaries. Conflicts of interest will inevitably develop between professional groups over the appropriate directions of policy:

> It is precisely in the planning process that political elements are likely to come to a head, both because of the planning process opening the operations of the health system to review, and because planning procedures change. Controversy is likely to become apparent even in the early stages of organizing and planning, as well as in the assigning of specific functions. Every major professional group and institution will seek representation in the planning group, will seek an effective veto power in the group's deliberations, and may even try to keep certain matters from being included in the planner's mandate.[14]

Even if the medical market were improved by the dissemination and understanding of medical intelligence and treatment costs, we could not make the comfortable assumption that there would be no disagreement about appropriate procedures. The development of a hard data base serves as a foundation for defining a consensus, but it hardly assures this will be realized. As Mark E. Schaefer points out:

> . . . the information available to expert opinion is limited and perhaps imperfectly perceived. At the present time, no one has impeccable data on the efficacy of various treatments classified by diagnosis and other appropriate variables. In the absence of hard data, it is natural for those active in the field to remember their personal experience selectively in a manner consistent with their self-image and with what they wish to be true. Moreover, in the absence of good information on the nonmedical services which the population consumed, it would be impossible for anyone to properly interpret the relations between medical service input and the resulting health status.

> . . . second, to the extent that the expert medical opinions are obtained from the providers of medical services, there will be an obvious conflict of interest. This may result in an estimate of need which is higher than it would be in the absence of such a conflict.

[14] Ibid., p. 1203.

Third, . . . even if exactly the same technical information is available to everyone, the evaluation of that information need not be unanimous. Tastes and preferences may differ among experts and between experts and consumers.[15]

The advance in planning will require a refinement of each unit's data base. But even if studies were able to identify the ideal cost–benefit ratios for alternative treatment options for health problems, agency valuations of its own effectiveness may not always prove particularly meaningful. More specifically, it will be very difficult for each planning unit to fashion specific standards to sustain normative judgments about relative needs. Patrick O'Donoghue explains the nature of the challenge:

. . . monitoring the quality of care on the basis of outcomes is not simply a matter of setting external standards at the Federal level which can then be enforced by relatively unskilled personnel at the state level. Instead, an effective system of quality regulations involves making relatively sophisticated judgments about not only the necessity for further surveillance and/or sanctions, but about how to best help a provider improve his quality assurance system and the quality of care it delivers.[16]

We should not underestimate the intensity of internal conflict over resource use, particularly if federal funding is reduced. The energies of many highly skilled persons can be drained off in internecine conflict over appropriate patterns of resource use. Funds for experimental or demonstration projects designed to cut across agencies to formulate innovative patterns are particularly suspect:

We learned that if you dangle a lot of Federal money in a community it is possible for them to set up an organization and accept it and to try to use it for purposes it thinks best. I spent some time looking at a community recently that accepted an experimental health-service delivery system—and this community has spent the bulk of its time fighting, quibbling and arguing with the other planning organizations, all of which were also set up with Federal funds, as to whose turf was whose, and what belonged to whom. In many places, the experimental health-service delivery system has further fragmented the planning efforts of agencies sponsored by the Federal government.[17]

[15] Mark E. Schaefer, "Demand versus Need for Medical Services in a General Cost–Benefit Setting," *American Journal of Public Health*, Vol. 65, no. 3 (March 1975), pp. 293–94.

[16] "An Alternative Approach to Assuring the Quality of Medical Care," Statement Submitted to the Subcommittee on Public Health and Environment of the Committee on Interstate and Foreign Commerce, House of Representatives, 92nd Cong., 2nd Session, *Health Maintenance Organizations*, Part IV, April/May 1972, p. 1205.

[17] Testimony of Eugene J. Rubel, Acting Associate Director for Health Resources Planning, Bureau of Health Resources Development, in *National Health Policy* p. 408.

Behind all concerns is a fundamental problem: the absence of a lucid definition of goals by the funding agencies. The political process obliged federal representatives to appear sympathetic to the convergence of pressures in Washington. As these pressures are transmitted, in turn, to agencies in the field, a sense quickly develops that priority must be given to "the world." Initial intentions are dissipated by more generalized statements of responsibility. The more encompassing the obligations of the agency, the more difficult the task of measuring goal achievement. Medical needs are not, as we have emphasized throughout, compartmentalized. It is natural, therefore, that the more sensitive the political process is to consumer interests, the more generalized becomes the definition of agency responsibility.

It is not surprising that the absence of goal definition has been identified as a source of frustration, as we see by the following complaints. Ronald Brand, Executive Director of Health Services Management, notes the assumption that

> . . . there are standards and criteria available to resolve the many issues the local health agencies will be faced with—if only they would use them. I would argue that, for the most part, such standards and criteria do not exist in usable form.
>
> . . . picture a group of providers, politicians and public members trying to decide which of three nursing home applicants in our community should be permitted to build one new nursing home. One of the criteria they should obviously consider is the location of the nursing home. Yet, when we consider location what are we talking about? Nearness to the physician, proximity to the hospital, distance from the patient's family, or location in relation to relatively low-paid workers and their ability to get to the nursing home to provide the necessary care? . . . This is the type of practical problem that the 200 local health agencies will face and we desperately need help in the form of usable criteria in order to do the job.
>
> . . . I am not saying anybody should dictate and say: We want to know the answer. Go then to the Federal government. Go to the experts. Nobody knows. Nobody has done their homework or the basic research.[18]

The dean of the medical school of the University of Arizona, Maurice DuVal, explains:

> We do not have a national health policy. . . . there is no single point of central intelligence operating anywhere within Government that is responsible for shaping policy which others could then in turn attack or support. . . .[19]

[18] *National Health Policy*, pp. 323–25.
[19] Ibid., p. 825.

The significance of setting priorities can be seen in more vivid form if a CHP is confronted with a series of competing demands. Let us, for purposes of illustration, imagine paired alternatives for resource use. In terms of benefit–cost criteria, which is the more rewarding investment?

1. a new sewage-treatment facility or a burn clinic?
2. renal dialysis transplantation equipment or free lunches for poor students?
3. additional jail facilities to incarcerate those convicted of drunken driving or more generous access to food stamps?
4. an antismoking campaign or additional training facilities for nurses?
5. funds for biomedical research or funds for birth-control information?
6. an ambulatory-care clinic or a trauma center?
7. prenatal-care facilities or a hospital-accessibility study?
8. construction of a mental-care center or a crippled-children facility?
9. extended-care facilities for the aged or purchase of an EMI brain scanner?

In reality, the choices do not involve paired alternatives, but perhaps as many as fifty program investments, all of which are ongoing. At the regional or local level, judgments about program quality will undoubtedly be colored by personal associations with staff, by assessments of staff dedication, and by a realization of the importance of sustaining the program. How does one discount the future-income stream of the crippled child compared with that of the middle-aged mental patient? The task of ordering the paired choices grows even more complicated, of course, with the obligation to order eighteen program investments in sequence of their "worth" to the community. It is easy to assert the need for objective criteria to simplify the task of resource use. It is tormenting, in contrast, to make those choices.[20]

THE FEAR OF FEDERAL CONTROL

As we have noted, local HSAs or planning groups forward their health plans to state councils, which in turn offer comment and forward these to the Secretary of Health, Education, and Welfare. The structure

[20] The above choices are even more complicated when one appreciates that the products of programs are not uniformly defined: a mental-health institution contains a mixture of patients, with varying degrees of response to varying treatment strategies. Some respond to treatment, others do not. How does one generalize about treatment effectiveness before the fact?

involves "bottom-up" planning, with initiatives and recommendations emanating from the local agencies. Even so, ultimate authority for funding rests with Washington. Because of this, there is concern that the planning process may be a pageantry, creating the illusion rather than the substance of local control. There is further concern that rigid federal mandates may indeed forestall the states' capacity to make effective use of their existing planning resources. In spite of the emphasis on local initiative, some fear that the Secretary of HEW has secured unprecedented power to direct the delivery of health care throughout the country.[21]

It is not surprising that existing state planning agencies should question the need for the duplication of their planning services. Why overlay one system with another?

The traditional oppressive influence of the federal bureaucracy was also cited in the debates over the appropriate form of the new planning structure. Steven C. Beering of the Indiana University School of Medicine describes the uncertainties of the RMP structure, with the inference that such oppressive influence is part of the pathology of the federal structure.

> In the research lab we can demonstrate that the quickest way to cause cancer is alternate stimulation and suppression of a tissue. This past week I had 11 different policy directives from Washington, all relating to what we should do with RMP. I think from studying RMP across the land that this start–stop mechanism, and the constant change of winds of policy, have caused the equivalent of socioeconomic cancer and chaos in this program. . . . I would welcome having the planning function coordinated nationally so I could pick up the phone and talk with one office and have one set of signals, whether I agreed with them or not.[22]

There is concern about elaborate reporting obligations; reporting costs seldom appear in federal estimates of their own operational costs. Ironically, these may so increase the clerical costs of the operating unit as to become a target for federal criticism. Walter Wenkert, director of an upstate New York Health Planning Council, describes the prospect: "We will receive a package of forms every Monday to be filled out by Friday afternoon. We have, for example, filled out fairly meaningless forms on health-scarcity areas whose eventual purpose remains as murky as the laborious and lengthy process that was needed to fill them out."

Critics have emphasized, too, the peculiarity of structure or the uniqueness of need in the health-care field. Federal guidelines have an inexorable tendency to require uniformity and conformity. Howard Ennis of the Equitable Life Insurance Company alludes to the risk of uniformity in eloquent terms:

[21] *National Health Policy*, p. 316.
[22] *National Health Policy*, p. 331.

. . . it will be a mistake of potentially tragic consequences if efforts to tidy up inherently complex interrelationships to fit some theoretical model have the effect of smothering much-needed sparks of community initiative, responsibility, and accountability.[23]

Diversity of form may, in reality, be required.

PROFESSIONAL STANDARDS REVIEW ORGANIZATIONS

Throughout, we have emphasized the conceptual need to define both the benefits and costs of medical care, and have provided evidence—often anecdotal—of the disappointing benefits of the system. Beyond this, we have provided a concept of analytic elegance to deal with the issue: benefit–cost ratios. Unhappily, there are enormous problems in applying the *technique* of cost-effectiveness analysis to the realities of societal needs. Affirmations of the excesses of quality care, of "moral hazards" and the inundation of the system have raised sober questions about our present strategy of reimbursing costs that providers consider reasonable. But what are the appropriate limits to expenditures? As Clark C. Havighurst and James F. Blumstein have observed:

. . . in health-policy debates perhaps more than anywhere else, the inevitable trade-off between benefits and costs is practically unmentionable. A policy dialogue in which a taboo surrounds any concession to the reality of limited resources is bound to be rich in posturing and assertion and, more seriously, is likely to produce programs whose marginal benefits are not worth their costs.[24]

We are, in effect, stumbling in a somewhat mindless fashion toward increased expenditures, which appear to be benefiting providers more substantially than the public. Undoubtedly the government's present program will be challenged by the allegation that we are collectively squandering an amount much more substantial than an individual would be willing to spend on health care for himself. Enriched providers and even satisfied patients are confronted with protests from angry taxpayers.

PSROs are self-regulatory organizations of physicians, sponsored by the government. They have the responsibility for monitoring individual physician decisions on use of health-care resources under some federal health programs. Congress concluded that cost escalation must be controlled. It concluded, too, that the persons best qualified to undertake this

---

[23] Ibid., p. 711.
[24] Clark C. Havighurst and James F. Blumstein, "Coping with Quality/Cost Trade-Offs in Medical Care: The Role of PSROs," *Northwestern University Law Review*, Vol. 70, no. 1 (1975), p. 7.

task would be physicians themselves. Just as we intimated that the HSA structure was a step toward a national health system, so the PSRO system is one that "is currently gestating . . . to be responsible for scrutinizing not merely a slice of the nation's medical services, but virtually the whole of the $100-billion-a-year health-care enterprise."[25]

The "trade-off" issue is, of course, fundamentally troubling, for in the search for standards of acceptable care for all, we have been drawn to the ideal of quality care, nurtured and sustained by the "spare-no-expense" syndrome of contemporary practice. The physician is less and less a prudent fiduciary agent, serving as custodian of the patient's pocket book, simply because it is not the patient who pays. If the increment of costs to the patient is close to zero, the increment of benefit is also close to zero. In effect, lacking an opportunity or need to determine "full-cost" pricing of services because of third-party payments, there is every economic incentive to push the volume of medical services well beyond the point where incremental benefits to society are equivalent to the incremental costs to society.[26] Havighurst and Blumstein make the point with appropriate force:

> There is, for all practical purposes, no one in the system of insured fee-for-service health care who has acted and can consistently act on an incentive to conserve resources; neither patient nor physician, nor institution, nor insurer, nor regulator, nor government faces, in any true sense, the cost of each procedure at a point where it can be effectively weighted against its benefit.[27]

What is required is the bringing together of individual needs and costs with societal perceptions and costs. That integration is critical simply because, with the move to third-party payments, it is the community more often than the individual that pays the bills.

Can the PSRO structure "solve" this problem? It appears doubtful. But society has few options but to rely on the technical expertise of the physician in determining appropriate treatment norms. The PSRO activity centers on review of service use, but that question inevitably must consider treatment norms. And definitions of what the appropriate treatment requires must, of necessity, consider outcomes. One cannot undertake a medical audit of what the effective treatment regimen has been until one can determine standards for effectiveness.[28]

[25] Daniel S. Greenberg, "PSRO: On the Way, but Where?" *The New England Journal of Medicine,* Vol. 290 (1974), p. 1493.

[26] For a discussion, and geometric explanation, see Havighurst and Blumstein, "Coping with Quality/Cost Trade-Offs in Medical Care," pp. 16–19.

[27] Ibid., p. 19.

[28] Studies of the British health system by A. L. Cochrane raise questions about the outcomes of widely accepted therapies. Widely used processes, whose superiority to cheaper alternatives is in doubt, include tonsillectomies, "Pap" smears, coronary-care

PSRO legislation reflected congressional concern with cost overruns for both the Medicare and Medicaid programs. In 1967, the Finance Committee noted that with the current rate of deficit, Part A of the Medicare program alone would produce a $240-billion deficit in 25 years. It is somewhat paradoxical that the use-review process mandated for hospitals under the Medicare program had not proved effective in curbing unnecessary services. In any event, the PSRO, again involving peer review, has been advanced as an "alternative" instrument to cost control.

The law's purpose is to promote the effective, efficient, and economical delivery of health-care services of proper quality. The PSRO has the responsibility to determine what services and items are medically necessary, to appraise the quality of services so that they might meet professionally recognized standards, and to determine whether outpatient care could be substituted—with no loss in quality—for inpatient care.

The American Medical Association has viewed such legislation with alarm. As a consequence, the Federal Office of Professional Standards Review (OPSR) was set up to explain the thrust of the new use-review program and to elicit the support of the medical fraternity. In this effort, it became necessary for the office to stress that quality (and not economy) was the prime concern of the program. Henry Simmons, Director of OPSR, avowed: "Quality control is the prime objective of Peer Review and cannot be allowed to become secondary to cost control."[29] Simmons also acknowledged that "the cost of medical care in this nation may well rise, and if it does, it will not mean that PSRO has failed. Total cost is not the key issue."[30] Simmons further identified the PSRO as a waste-control, rather than cost-control program, which now provides good physicians with a fresh opportunity to correct unethical practices and to remedy poor-quality care they see going on about them.

The fear expressed by physicians was clear enough. Some fear the prospect of "cookbook" medicine, with imposed standards of treatment that would restrict their discretion. The AMA has charged that local guidelines would inevitably became national guidelines, with treatment procedures so rigidly specified as to thwart consideration of the complexities of individual cases. It also charged that such intrusion by the federal government in sponsoring local peer review sets the stage for federal regulation of individual physician practice. It charged further that the standardization process would have the perverse consequences of reducing innovations and experimentation in the treatment process.

---

units, and hospitalization for routine childbirths rather than home midwife care. See A. L. Cochrane, *Effectiveness and Efficiency: Random Reflections on Health Services*, Nuffield Provincial Hospital Trust, 1972, chapter 6.

[29] American Medical Association, *Peer Review Manual*, no. 16, 1972.

[30] "PSRO and the Quality of Medical Care," Address by Henry Simmons before the Indiana Medical Association, May 16, 1974, p. 122.

Outside the medical academy, the public, too, expressed their concerns. First, if the committees reviewing hospital use were unable to control overhospitalization should peer review, intended to establish standards for use and care, be expected to do any better? Second, with the cultural emphasis on quality, is it not likely that the institutionalization of treatment standards would simply make the quality bias more explicit? As physicians within PSROs press for even higher levels of quality care, these raised standards become part of the review mechanism. The result might be, as Scott Fleming, HEW Deputy Assistant Secretary for Policy Development, has acknowledged, that "the most expensive levels of care would become the norms."[31]

SUGGESTED READINGS

ANDERSON, ODIN W., "PSROs, the Medical Profession and the Public Interest," *Milbank Memorial Fund Quarterly*, Vol. 54, no. 3 (Summer 1976), pp. 379–88. A discussion of the issue in practical terms, emphasizing the technique as a performance-valuation mechanism in the context of moves toward comprehensive medical services.

BEAUCHAMP, DAN E., "Public Health As Social Justice," *Inquiry*, Vol. 13, no. 1 (March 1976), pp. 3–14. A review of major problems in the medical sector, including a discussion of issues of equity.

BLUMSTEIN, JAMES F., "Coping With Quality/Cost Trade-Offs in Medical Care: The Role of PSRO's," *Northwestern University Law Review*, Vol. 70, no. 1 (1975), pp. 6–68. A comprehensive review of the entire subject of program evaluation, including both economic and legal aspects.

BRAUNWALD, EUGENE, "Future Shock in Academic Medicine," *The New England Journal of Medicine*, Vol. 286, no. 19 (May 11, 1972), pp. 1031–35. A study of the shattering stress and disorientation in the medical field.

CAMPBELL, RITA RICARDO, "National Levels of Health," *Economics of Health and Public Policy* (Washington: American Enterprise Institute, June 1971), pp. 41–52. An attempt to provide evidence to explain disparities in health performance between the United States and other developed nations.

KAVET, JOEL and HAROLD S. LUFT, "The Implications of the PSRO Legislation for the Teaching Hospital Sector," *Journal of Medical Education*, Vol. 49, no. 4 (April 1974), pp. 321–30. A commentary on the PSRO from the professional and institutional viewpoint.

KISSICK, WILLIAM L., "Health Policy Directions for the 1970's," *The New England Journal of Medicine*, Vol. 282, no. 24 (June 11, 1970), pp. 1343–54. An overview of the health-care system and an accompanying prognosis regarding its future.

KLARMAN, HERBERT E., "National Policies and Local Planning for Health Serv-

31 *American Medical News*, February 26, 1973, p. 3.

ices," *Milbank Memorial Fund Quarterly*, Winter 1976, pp. 1–28. A critical commentary on health-care planning.

KLEINMAN, KENNETH W., "PSRO: Malpractice Liability and the Impact of the Civil Immunity Clause," *The Georgetown Law Journal*, Vol. 62 (1974), pp. 1499–1513. A consideration of the relevance of PSRO standards for adequate care to the malpractice issue.

LAVE, JUDITH R. and LESTER B. LAVE, "Medical Care and Its Delivery: An Economic Appraisal," *Law and Contemporary Problems*, Vol. 25 (Spring 1970), pp. 252–66. A diagnosis of where the health-care industry is and where it might go.

O'CONNOR, JOHN T., "Comprehensive Health Plannings: Dreams and Realities," *Milbank Memorial Fund Quarterly*, Fall 1974, pp. 391–413. A discussion of the planning process and implementing mechanisms.

PICKETT, GEORGE, "Toward a National Health Policy: Values in Conflict," *American Journal of Public Health*, Vol. 65, no. 12 (1975), pp. 1335–38. A critical essay on the current health-care delivery system.

PSRO Program Manual (Washington, D.C.: GPO, USDHEW, Public Health Service, Health Services Administration, Bureau of Quality Assurance, 1976). Discusses the practicalities, guidelines, and institutional form of the PSRO structure.

RAPP, MICHAEL, "Federally Imposed Self-Regulation of Medical Practice: A Critique of the Professional Standards Review Organization," *George Washington Law Review*, Vol. 42, no. 4 (May 1974), pp. 822–49. Analyzes the intended thrust of the PSRO program and some of its problems in practical terms.

REINHARDT, UWE E., "Proposed Changes in the Organization of Health Care Delivery: An Overview and Critique," *Milbank Memorial Fund Quarterly*, Vol. 57, no. 2 (Spring 1973), pp. 169–222. A survey that identifies related research materials concerning the organization of the health-care system.

14
THE CASE FOR
HEALTH-MAINTENANCE
ORGANIZATIONS

The prepaid group practice or health maintenance organization movement has been described as a technological and organizational revolution now sweeping the health-care industry. Apostles of the movement truly display a religious fervor and are inclined to the view that disbelievers are not corrupted by the devil, but have not read the scriptures. The problem in securing the conversion is one of education, not of confrontation. In this section, we will outline themes that are important to the movement. Our purpose is to identify reasons that the movement has achieved success and is gaining momentum.

PRELIMINARY PHILOSOPHICAL PERSPECTIVES

The HMO movement enjoys support because it is philosophically and ideologically "clean." By that we mean it is not a program that conjures up images of disruption or demolition of the existing system, the enslavement of physicians, the extension of federal bureaucracy, the entrapment of patients, the centralization of services, the socialization of the industry, or the erosion of health-care services. The program is "for" diversity of form, local autonomy, self-sufficiency, minimal government intrusions, and physician definition of quality care. But most importantly, the program is "for" health. Economic incentives are inverted in that rewards are provided for the *prevention* of illness, for the *maintenance* of health.

To be "for" health under a new reward system creates the inference that, under traditional fee-for-service, providers profit from affliction and are thus "for" disease. This, in the mind of many physicians, is a cruel and unwarranted dichotomy. In their view, their remediation activities are designed to restore health. To expiate the evil of illness is equivalent to being "for" virtue. But not so, say HMO apostles. As one explains:

> Changes come slowly in the medical system because the system works for everyone but the patient. The sicker you are, the better off I, as a health-insurance salesman, am, the better off the doctor is, and the better off the hospital. Under the health maintenance concept, the better off you are, the better off I am.[1]

If this be regarded as yellow journalism or an unfair assault on physician practices, the President's health message of November 18, 1971, captured the same view:

> Under traditional systems, doctors and hospitals are paid, in effect, on a piecework basis. The more illnesses they treat—and the more service they render—the more their income rises. This does not mean, of course, that they do any less than their very best to make people well. But it does mean that there is no economic incentive for them to concentrate on keeping people healthy.[2]

The physician feels that his obligation to serve transcends the pricing mechanism, and that the profession is vulgarized, in effect, by intimations that service can be improved by rewarding the maintenance of health rather than the remediation of disease. As we noted earlier, preventive and maintenance functions require, almost totally, motivations to improve the individual's lifestyle. The technical virtuosity of the physician cannot affect that issue. The challenge confronting the HMO movement is to bridge the gap. "Health" is no longer defined only as the successful removal of a cancerous lung: it is also the prevention of lung cancer. Health is no longer defined in terms of the antiseptic operating room: it is defined as an individual's capacity to function—and survive—in a society that is less than antiseptic. This is the philosophic taproot of the HMO movement.

As we have made the point above, few physicians are opposed to preventive medicine, but may speak scornfully of its feasibility. The arguments can be reduced to the basic proposition that people simply don't care: they discount long-term survival in pursuit of short-term pleasures; they cultivate the illusion they are immortal, no matter what they do.

The HMO movement is not discouraged by the frequent charge that individuals—and not the health industry—are to be faulted for our poor health. We need preventive strategies, and certainly fall-back remedies when preventive techniques fail. Consumer education on personal body care is not an unnatural, illogical, or unreasonable extension of activity for those who "manufacture" health. The ingenuity of the HMO

[1] Jay Kobler, "A Reasonable Alternative," *Best's Review*, no. 75 (June 1974), p. 34.
[2] U.S. Congress, House Document 49, 92nd Congress, *Health Message from the President of the United States*, February 18, 1971.

movement is the rewards it places on maintaining health and the penalties placed on both the system and the individual when good health fails. Whether consumer attitudes can, in fact, be affected if major portions of the health industry would have a vested interest in sustaining health remains to be proved. To charge that most individuals display an appalling indifference to health does not logically prove the point that public attitudes cannot or should not be changed.

In our search for criticism of the HMO movement, we classified sources of anxiety for the physician and the consumer. Let us maintain that classification system in viewing the inducements of the HMO to both the physician and the consumer.

PHYSICIAN ATTRACTIONS TO THE HMO

We have previously noted that the prospects for the HMO movement would reflect the willingness of physicians to participate in this venture. Physician attitudes, though critical to the growth of the movement, have not been subject to much systematic study. Objective evidence of physician satisfaction may be inferred from the ease of their recruitment into group practice and their modest turnover rates. Discussions of physician satisfaction (and dissatisfaction) have been largely confined to the Kaiser-Permanente experiences, and even here the narrative tends to be intuitive and suggestive, rather than formal or statistical. Such paucity of data may indicate a reluctance of physicians to reveal innermost thoughts about the satisfactions of practice; it may reflect the reluctance of some to speak "for the record" about the HMO innovation. Criticisms may offend their peers in group practice; adulation may offend their peers in the AMA. Or it may simply reflect the physician's preoccupation with his medical practice, with little time for reflection about sources of satisfaction.

In a University of Illinois study of 584 medical students, students were asked whether they would like to practice with an HMO (prepaid group) practice. Forty-four percent indicated yes, 10 percent no; the remainder were uncertain. When asked about career interests or service in a foundation plan (involving prepayment but fee-for-service), students expressed less interest: 10 percent favored such participation, 24 percent did not. The rest were uncertain.

A follow-up study of interns and residents was made to determine whether the completion of schooling had changed attitudes about the desirability of group practice. The evidence indicated essentially the same attitudes.

A further study involved views of those attending the University of

Florida Medical School and those attending Duke University and the University of Chicago Medical Schools. There was consistency with the earlier studies. Fifty-five percent of the students indicated a preference for a group-practice setting. Forty-five percent indicated no.[3] Thus, the balance of interests favored prepaid group practice, a remarkable measure of support when one considers the frequent allegations of physician ignorance of prepayment plans and their concerns about the restrictive nature of such group practices.[4]

A more significant index of physician support can be found in the problems of recruiting staff for group-practice plans. Problems of recruitment, though they have become less difficult in recent years, reflect the attractive earning opportunities elsewhere for particular specialties. The liberalization of abortion provisions has, for example, created a strong demand for gynecologists. There has been a persistent difficulty in recruiting anethesiologists, some of whom are making well over $150,000 annually. Matching these salaries poses obvious challenges to the relatively fixed budgets of an HMO program.[5]

One field report on the problem of staffing group plans is offered by Greer Williams. He notes that all regions feel the national medical manpower pinch, some groups and some specialities far more than others. One northern California physician-in-chief said, "Recruiting is the major stumbling block in our growth. Doctors are leaving our group for more money." Another northern California physician-in-chief said his hospital did not suffer any shortage but added, "We could use another neurologist,

[3] These data are provided by Paul M. Ellwood, Jr., Hearings before the Subcommittee on Public Health and Environment of the Committee on Interstate and Foreign Commerce, House of Representatives, 92nd Congress, 2nd session, April and May 1972. Part 2: *Health Maintenance Organizations*, p. 395. This source is hereinafter represented as Hearings, *Health Maintenance Organizations*.

[4] Russell B. Roth of the American Medical Association reported a contrasting view. At the University of Indiana School of Medicine, he discussed various administration proposals on health care with medical students. One posed the following concern. "I am a graduate. I have a college degree and I am now in medicine. I have to finish medical school. I have to take an internship and probably a residency. I am doing it all on borrowed money. I am not the smartest person in the university. What is the future of medicine? As you paint it, under the conditions in which it is proposed that I practice, I fear I'll become like a technician in a public utility. Is it worth my time to go through with this?" The room broke out in applause. Hearings, *Health Maintenance Organizations*, 1972, Part 2, p. 346.

[5] The reports from medical directors of group practice organizations in the 1950s and early 1960s acknowledged the difficulties of recruiting an adequate number of physicians; recent reports indicate that the only difficulty arises from the present inadequate supply of physicians and that recruitment for PGP (prepaid group programs) has become relatively successful. Merwyn R. Greenlick, "The Impact of Prepaid Group Practice on American Medical Care: A Critical Evaluation," *The Annals of the American Academy of Political and Social Science*, Vol. 399 (January 1972), p. 107.

otolaryngologist, ophthalmologist, and a radiologist." These specialities appear to be in short supply everywhere. Orthopedic surgeons are among the hardest to recruit, for resident training in this field has been highly restricted and income opportunities exceed the Permanente income scale. There is a brisk demand for internists and pediatricians, who carry the bulk of primary-care load, and also for general practitioners to run satellite clinics. There are standard shortages of radiologists and anaesthesiologists; much less so of urologists and pathologists.[6]

A second piece of objective evidence is the turnover of physicians in group practice. One would reasonably conclude that if job attractions were minimal, the tight labor market would encourage physicians to seek out more favorable alternatives. In the Permanente plan, recruitment involves seeking out evidence of technical competency and a capacity for verbal facility in communication with patients and associates. Preferred candidates are those who are articulate and have an outgoing personality. There is a probationary period for accepted candidates from one to three years, depending on the region.

The regional Medical Group's executive committee periodically reviews the work of each staff member. The doctor can judge how well he is viewed in the eyes of the committee by whether he gets raises in pay. If he doesn't his opportunity for partnership is delayed or foreclosed. The turnover in the first year is from eight to fourteen percent, but falls to under one percent annually after partnership is achieved.[7]

In one view, the physician most likely to be attracted to group practice is one whose professional interests take priority over top income. Group plans can appeal to one's sense of altruism. Robert Gumbiner, Executive Director of the Family Health Program of Long Beach, California, complains of the lack of social responsibility in many medical school graduates.

> Through our ongoing recruiting of doctors and after discussing this with several deans of medical schools, I have come to the conclusion that not more than 3 to 5 percent of the physicians will, after finishing their residencies, retain a sense of social responsibility. Why should they? Until the reward system changes, the type of emerging physician will not change. We are faced with working with what we have. It would be naive to think that we have a supply of a different kind of doctor.[8]

Gumbiner did not indicate whether the distortions of the existing system reflected excessive pay of solo practice or inadequate pay in group prac-

---

[6] Testimony provided in Greer Williams, "Kaiser: What Is It? How Does It Work?" *Modern Hospital*, Vol. 116 (February 1971), p. 78.

[7] Ibid., p. 75.

[8] Hearings, *Health Maintenance Organizations*, Vol. 2 (May 3, 1972), p. 602.

tice, or whether the fault of the value structure was with the interest in pay in both systems.

Some physicians attest that one of the most desired features of group practice is the opportunity to set aside the calculus of patient income in defining an appropriate treatment program. They dislike the fact that in solo practice "economic realities" may come between them and their patients. They are discomforted with the obligation to adjust service patterns to the patient's ability to pay. Economic constraints also operate in group practice because of the obvious need to keep operating costs within the limits of revenues. Rationing in this context should center on medical needs, constrained by the group's resources.

It has also been suggested that young physicians "not too far in debt" may find group practice more attractive, mainly because there is less pressure to earn immediate and substantial fees. Another possible explanation is the setting for the medical training itself. If the graduate has been educated in the equivalent of a clinical or group practice, he may be attracted to continued service in such a setting. Significantly, three major medical schools, Harvard, Yale, and Johns Hopkins, have set up their own HMOs. In each case, medical services are separated from the academic functions of the university. It is not clear whether this separation of staff and budget impedes opportunities for student training in the school's HMO practice. Such separation, it appears, is to avoid comingling revenues.[9]

When a Kaiser Group elects a physician to partnership, he receives a substantial income. With continued service, he is assured of financial security and of disability and retirement income. His monthly pay reflects monthly drawings of salary, along with his annual share of the group's net earnings. There is no contract binding the physician to the Kaiser plan, and this gives credence to "turnover" statistics as an index of morale. The Kaiser operation has attracted doctors from 90 medical schools and 350 teaching hospitals throughout the country. The most prestigious are heavily represented in the staff. A third of the doctors have been in

[9] "We have three medical schools involved at the moment in the development of HMOs. We have been very careful to set them aside organizationally from the academic enterprise . . . so that the financing of the HMOs is not involved in any way with the financing of the medical schools. . . . Setting up an HMO as part of a medical school is perhaps too restrictive. Harvard, Yale, and Johns Hopkins are very much in control of their HMOs but they are not managed through the usual academic enterprise, that is, through the dean's office, as an example. They are set aside as separate corporate entities and the physicians' groups are separate groups from the faculty payment mechanisms. . . . They have their names and reputations on the line, but they don't have their fiscal lives on the line for these institutions; nor is the HMO supporting the academic enterprise." Robert M. Yeyssel, Hearings, *Health Maintenance Organizations*, 1972, Part 2, pp. 925–26.

the group practice for less than 3 years, another third from 4 to 8 years, and a final third, 9 years or more. The majority enter group practice in their 30s, and the majority of physicians-in-chief and chiefs of services are in their late 40s and 50s.[10]

There is considerable evidence of physician satisfaction with the Kaiser plan. This probably reflects the view of most physicians that they are part of an operation that has professional stature. They take pride in their affiliation and in their colleagues. Many are instructing in area medical schools, and the plan has its internal educational program to update skills of its staff. Data for 1966 to 1970 in northern California indicate an average annual turnover rate of less than ten percent for employed physicians and less than two percent for the partners.[11]

A 1970 national survey by Laurence D. Prybil found that physicians in private multispeciality group practices experienced an annual turnover rate of less than five percent, and there is evidence that this rate is becoming even lower.[12] Those who may be most inclined to leave the service are physicians under the age of forty-five, who, for the most part, do not take up solo practice, but a position in another organized setting. Austin Ross attributed turnover to the inadequate pay of group practice,[13] and in an unpublished study, David Mechanic found that ninety-five percent of a national survey of physicians in group practice were "very" or "fairly" satisfied. Over half of all respondents were "very satisfied."[14]

Roemer and Schonick, in their review of studies of physician satisfaction, have pointed to methodological problems: seldom does research compare relative satsifaction of solo and group practice, either by interviewing persons with both experiences or by using control groups; and it is possible that the favorable attitudes to group practice reflect personality traits that attract individuals to group practice to begin with. The latter, it seems, is hardly a consideration that should discount "true" measures of satisfaction, even though it does suggest that we should not be surprised that individuals who seek out group practice are satisfied with their choice.[15]

[10] Williams, "Kaiser," p. 77.
[11] These statistics are provided by Wallace H. Cook, "Profile of the Permanente Physician." In Anne R. Somers (ed.), *The Kaiser-Permanente Medical Care Program* (New York: Commonwealth Fund, 1971), p. 104.
[12] Laurence D. Prybil, "Physician Terminations in Large Multi-Speciality Groups," *Medical Group Management*, no. 18 (September 1971).
[13] Austin Ross, Jr., "A Report on Physician Terminations in Group Practice," *Medical Group Management*, no. 16 (1969), pp. 15–21.
[14] David Mechanic, "Physician Satisfaction in Varying Settings," University of Wisconsin, mimeographed, 1972.
[15] For an excellent review of this and related features of HMO activities, see Milton I. Roemer and William Schonick, "HMO Performance: The Recent Evidence," *Milbank Memorial Fund Quarterly*, Summer 1973, pp. 271–317.

Let us now turn to some of the more subjective appeals of group practice. First, there is a clear advantage in walking into group practice with established facilities, overhead, and operating procedure. The physician is not under pressure to penetrate a new market; he need not increase the debts created through medical school by absorbing the very substantial costs of equipment purchases, hiring supporting personnel, paying for office facilities, and so on. Further, the physician has an opportunity to carry his weight or justify his salary almost immediately. In solo practice, there is some loss to society in the "underemployment" of the physician during this start-up period, and the possible duplication of facilities in population centers where physicians are heavily represented. The physician who needs an immediate income flow to cover the costs of previous education may find the salary of group practice attractive.[16]

A second attraction is the affiliation with a distinguished physician panel. It is perhaps tautological to assert that skilled or promising graduates have an affinity with skilled staffs. If the group team is made up of highly respected practitioners, there is every reason that the plan will attract capable physicians. Again, about eighty-five percent of the Permanente Medical Group's physicians are certified specialists and ten percent hold university teaching-hospital appointments. In many groups, board-certified or board-qualified specialists predominate, and participation in clinical research and in continuing-education programs and teaching is common.[17]

Related to this is the possibility of some specialized services. Although general-practice responsibilities dominate group-practice plans, there are divisions of labor within the larger systems that offer single-focus opportunities not available to the solo practitioner. The new candidate may, as a consequence, see the group practice as a means of providing instant service. Establishing a specialty solo practice may prove much more difficult than establishing a solo general practice.

A further initial attraction is the prospect of affiliation with a group of experienced professionals who will be willing to share responsibilities and experiences during such service. During a period of rising concern about malpractice suits, the opportunities for curbstone conferral with as-

[16] Joseph P. Newhouse has raised a somewhat strained point in asking whether the full use of the new physician in group practice is made at the expense of other physicians in the group and questions whether, in fact, the total supply of medical services is actually increased when the physician joins a group. He contends, "There is no evidence on this point." Logic certainly suggests that the immediate effect is the prompt matching of supply with demand, increasing the community-welfare function. For discussion, see Joseph P. Newhouse, "The Economics of Group Practice," *The Journal of Human Resources*, Vol. 8, no. 1, p. 52.

[17] Jerry Phelan, Robert Erickson, and Scott Fleming, "Group Practice Prepayment: An Approach to Delivering Organized Health Services," *Law and Contemporary Problems*, Vol. 35, no. 4 (Autumn 1970), p. 798.

sociates is a major advantage of group practice. Of all the advantages of group practice, the most frequently mentioned feature is this opportunity for conferral with associates. A sampling of observations is appropriate:

> Many HMOs emphasize multispeciality practice and centralization of facilities. Physicians can send down the hall for a diagnosis or quickly secure the advice of another specialist.[18]

> I have all my consultants right next door. It's also a great advantage to the patient because if I knew another opinion was going to cost him $75, I might be hesitant to send him.[19]

> Conceptually, at least, the group-practice system is one well designed to increase physician satisfaction. The freedom from concern with the mundane business operations of medical practice, the ability to arrange hours and to limit the excessive burdens of long night and weekend calls, the ready availability of various fringe benefits, and the easy access and social support of working with a group of esteemed colleagues combine to make PGP an apparently favorable work environment.[20]

The camaraderie of group practice, while an obvious source of social and technical support, may also have somewhat perverse effects when one considers the discipline and control of peer review upon which the group-practice system is built. The case has been made that the social pressures of the group can operate to "cover" a colleague's flaws of judgment as much as they might expose such deficiencies. Merwyn Greenlick observes:

> It is easy to imagine the problems that would be created by a group of physicians which is tightly controlled and operating under norms that motivate it in an antisocial direction. In the highly structured situation of many group-practice organizations, the consensus position, good or bad, concerning quality and appropriate utilization of services will be reflected in the practice pattern of the physicians.[21]

Similarly, Freidson has noted that group organization means that the doctor practices in a context with other doctors and is, as a consequence, less dependent on his individual patients. In effect, the doctor is oriented more to the standards of his colleagues, less to the demands and wishes of his patients.[22]

---

[18] Paul Snider, "Health Maintenance Organizations," *Personnel*, Vol. 51 (November 1974), p. 42.

[19] Stephen Taller, quoted by Williams "Kaiser," p. 87.

[20] Merwyn R. Greenlick, "The Impact of Prepaid Group Practice on American Medical Care: A Critical Evaluation," *The Annals of the American Academy of Political and Social Science*, Vol. 399 (January 1972), p. 107.

[21] Ibid., p. 105.

[22] Eliot Freidson, *Patient's View of Medical Practice* (New York: Russell Sage Foundation, 1961) and David Mechanic, "Human Problems and the Organization of Health Care," *The Annals*, p. 6.

The more obvious advantage to the physician is the regularization of the work day. Rhythms of work are largely predictable, allowing one to rationally plan attention to home life, recreation, vacations with pay, hobbies, and participation in cultural events of the community. The individual is able to maintain a balance between work and leisure. The job becomes a means to an end—the enjoyment of life—and not an end in itself. Although a case has been made that many physicians enjoy an eighty-hour work week, it seems improbable that the frantic pace of private practice (despite all of its pecuniary rewards) proves to be fully satisfying. Cases are common of physicians who cannot "afford" a vacation because of the cost of foregoing work. To some, paying for an elegant dinner in a fashionable supper club is not nearly so painful as the revenues lost in the time of its consumption.

Related to this is the enormous relief achieved with the understanding that patient difficulties are being cared for by physician associates around the clock. One need not be harnessed to a portable receiver, with its unpredictable beep interrupting social functions. Vacations out of town need not be overshadowed by lingering concern about patient welfare, for one has capable colleagues taking care of the patient load.

Overall, not only are hours regularized, but there are fewer hours of required service. The forty-hour work week becomes a norm, not an unusual event. There are often provisions for sabbaticals and leaves to attend professional meetings and seminars to update skills. There is, in addition, group life insurance, group health insurance, and provision for sick leaves with pay. Some plans provide technical consultation on tax-shelter programs and other issues of portfolio management to maximize lifetime income for participating staff. The collegiality of a well-defined work day need not terminate with retirement for some plans encourage a consulting relationship of retired staff.

Delegating task functions to paramedical professionals has not been realized, but much less physician time has been absorbed in clerical services, report making, and other nonmedical services.

> Because of the volume of work, outside experts can be hired in medicine's housekeeping and supportive activities such as accounting, billing and collections, public relations, finance and investing, office structures, nursing, laboratory and x-ray services, parking, hospital relations, investing, patient records, and malpractice and other insurance.[23]

Although the critics of group practice have raised the haunting specter of medical teams denying services to the needy (even to the point of permitting death because of the unhappy state of the group's profit-and-loss statement), there is every reason to believe that the group practice

[23] Anthony J. Rourke, "Doctors Who Practice Together Earn These Advantages," *Modern Hospital* (June 1971), p. 128.

itself would represent a cooperative collegium rather than an entrepreneurial effort. The physician constantly makes decisions that affect life and death, regardless of the setting. Few have suggested that the tenacity of physicians in providing for elaborate artificial support systems to sustain life (where brain damage indicates recovery is impossible) is the perverse enthusiasm to increase personal income. By the same logic, it would seem unreasonable that group-practice physicians would prematurely "pull the plug" on support systems.

We have given unusual attention to the physician's perceptions because of his strategic position in the medical industry. The physician can "break or make" the HMO movement. Yet even though his participation is necessary, it is not a sufficient condition to ensure success. In the final analysis, sanctions for the program must be found in their performance ratios and patient satisfaction.

PERFORMANCE EVALUATIONS OF PREPAID GROUP PRACTICE

Senator Edward Kennedy, in advancing the Health Maintenance Organization and Resources Development Act of 1972 (S. 3327), saw the HMO as a forward step in universalizing medical care for the American citizen. After some thirteen months of study, he reported on the "striking evidence of the disorganization, waste, and inefficiency inherent in our fragmented system of health care. . . . *At the present time, we are spending almost enough money on personal health services to purchase two memberships in Kaiser or any other of the major prepaid group practices for every resident of the United States.*"[24]

Consumers have reason to object, too, because of the disparities of services that reflect not only the income of consumers, but also their geographic location. Existing private insurance programs favor not only those who can afford premiums, but also those who are less likely to need attention. As Senator Kennedy charges, experience rating has the effect of leaving those with the most serious need with the highest bills. "Skimming" is encouraged to improve the profit rates for private carriers. Would-be consumers, disenfranchised because of inadequate income and/or poor health, do not always get into the data bank of the treatment center, for they do not always gain access to the center.[25]

[24] Introductory Remarks, *Health Maintenance Organization and Resources Development Act of 1972*, S. 3327, Bill Text, section by section analysis and background material, prepared by the Subcommittee on Health of the Committee on Labor and Public Welfare, U.S. Senate, March 1972, GPO, p. 117.

[25] For vivid testimony from many who are disenfranchised, see the monograph, *Heal Thyself*, a Report of the Citizens Board of Inquiry into Health Services for America, 92 pages, undated.

It is, in the final analysis, the consumer (or taxpayer) who must pay the bills for spiraling health-care costs. During a period of serious inflation, sensitivities to price increases (not always matched by income increases) sharpen awareness and resentment.

Many insurance plans have contracts signed by major institutions, with joint contributions by employer and employee. Many of these plans appear complex, both in the manner of funding and in services provided. The renegotiation of annual benefit and cost packages is typically left to technicians, though companies sometimes attempt modest educational programs to alert the insured of such changes. Somewhere in that process, individual control of premium costs is lost. Employees are typically confused by the complexity of the insuring process, and some placidly accept annual premium increases as a ritual to invoke the diety for good health. The employee draws small comfort from the fact that the employer has to pay his share of the increase. For the employer's part, such fringes represent an alternative form of wage payments, a necessary cost of doing business. Increased health-care premiums, even if not accompanied by liberalized coverage, simply mean less liberalized wage payments. And to providers, with services reimbursed on a cost-plus basis, there are few inhibitions in expanding activities to absorb the surprising (and seemingly endless) flow of expenditures. As Walter J. McNerey, President of the Blue Cross Association, has explained: "Use tends to follow prepayment. The whole pattern of medical care is warped in favor of providing treatment in those expensive hospitals."[26]

> Speaking for the public sector, Weinberger acknowledged that with the introduction of Medicare we guaranteed payment of almost any bill submitted in any amount, and we had a considerable shortage of medical personnel at that time; and with those factors coming together and with no cost control, the costs went virtually perpendicular on all of the indexes.[27]

The Committee for Economic Development, respected for its neutral philosophic perspective, studied the health-care field and confirmed the need for reorganization of delivery systems. Project director Joseph C. Wilson (previously chairman of the Xerox Corporation) noted that "health care, as an industry, is not unlike many other American industries which are equally far-flung, extraordinarily complex, and yet are susceptible to rational managerial evaluations."[28] The CED concluded that

26 Edmund K. Faltermayer, "Better Care at Less Cost Without Miracles," *Fortune*, January 1970, p. 81.
27 Testimony of HEW secretary, Caspar Weinberger, January 31, 1974. Hearings before the Committee on Finance of the U.S. Senate, 93rd Congress, 2nd Session, January 31, 1974, *Administration Health Proposals*, p. 2.
28 Testimony of Alfred C. Neal, "Health Care Costs," to the Subcommittee on Consumer Economics of the Joint Economic Committee, *Medical Policies and Costs*, 1973, GPO, p. 81.

"even if vastly greater resources are poured into the health-care system, the goal of providing adequate health care for all will continue to elude the nation unless the delivery of health-care services is substantially restructured."[29]

Emphasizing the importance of access, the report noted that,

> while medical care was only one factor contributing to health, ". . . it can be literally a matter of life and death. Self-denial because of low income is not the same in this situation as in rationing one's income when purchasing cars, clothing, or television sets."[30]

We are confronted with alarming data involving disparities of treatment between individuals who are commercially insured and those covered by group insurance plans. To the critics, these disparities reflect the widespread overprescribing of drugs, extravagant overhospitalization, a proliferation of overtesting, and excessive surgery. One study of government employees covered by Blue Shield showed that they have four times as many tonsillectomies as those covered by group health plans. They have twice as many appendectomies and twice as much female surgery, including mastectomies and hysterectomies.[31] The evidence is fairly persuasive that fee-for-service insurance plans encourage expensive medical services and an unusual amount of surgery. For example,

> Federal employees enrolled in prepaid group practice programs use 60 percent less hospital days than those enrolled in Blue Cross or indemnity programs. . . . Federal employees use less than 400 days per 1,000 people at Kaiser and more than 800 days per 1,000 population under the Blue Cross, Blue Shield program.[32]

> Kaiser's Medicare population used slightly more than 1,500 days [of hospitalization] per 1,000 [persons] as opposed to the national average of 2,700 days per 1,000.[33]

Studies conducted by the United Mineworkers and the Teamsters to evaluate quality of service provided for insured members both allude to a flood of unnecessary operations.

Health-care providers contend that these high ratios for hospitalization and surgery for the privately insured reflect the laudable purpose of providing quality health care. Low-service indices for those in group pre-

29 Ibid., p. 81.
30 Ibid., p. 82.
31 For discussion, see Victor R. Fuchs, "Improving the Delivery of Health Services." In Fuchs (ed.), *Essays in the Economics of Health and Medical Care* (New York: Columbia University Press, 1972), pp. 52–53.
32 George S. Perrott, *Group Health and Welfare News*, Special Supplement, March 1964, pp. 2, 3.
33 Ernest W. Saward, *New Physician*, Vol. 18, no. 41 (1969), p. 42.

capitation plans (by this same line of reasoning) are suffering inadequate attention because of cost economies. It is irrational, therefore, to hold up ratios of service under prepaid plans as a standard for "quality" service.

Clearly much work has yet to be done to establish and refine performance indicators. Some studies suggest, however, that in this area price does not always equal value, that expenditures do not always ensure good health. The 1967 Report of the Advisory Commission on Health Manpower observed that the Kaiser medical services were "equivalent, if not superior, to that available in most communities."[34] With the Health Insurance Plan of New York (HIP), all insured infants were immunized against whooping cough, diphtheria, tetanus, and smallpox during their first year of life.[35] A Columbia University study showed that eighty-three percent of surgical procedures in HIP were performed by recognized specialists in surgery, compared with sixty-two percent under Blue Shield and fifty-seven percent under group health insurance. Another study observed:

> Quality and the question of the improvement of health tend to merge in the finding that the infant death rate in HIP from 1955 to 1957 was 23.1 per thousand births compared with 27.9 for other New York City babies delivered in hospitals by private physicians. A greater proportion of HIP mothers were receiving prenatal care during the first three months of pregnancy. Moreover, HIP deliveries were by specialists.[36]

One remarkable statistical study evaluated HIP's enrollment of 13,000 of the city's Medicaid patients who were on old-age assistance. Studies were made of these 13,000 patients compared with 13,000 patients outside HIP. After the second year, those served by HIP showed 14 percent less mortality than the other group.[37] Other studies reveal that infant and maternal mortality for HIP enrollees is lower than for the rest of the city, including persons using private fee-for-service practitioners.

Further, the state of California contracted with the San Joaquin Valley Medical Society to give all necessary care for one year to those eligible for Medicaid. The participating physicians received funds reflecting the anticipated expenditure for the population. The physicians

[34] *Report of the National Advisory Commission on Health Manpower,* Vol. 11 (November 1967), p. 206.

[35] Edwin F. Daily, "Medical Care Under the Health Insurance Plan of Greater New York," *Journal of the American Medical Association,* no. 70 (1959), pp. 272–76.

[36] Sam Shapiro, Harold Jacobziner, Paul M. Densen, and Louis Weiner, "Further Observations on Prematurity and Perinatal Mortality in a General Hospital and in the Population of a Prepaid Group Practice Medical Plan," *American Journal of Public Health,* Vol. 50, no. 9 (September 1960), pp. 1304–17. The above statistics have been gathered by Richard A. Berman, Hearings, *Health Maintenance Organizations,* Part 4, pp. 1374–76.

[37] Roul Tunley, ibid., p. 12.

cared for all seeking help and returned $200,000 to a startled state finance department.[38]

The charge is also made that each hospital strives to acquire the most recent technology, without carefully considering equipment use. In New York City, for example, there are eighteen open-heart surgery teams in eighteen different hospitals. Studies show that nine of these teams provide ninety percent of all such surgery. This is, of course, a costly investment in overhead, and it has also been considered dangerous. In one view, the most successful surgery teams are those that work together regularly. Unless such teams perform at least one operation a week, success ratios for surgery tend to decline.[39]

Fortune has estimated the costs of an average family of two adults and 1.9 children under the group-practice plan affiliated with Johns Hopkins Hospital of Baltimore and under "typical" insurance coverage. The annual costs of private insurance for the prescribed package of coverage, is $527. Under the Columbia (Maryland) Medical Plan, affiliated with Johns Hopkins Hospital of Baltimore, coverage is $358. The consumer saves, in this group-practice arrangement, $170 a year, or 32 percent of what comparable private insurance would cost.[40] A survey of federal employees and their dependents enrolled in prepaid medical plans showed they spent only 222 days in the hospital per 1,000 members each year, whereas those in Blue Cross spent 924 days per 1,000 members. Those insured under commercial health plans spent 987 days in hospital for each 1,000 members.[41]

The study of federal employees is authoritative, for it undertook well-controlled examination of data that might influence the results. The Federal Employees Health Benefits Program covers medical and hospital services for 8 million employees, annuitants, and their dependents. Employees have 3 options for health service: nonprofit health insurance, proprietary health insurance, and HMOs. When adjustments are made for the age structure of the participants in each category, Table 14-1 shows the hospital use by annuitants, employees, and dependents in 1968. There are, as we can see, sharp disparities: hospitalization was 420 days for 1,000 employees covered by the HMO, compared with 934 for proprietary insurance companies. Perrott found that although the average length of hospital stay was about the same for both systems, the proportion of HMO enrollees admitted for hospital care was only about one-half of that for persons covered by commercial insurance.

In Table 14-2, we have data showing the results of surgical care for

38 Ibid., p. 12.
39 Ibid., p. 13.
40 These data are reproduced in J. Wandres, "HMOs: The Answer to Spiraling Medical Costs?" *Retirement Living* (September 1974), p. 26.
41 Ibid., p. 27.

Table 14-1.   Hospital Use by Annuitants, Employees, and Dependents Under the U.S. Federal Employees Health Benefits Program, 1968

(days per 1,000 covered persons)

	Type of plan		
Type of enrollee[1]	Nonprofit insurance company	Proprietary insurance company	HMO[2]
All enrollees	924	934	420
Annuitants	3,180	2,675	1,530
Active employees	1,085	1,080	560
Dependents	715	765	305

[1] Rates are adjusted for age and sex within each category.
[2] Statistical sample drawn from over 85 percent of federal beneficiaries enrolled in HMOs.

Source: George S. Perrott, *Enrollment and Utilization of Health Services 1961–68: The Federal Employees Health Benefits Program* (Washington, D.C.: U.S. Dept. of HEW, 1971).

Table 14-2.   Surgery Rates of Persons Covered by Nonprofit Insurance and HMOs Under the U.S. Federal Employees Health Benefits Program, 1968

(surgical procedures per 1,000 persons)

Type of surgery	Nonprofit insurance (fee-for-service practice)	HMOs (multispecialty group practice)
All surgery	75	34
Tonsillectomy and/or adenoidectomy	6.9	2.4
Female surgery	9.2	4.8
Appendectomy	2.1	1.1
Cholecystectomy (gall-bladder surgery)	2.1	1.5

Source: Perrott, *Enrollment and Utilization of Health Services.*

the three groups. Again, surgery was performed on 34 persons per 1,000 covered by multispecialty group practice, compared with a ratio of 75 per 1,000 for those participating in nonprofit insurance company programs. This analysis is particularly authoritative, for it covers 8 years of statistics, with population characteristics of each group that can be assumed to be relatively uniform.[42]

In further studies of federal employees, George S. Perrott and Jean C. Chase provide insight into the volume of care provided by group-

[42] George S. Perrott, *Enrollment and Utilization of Health Services, 1961–68: The Federal Employees Health Benefits Program* (Washington, D.C.: U.S. Dept. of HEW, 1971). For discussion, see Gordon K. MacLeod, "Health Maintenance Organizations in the United States," *International Labour Review*, Vol. 110 (October 1974), pp. 335–50.

practice programs. The Blue Cross rate for inpatient treatment in 1966 was 9.8 percent of enrollees, compared with 4.6 percent for those in group practice. But in terms of "total benefits" provided by the plan, the Blue Cross percentage of service was 25.3 percent of its members, compared with 84.6 percent for group practice.[43] Clearly, the latter provided extensive ambulatory care.

Further evidence and testimony on the advantage of prepaid group practice points to a significant improvement in the quality of medical care for subscribers.[44] Shapiro indicated a decrease in infant mortality among subscribers to the Health Insurance Plan (HIP) in a comparative study with nonaffiliated residents of New York City.[45]

Economies in program costs have also been reported by the California State Department of Health Care Services. When Medicaid patients were shifted from fee-for-service to prepaid group-practice plans or HMOs, costs dropped by 10 to 20 percent. In a 7-year study of 3,200 southern California families Milton Roemer found that out-of-pocket medical expenses and total costs were much lower for families in HMOs than for those covered by Blue Cross or Blue Shield, even though average HMO fees were somewhat higher than the premiums for the other plans.[46]

The figures cited consistently support the hypothesis that there is an improvement in health care for HMO subscribers or, at the very least, that there is no decline in the quality of service for members. The obvious disparities in the number of hospitalizations for group and nongroup members raise serious questions about excessive surgery and overhospitalization. An AMA spokesman challenged the statistical reports about overhospitalization before the House Committee studying HMOs. (He was invited to submit empirical information to support his criticisms, but

[43] George S. Perrott and Jean C. Chase, *Group Health and Welfare News Supplement,* October 1968, and quoted by Anthony J. J. Rourke, "Study Indicates Group Practice Lowers Hospitalization Rates," *Modern Hospital,* Vol. 113 (August 1969), p. 120.

[44] Eugene Vayda, "The Potential of Prepaid Group Practice in Community Medicine Teaching Programs," *Milbank Memorial Fund Quarterly,* Vol. 47 no. 2 (April 1970), p. 131.

[45] Sam Shapiro, Louis Weiner, and Paul M. Densen, "Comparison of Prematurity and Perinatal Mortality in the General Population and in the Population of a Prepaid Practice Medical Care Plan, *American Journal of Public Health,* Vol. 48 (January 1958), pp. 170–87.

Further statistical outputs, supporting the above trends, can be found in Perrott, "Federal Employees Health Benefits Program: III: Utilization of Hospital Services, *American Journal of Public Health,* Vol. 56 (January 1966), pp. 57–64 and P. M. Densen, E. Balamuth, and S. Shapiro, *Prepaid Medical Care and Hospital Utilization,* Hospital Monograph Series No. 3 (Chicago: American Medical Association, 1958), pp. 6–34.

[46] As noted by Michael B. Rothfeld, "Sensible Surgery for Swelling Medical Costs," *Fortune,* Vol. 87 (April 1973), p. 116.

at the date of publication of the Hearings, that information was not forth-coming.) The most charitable view that can be offered is the impulse of physicians to treat in a hospital setting. This may be an educational re-flex, or it may reflect concerns of malpractice suits. Critics of HMOs have contended, however, that the HMO restriction of hospital use reflects limits of hospital beds made available to group plans. Although this may explain some of the moderated use of hospitals, it certainly cannot ex-plain all such disparities. The HIP plan, as a case in point, does not own any hospitals, but contracts for services for its clients. Even if the data were not used to support the HMO, they stand as a large question mark for the health-care system today.

The disparities of service are typically dismissed by references to the high quality of service under traditional delivery modes or, at the very least, by references to the "untested" hypothesis of quality mainte-nance under group practice. What restrictions are imposed by the "skimp-ing" hypothesis that encourages group practitioners to deliberately neglect the health needs of enrollees because of a declining P&L statement?

There are several reasons that such neglect may be imprudent for the HMO. There is the possibility of well-advertised consumer resent-ment of such treatment and the consequences of such neglect. Within the HMO movement, "the word gets around." It is, as a consequence, an ob-ligation of the staff to persuade clients that they are getting first-class treatment. There is also a more compelling consideration, which builds on the reality that neglect of minor difficulty may well create major con-tractual obligations for the group. Both the system and the patient tend to suffer the consequences of such neglect. A review process examines at least three stages of physician effectiveness.

When Representative William R. Roy of Kansas asked what provi-sions the administration had in mind to avoid skimping, HEW Secretary Richardson replied:

> Of course, the theory of an HMO is that it has an economic incentive to keep people well, therefore not skimping. We agree that there is needed some greater assurance than reliance on economic theory from the point of view of subscribers.
>
> Our best thought, at the present, is that we should rely, in part, on the kind of professional standards review that has been the subject of con-siderable discussion as it applies to medicare, medicaid, and other legislation.[47]

One example of internal review procedures operates within the Har-vard Health Plan. In this group operation, computers tabulate the proce-dures, drugs, and tests used by every physician. This information, includ-ing a randomly selected sample of more detailed diagnosis, is reviewed

[47] Hearings, *Health Maintenance Organizations*, April 1972, Part I, p. 109.

by a committee of physicians in each department. This review procedure found that some tests and drugs were ineffective, and these were dropped from the treatment schedule. A *Fortune* study noted that a number of other HMOs were using the review process to identify doctors who were putting an exceptionally high or low number of patients in hospitals. In this peer-review situation, doctors are required to explain or justify decisions.[48]

In some of the major prepaid groups, including Kaiser and HIP, internal research teams are designated to assess various aspects of system performance and feed results back into the system. "Such systematic research is rarely attempted in other segments of the medical care system because neither a defined population base nor an integrated unit record system are available." As Saward and Greenlick observe, "This type of research provides at least the potential for assessing and therefore affecting quality."[49]

CONSUMER PERCEPTIONS

Although we have noted consumer complaints about the lack of accessibility to and absence of informality of service from group practices, the evidence collected from subscribers offers strong evidence of support for these plans. We have noted the challenge of improving the efficiency of a delivery system by reducing doctor–enrollee ratios, multiphasic screening, and the like. But there is always the risk that a technically excellent service might seem less than adequate to the consumers of that service. Nonetheless, in 1964 Weinerman noted the high degree of overall satisfaction with group-practice service in spite of many complaints about the impersonality of the doctor–patient relationship in its "clinic setting."[50] More recently, Donabedian also found a relatively high degree of consumer satisfaction with health services associated with the HMO pattern.[51] In a 1973 publication of 1968 data, Roemer identified the two major aspects of consumer concern with enrollment in a health-care group plan: satisfaction with service and financial protection. Within all religious categories, all social classes, and all levels of geographic mobility, there

48 Rothfeld, "Sensible Surgery for Swelling Medical Costs," p. 117.
49 Ernest W. Saward and Merwyn R. Greenlick, "Health Policy and the HMO." In John B. McKinlay (ed.), *Politics and Law in Health Care Policy, Milbank Memorial Fund Quarterly,* p. 386.
50 See E. Richard Weinerman, "Patients' Perceptions of Group Medical Care," *American Journal of Public Health,* no. 54 (June 1964), pp. 880–89, and "Problems and Perspectives in Group Practice," *Group Practice,* Vol. 18 (April 1969), p. 30.
51 Avedis Donabedian "An Evaluation of Prepaid Group Practice," *Inquiry,* no. 6 (September 1969), pp. 3–27.

was praise for the financial protection of the PGP pattern. "Definite dissatisfaction was reported by 8.6 percent of PGP plan families, compared to 17.4 and 20.3 percent in the commercial and 'Blues' plan-types."[52]

Although the evidence of support is persuasive, it is not unanimous. In 1959, Anderson and Sheatsley found significantly more dissatisfaction among prepaid group-practice consumers than among those of more traditional health insurance.[53] In 1975, Tessler and Mechanic noted a slight preference of subscribers for Blue Cross rather than for group plans.[54] In a 1973 study of Medicaid recipients and those enrolled in a prepaid group practice, there was no significant difference in satisfaction uncovered.[55]

In viewing this evidence before a congressional committee, Paul M. Ellwood, Jr., has observed, "I have not seen a single study of the performance of HMOs in a qualitative sense, as compared to the existing system, that shows that the quality of care was any lower than that of the existing system."[56]

Let us view a complementary set of HMO subscriber benefits with brief treatment to each. In many group plans, subscription or enrollment begins because of the participation of both employers and unions in a collective-bargaining agreement. In many plans, the termination of employment under that contract need not terminate participation in the health-insurance plan. The individual can maintain membership by meeting the full subscription fee, usually with no penalty or a modest increase of premium rates. Some plans provide for physician house calls. In the Kaiser plan, house calls require an extra charge of from three to five dollars per call, depending on the amount of travel. Access to physician home visits is limited or nonexistent in most commercially insured plans. In many group plans, the patient has the opportunity to select the physician of his choice, and loyalties are frequently cultivated because of the continuity of that relationship.

Because physician members of a group practice have a scheduled work day a patient cannot expect around-the-clock access to his service.

[52] Roemer and Schonick, "HMO Performance: The Recent Evidence," p. 305. See also Milton Roemer, Robert W. Hetherington, Carl E. Hopkins, Arthur E. Gerst, Eleanore Parsons, and Donald M. Long, *Health Insurance Effects: Services, Expenditures and Attitudes under Three Types of Plan* (Ann Arbor: University of Michigan School of Public Health, 1973).

[53] Odin W. Anderson and Paul B. Sheatsley, *Comprehensive Medical Insurance: A Study of Costs, Use, and Attitudes Under Two Plans*, Research Series No. 9:61-62 (Chicago: Health Insurance Foundation, 1959).

[54] Richard Tessler and David Mechanic, "Consumer Satisfaction with Prepaid Group Practice: A Comparative Study," *Journal of Health and Social Behavior*, Vol. 16, no. 1 (March 1975).

[55] F. E. Gartside, C. E. Hopkins, and M. I. Roemer, *Medicaid Services in California Under Different Organizational Modes* (Los Angeles: University of California, School of Public Health, 1973).

[56] Hearings, *Health Maintenance Organizations*, April 1972, p. 389.

Proponents of the HMO structure have reminded us that such access is also not typically available to those being served by solo practitioners. Some group plans provide allowances for transportation to the service center or a flat sum to subsidize travel to a hospital. For low-income groups, transportation can be a major problem. A further advantage to the consumer is the realization that the physician panel members do, in fact, confer with one another on problematic issues. Having noted the convenience of group practice to the physician, we should also note the advantage of speed and economy for the enrollee.

Related to this consideration is the "one-stop" (or "one-step"), "single-doorway" feature of most HMO plans. "Patients would be 'plugged in' to a specific source of care, a single doorway and telephone number, and this might help many persons who would otherwise feel medically disengaged and insecure."[57] In one interpretation, the HMO movement can fulfill its promise of delivery only if it is hospital based, with inpatient and outpatient services integrated in one setting.

> Equipment and supporting personnel which often would be prohibitively expensive for solo practitioners or small groups can be shared and more fully utilized at medical centers serving large and coordinated groups of physicians.[58]

Even so, the HMO movement is tied, of necessity, to geographic areas of population density. The needs of rural Americans can only be served with the extension of a network of outreach offices. Here, skilled paramedics would be involved in routine primary-care functions and would maintain constant communications with the "heart" of the service center through telephonic and television communication. Where population density cannot support an outreach clinic, it will be necessary to rely on mobile medical units, which will periodically visit areas to offer diagnostic and other treatment. Behind this plan must be facilities for the speedy transport of patients requiring hospital care, including access to private airplane, helicopter, and (for shorter distances) ambulances. Some have expressed legitimate concern that the development of service centers in a group-practice delivery mode may actually complicate the problem of geographic access to the center. In most studies, a twenty- to thirty-minute commutation is considered the maximum. If the minimum "break-even" point for a plan is thought to be twenty thousand enrollees, clearly the HMO will require a unique design to serve sparsely populated areas. In extolling the virtues of one-stop service, one must also be aware of the problems of reaching that doorway.

[57] Ray E. Brown, "Symposium Hears Criticism, Defense of HMO Concept," *Modern Hospital*, June 1971, p. 41.
[58] Jerry Phelan, Robert Erickson, and Scott Fleming, "Group Practice Prepayment: An Approach to Delivering Organized Health Services," *Law and Contemporary Problems*, Vol. 35, no. 4 (Autumn 1970), p. 798.

It is difficult to exaggerate the significance to the consumer of knowledge that he has access to a system. Even with a twenty-minute "hold" on a telephone line, it is reassuring that somewhere out there is a system with legal, economic, and moral obligations to respond to your problems. This is not always the case in solo practice. There is no lack of evidence of solo practitioners who simply refuse to "take on" additional patients, and often that refusal may reflect modest reimbursement fees provided by government ceilings in Medicare and Medicaid. Proof of patient frustration is the fact that, increasingly, the emergency room is an entry point to the system. Approximately sixty percent of all emergency-room visits are nonurgent, reflecting the breakdown of consumer access to the existing system.[59]

In concluding our diagnosis of consumer benefits, we should look briefly at two interrelated themes. The first is the appeal of the egalitarian ideal represented in the HMO movement, reflecting community ratings rather than merit ratings. The second is the persuasiveness that investments in preventive programs of health maintenance are much to be preferred to the episodic intervention of the physician to repair serious (and sometimes irreparable) damage.

The HMO movement is not designed to provide quality care for all Americans. There is the remaining problem of limited health services to the poverty groups in the central cities and to rural Americans. Neither the HMO movement nor the House version of HMO legislation adopted by Congress addresses itself to this issue. But the decision to require community rating rather than merit rating in certifying HMOs eligible for federal aid represents a determined effort to apply the insurance principle to health care. The HMO, in effect, is built on the proposition that there is financial protection for all members when confronted with unanticipated illness. But it is also built on the proposition that, through such insurance, those who are not afflicted should be expected to pay for medical care for those who are. From the consumer's viewpoint, there is considerable relief in belonging to any plan that protects him from the financial disaster of major or catastrophic illness. The cost of such protection provides its own rewards in the security of the customer. Certainly there must be satisfaction, too, in knowing that other members are not subject to economic disaster when confronted with ill health. With community ratings, there is one benefit package at one price to all members. Under existing insurance arrangements, many older people could no longer purchase insurance at a price they could afford. A private insurance plan, based on community rating, represents a first stage in forestalling or at least minimizing, the income transfers necessary with a national insurance plan. The degree to which private HMO plans can, in reality, afford to absorb substantial

[59] See Vayda, "The Potential of Prepaid Group Practice in Community Medicine Teaching Programs."

numbers of the chronically ill remains an issue of serious concern to all. The government is understandably reluctant to issue blank checks for cost reimbursement to HMOs, with the rapid spiral of costs confronting both the Medicaid and Medicare programs.

A second principle that has appeal to members of the HMO delivery system is the attention provided, at least in principle, to preventive health care. Although the consumer can properly be criticized for his neglect of body care, he seeks assurances that the options of examination, diagnosis, and prescription are available to him without additional costs. The evidence does not establish HMOs as a major provider of preventive care, but they do administer more such care than traditional group practices.

> . . . preventive services are used more frequently by members of prepaid group practice programs, particularly higher utilization for cervical cytology examinations and more appropriate use of general and prenatal checkups among members of the group practice plans. A higher proportion of group practice members make contact with a physician each year, thereby increasing the probability of preventive care.[60]

And even if such service is not typical today, the HMO structure creates the opportunity and the incentive for expanding such care. Again, as Paul Ellsworth explains:

> The performance of existing HMOs in providing health-maintenance services is less well understood and less impressive than their selective reduction of hospitalization. It's true that multiphasic screening has seen its highest development in HMOs and that their subscribers are more likely to be immunized and to receive preventive procedures such as Papanicolaou smears. However, in view of the inherent economic incentive they have for maintaining the health of their subscribers—they can take the premium money and spend it in any number of ways to do the difficult job of influencing their subscribers' behavior to live better, and so forth—their performance in this regard is not exceptional. In fact, I feel their record in introducing innovation in medical practice is far below their potential. The prototype HMOs are good, but rather conventional group practices.[61]

SUMMARY AND CONCLUSIONS

Throughout the country, advocates of the HMO movement are constantly reminded that employers, citizens, medical personnel, and even medical schools have only a casual knowledge of prepaid group practice. As we mentioned at the outset, resistance to change does not reflect hostility, but ignorance.

[60] Saward and Greenlick, "Health Policy and the HMO," p. 386.
[61] Hearings, *Health Maintenance Organizations*, Part 2, p. 388.

The struggle to ensure minimal medical care to all Americans will require some modification of our existing delivery system, particularly because of the geographic and occupational imbalances in the distribution of our physicians. The HMO movement, unfortunately, is not well structured to solve the problems of rural Americans and of the poor in the central cities. A coalition of group-practice specialists must exist among a predetermined minimum number of subscribers. To serve thinly populated areas, these coalitions must also have outreach activities, clinics, and communication and transportation networks linking medical services in the frontier to the heart of the service center. Existing self-help models do not appear effective for the urban poor, for they identify neither the incentives to physicians to serve in the core city nor the income sources that will pay for services rendered to the poor. The Kennedy version of the HMO legislation that did not secure congressional support gave much more attention to provisions designed to avoid a two-track system or continued contrasting service patterns for the poor and the affluent. With the racial segregation of much of our population, it is difficult to integrate medical services. Nevertheless, the problems, at the outset, are logistical (mainly involving transportation and money) rather than racial.

The federal government appears cautious about giving support to the HMO movement, fearing another raid on the treasury characterized by its Medicare and Medicaid programs. To qualify for federal funds, an HMO must provide a broad and expensive range of services, creating serious impediments to the prospect of fiscal solvency. The Kennedy version of HMO legislation would have provided for staged subsidies for the HMO to cover deficits during its first three years of operation, but there are no such provisions in the HMO Act of 1973. If the HMO movement is going to "take off" as a form that will serve any major segment of American society, it will require much stronger support than is now available in federal legislation.

It seems clear, however, that the HMO structure is a feasible and attractive mode of operation for almost all parties. The physician has at least as much to gain as the consumers. As the potential flexibility of various operations become better known, we would expect opposition to diminish and interest and support to increase. It is reasonable to conclude that the HMO's "time has come." Its gradual growth does not require federal funds, for the movement has a logic and momentum of its own. Its rapid growth will, however, require much more generous federal funding.

SUGGESTED READINGS

BAUMAN, PATRICIA, "The Formulation and Evolution of the Health Maintenance Organization Policy, 1970–1973," *Social Science and Medicine,*

Vol. 10 (March/April 1976), pp. 129–42. An exposé of the circumstances leading to President Nixon's acceptance of the HMO concept. Observers have often expressed some surprise at the strength of Nixon's apparent support.

EASTON, ALLAN, *The Design of a Health Maintenance Organization: A Handbook for Practitioners* (New York: Praeger, 1975). A collection of essays on the planning of HMOs. Chapters provide various organizational plans for the HMO and requirements for securing profitable operations and financial planning.

GAUS, CLIFTON R., BARBARA S. COOPER, and CONSTANCE G. HIRSCHMAN, "Contrasts in HMO and Fee-for-Service Performance," *Social Security Bulletin*, Vol. 39, no. 5 (May 1976), pp. 3–14. A statistical analysis of the relative performance characteristics of HMOs in contrast to solo practice and commercial insurance coverage.

GREENBERG, IRA B. and MICHAEL L. RODBURG, "The Role of Prepaid Group Practice in Relieving the Medical Care Crisis," *Harvard Law Review*, Vol. 84 (February 1971). An overview of the key issues of prepaid group practice.

GUMBINER, ROBERT, *HMO: Putting It All Together* (St. Louis: Mosby, 1975). A consideration of the organization of HMOs, including marketing, recruiting physicians, and determining breakeven points and costs.

KENTON, CHARLOTTE, *Health Maintenance Organizations, January 1969 to January 1973* (Literature Search No. 73–5 for National Library of Medicine, U.S. Department of Health, Education and Welfare, Public Health Service, National Institutes of Health. Address: 8600 Rockville Pike, Bethesda, Maryland, 20014). A literature search on health-maintenance organizations and prepaid group plans.

MACCOLL, WILLIAM A., *Group Practice and Prepayment of Medical Care* (Washington, D.C.: Public Affairs Press, 1966). A discussion of facilities for family care, of legal issues, and of the organization of group plans in terms of costs, resources, and use.

McNEIL, JR., RICHARD and ROBERT E. SCHLENKER, "HMOs, Competition, and Government," *Milbank Memorial Fund Quarterly*, Spring 1975, pp. 195–224. A progress report on the HMO movement, comparing activities from 1970 to 1973 and looking at the content of the 1973 HMO Act.

STARR, PAUL, "The Undelivered Health System," *Public Interest*, no. 42 (Winter 1976), pp. 66–85. Describes the high hopes for the benefits of HMOs and the subsequent disappointment.

15
THE CASE AGAINST
HEALTH-MAINTENANCE
ORGANIZATIONS

Group practice, which includes the prepayment of a fixed fee by a consumer group, is not a dominant institutional reality in America today. However, it is a dominant issue and it remains the centerpiece of the federal government's efforts to reform and improve health-care delivery. Because the implications of group practice are so important, and because high hopes have been raised about the potential of the HMO, this chapter will review selected problems posed by group practice. Clearly, those who support the HMO movement do not consider it a panacea for all health-care problems. But both aspirations and enthusiasm have soared; consequently, there is some risk that the unwarranted pessimism that characterizes much of the present view of the health scene is being supplanted by an unwarranted optimism about the potential of group practice. In this section, we will review some of the chilling realities confronting the prepaid group-practice program.

Much of the discussion will center on attitudes and perceptions, rather than on statistics. The narrative will attempt to capture the essence of anxieties—indeed, to stereotype the concerns of physicians, consumers, and economists. Even if popular attitudes or perceptions are not thoroughly rooted in reality, their existence constitutes a reality that will determine the fate of the HMOs. It is natural to focus attention on the physician and the health-service consumer, for the supplier and the buyer are the leading actors in this play. This "warts and all" portrait of the HMO prospect is not, of course, intended to fault the play's trial run, nor to discourage public attendance at its gala opening. Playwrights are still amending the script, and this chapter will attempt to explain why. The debate involves both philosophy and practicalities. As Uwe E. Reinhardt explains:

> . . . the lack of agreement [over the appropriate form of health care] . . . reflects deep-seated ideological differences and conflicting views on what constitutes "quality" in health-care delivery. But there is also a

dearth of information on the socioeconomic and medical characteristics of alternative provider systems, existing or imagined. If the choice of a new provider system had to be made at this time, it would have to be made essentially on the basis of conjecture.[1]

Our purpose is to reduce that conjecture.

THE CONCERNS OF THE PHYSICIAN

All sides acknowledge that the HMO movement cannot get off the ground if programs do not enjoy the support of the physician. According to Robert Gumbiner:

> It is hard to believe, but many physicians haven't got the foggiest idea of what an HMO really is! As a matter of fact, just recently a doctor asked me if I would help him put an HMO together for plastic surgeons. A hard-hitting, far-reaching educational campaign to move some of the physicians out of their present mode of practice is going to be a necessity.[2]

The issue is much more serious than simply securing AMA endorsement of the principle. It involves the very lifestyle of this strategically located professional. It is not surprising, therefore, that proponents of HMOs approach the physician with diffidence and caution.

Physicians are quite properly puzzled about invitations to support a sharply different system for delivering their services, without a clear delineation of what form such a system would take. This paradox reflects two realities: First, there is no prototype of the HMO structure, no agreed-upon size. As Robert V. Sager testified:

> An HMO may be public at any level, federal, state, local, regional; non-profit private, including consumer and neighborhood sponsored groups; medical-society foundations which are associations of solo physicians and not groups at all; and Blue Shield and Blue Cross insurance associations; and finally, profit-making private organizations under a variety of sponsorships, singly or in consortiums; commercial insurance companies, electronic and industrial firms, drug houses, banks, management companies, and so on.

[1] Uwe E. Reinhardt, "Proposed Changes in the Organization of Health Care Delivery: An Overview and Critique," *Milbank Memorial Fund Quarterly*, Vol. 51, no. 2 (Spring 1973), p. 170.

[2] Hearings before the Subcommittee on Public Health and Environment of the Committee on Interstate and Foreign Commerce, House of Representatives, 92nd Congress, 2nd Session, April–May 1972, Health Maintenance Organizations. Testimony provided May 3, 1972, Vol. 2, p. 602.

Physicians in these organizations may be full time or part time, paid by salary, partnership share, or fee-for-service. The HMO may give most of the health services directly or contract out for them; they may operate from an institution, an ambulatory health center, a neighborhood health center, a number of scattered centers, or from solo private offices. A glance at the first grants to HMOs indicates that almost all of these varieties are at present in gestation.[3]

In addition to the different systems there are often undefined or unresolved issues of lay versus physician control, quality standards in the recruitment of staff, anticipated earnings, the structure of administrative authority, and so on. Will registration be open to all or be selective? One can hardly articulate reasons to support (or oppose) a new program of ill-defined form. Initial discussions with physicians can run aground on such ambiguity. On the other hand, there may be some hesitancy in arbitrarily specifying one form out of respect for the proposition that participating physicians should have a major influence in designing their group practice.

A second related issue involves the uncertainties of economic reality. Most experts contend that an HMO cannot be organized casually, on a piecemeal basis, served by physicians on a part-time basis. But a new program cannot offer instant comprehensive services because of the logistics of launching it. Related to this is the critical issue of market penetration: what is the market size or market penetration that will provide an HMO with fiscal solvency? If short-term losses are anticipated because of heavy start-up costs, who will absorb those costs? To what extent will the physicians' salaries be adjusted to marketing success? Will the physician receive guarantees that he will not suffer an interruption of income should the HMO falter?

In the first category of concerns we have the chicken-or-egg puzzle: Should the conceptualization of the model precede or follow physician support? And, in the second, what warranties do we have for the benefits of a system, when we have no warranties about its market penetration? Too, how can we speak convincingly to consumers about the array of available physician services if the physician himself is awaiting evidence of consumer interest?

The 1973 HMO Act provides $325 million in grants to assist the organization of between 300 and 500 HMO groups.

The government's goal is to encourage growth of HMOs to the point where 90 percent of the population will have access to at least one prepaid group by 1980. In that year, according to official estimates, some

[3] Hearings, *Health Maintenance Organizations*, Part 3, May 9, 1972, p. 876.

40 million people will be prepaying their medical bills. Enrollment in HMOs is expected to double to 16 million in just the next two years.[4]

The act specifies an exhaustive list of basic services that must be provided by any organization seeking to qualify for federal aid. There is no provision to support programs that begin modestly until such time as their services (and, consequently, their revenues) can increase. Teams considering a gradualist approach are properly concerned about recovering very substantial start-up costs.

But creating such an instant network of physician services is difficult. Some have held, however, that the federal government should provide initial support until the HMO can increase the number and effectiveness of its services.[5]

The most serious concern to the physician must ultimately be economic. The young physician has invested heavily in his education and is eager to recover some of this investment. In private practice, his earnings curve is likely to be a rising arc, peaking as he approaches retirement. Thus, the earnings schedule under an ongoing prepayment plan must reflect competitive realities and be able to meet the market demand if it hopes to recruit and maintain a medical team of first-rate quality. The physician considering an HMO must, however, discount the possibility of soaring increases in earnings. Association with an HMO will probably provide him with a more predictable (but perhaps more moderate) level of earnings than otherwise available with private practice. The physician, in making these comparisons, must also consider the risk that the widespread popularity of the HMOs might narrow his market for private practice, thus reducing his private-practice earnings. He may conclude that it is more prudent to join the movement than compete with it.

But certainly the physician might not be enthusiastic about a "high-risk" venture that requires heavy investment of his service in a group-practice program that might falter. Recent evidence of failing plans only compounds that anxiety. Just as the risk of the default of New York City debts has raised the risk premium required in marketing all major city debentures, so physicians who consider joining new plans will have to be wooed by the prospects of more substantial lifetime earnings. John R. Kernodle of the AMA pointed out:

> Closed-panel prepaid groups today attract only some 2 percent of practicing physicians and less than 4 percent of the populations. So there is question as to acceptance. HMOs as we now know them have achieved

[4] "Coming on Fast: One Stop Health Care," U.S. News and World Report, Vol. 74 (May 21, 1973), p. 54.
[5] For discussion, see "Prescription for an HMO: Muscle, Doctors and Millions of Bodies," Modern Hospital, Vol. 117 (November 1971), p. 10.

something less than universal acceptance by both consumers and physicians.[6]

What are some of the noneconomic aspects of group practice that are sources of physician concern? Certainly, much of his medical-school experience has been oriented to solo practice in a field specialty. Hospital-based medical training tends, as noted throughout, to focus on the pathology of "interesting" or rare medical cases. It does not encourage general practice or family-care specialties and, for the most part, is not community-based. His service in a group plan, while technically providing for a division of labor, may not in reality allow him the undivided attention to a field specialty reflecting that training. Inevitably, his obligations to serve the needs of all clients will demand attention to the flow of routine medical problems. He will have to deal with the "worried-well" and on occasion with the aggressive patient (sick or not) demanding attention.

This contrasts sharply with solo practice. There, the stream of patient problems is not always congruent with the physician specialties, but there is the opportunity in the patient's selection of his physician to secure some relationship between patient needs and physician interests. The obligations of a group plan to provide a complete package of services may appear tedious to the specialist hoping to establish his credentials through unusual medical feats.

We tend to forget that under solo practice, the physician chooses his own hours and determines quality standards for personal service. The AMA is, as one would expect, strongly committed to the principle of free choice as it applies to the physician, and makes the assumption that consumers are equally free in matters of opting for medical care. John R. Kernodle explained:

> For many reasons—among them the diverse geography of this country, varying traditions, and a long history of individualism—we favor a pluralistic system of medical care. We believe different methods of medical care should be allowed to compete freely in the marketplace to satisfy varying public demands. We assert that a physician is entitled to the freedom to choose the form of practice most suitable to his individual talents, just as the patient is entitled to the freedom to choose the type of service most suitable to his individual desires.[7]

Although much is made of the sixty-hour work week and the burden of around-the-clock responsibilities for patient care, the physician is much less likely to resent a work regimen if it reflects his—not the organization's—choice. Under solo practice, he has an opportunity to adjust his level of service with his own energy level and motivation to improve earnings. Such variation in personal planning is more restricted under group

---

[6] Hearings, *Health Maintenance Organizations*, p. 334.

[7] Hearings, *Health Maintenance Organizations*, Part II, April 13, 1972, p. 333.

practice. The benefits, the vacations, the work day, all tend to be formally prescribed. The stability and shorter length of the work day may well prove a much more attractive lifestyle to some, but certainly not to all. Anthony J. J. Rourke explained:

> Depending on the group, the doctor is not always able to practice exclusively within his specialty. Without general practitioners in the group, doctors may have to take turns providing night and weekend coverage and serving as the admitting physician. If the group is the sole staff of a hospital, each doctor must take a turn working in the emergency department.[8]

Concern has also been expressed that the growth of the group practice may tend to polarize physicians into two groups. The collegiality within the profession may be diminished, reflecting the difference in value structures and lifestyles between solo and group practice. The opportunities for reciprocal service in consulting will be altered. Those within the group system may feel a primary obligation to confer with colleagues within the system, or perhaps even within their own panel. "Physicians who remain in solo practice have been known to negatively label and identify the group physician, which can affect both the volume of his referral work and his social life."[9]

A physician beginning medical service with an established group will probably have to start at the bottom of a pay scale, with increments of pay reflecting years of service. The salary structure is likely to be rationalized according to definitions of internal equity, rather than the market. Group-plan administrators may be confronted with some of the problems of a monopsonist: efforts to improve, unilaterally, the salary of one physician may have adverse morale effects for the rest of the physician team; yet to generalize the salary increase (made necessary to satisfy one physician) may involve prohibitive costs to the plan. Some physicians may well resent the lockstep path of salary progressions. The spirit of individualism, with the corollary that each physician should be paid according to his individual productivity, is a conspicuous physician trait. Will most talented and productive physicians be content with obligations to serve group needs, with the rewards centered on group rather than individual productivity?

The problem of motivation is general, not specific. The axiom has been advanced that the larger the physician panel, the more difficult it will be for the physician to impute any direct payoff for unusual services rendered. Similarly, the larger the group, the less the individual penalty for declining service to the group practice. The loosening of the ties be-

[8] "Group Practice Affects M.D. Hours, Standards, Relationships, Finances," *Modern Hospital,* Vol. 116 (June 1971), p. 128.
[9] Ibid.

tween individual service and reward will, as a consequence, have deleterious effects on both the volume and quality of work. Further, the larger the group, the more difficult the definition (and policing) of service norms for the individual.[10]

Still another concern is the possible commercialization of medical services, particularly in marketing the product. Marketing is the key to group-practice success. Although marketing can take the form of dignified education, any advertising can offend the American Medical Association. When conducting feasibility studies it is essential to determine whether advertisements of the HMO violate state statutes. A state's medical-practice act may forbid solicitation of patients by physicians and the publishing of physician fee schedules. In some states, however, Blue Cross and Blue Shield programs have been allowed to advertise. With the growth of such plans, a state or county medical society may have prepared itself to enforce advertising prohibitions contained in their code of ethics.[11] The AMA strongly opposes a doctor's selling his services to a consumer group, for fear that commercialization in the marketing process may erode quality standards for care.

A shadow has been cast over the entire HMO movement following the efforts of state governments to utilize incentives implicit in the prepayment system to economize in health-care services for the medically indigent. Newspaper accounts have criticized the marketing techniques of medical panels because these appear more interested in penetrating a designated market of a poverty area rather than providing comprehensive medical care. The appearance of shoddy merchandising may emerge when a panel of physicians decides to incorporate as a formal Prepaid Health Plan (PHP). The solvency of such an operation requires an immediate subscribing population, the breakeven point variously designated from 3,000 to 9,000 persons. The greater the time span required to secure the revenue flow—payments made directly by the government on a capitation basis—the greater the risk that the overhead cost of the medical panel will be more substantial than the revenue flow.

[10] For an illuminating discussion of the economic theory of incentives for groups, see Joseph P. Newhouse, "The Economics of Group Practice," *The Journal of Human Resources*, Vol. 8, no. 1, p. 39 and Mancur Olson, Jr., *The Logic of Collective Action*, rev. ed. (Cambridge, Mass.: Harvard University Press, 1971), esp. pp. 54–55.

[11] For discussion, see HMO Feasibility Study Guide, HEW, Publication No. (HSA) 75-113020 (Washington, D.C.: GPO, February 1974), p. 28. Frank H. Seubold, HMO director of the Department of HEW, explained that the federal act still requires HMOs to organize under state charters and be subject to state legislation. But later provisions of state law under Section 1311 include: state requirements that the medical society approve HMO services, that physicians constitute all or a specific percentage of the governing body, and that all physicians or a certain percentage of them must participate (or be permitted to participate) in the HMO. See "Commissioners Ponder: Does New Federal HMO Statute Usurp State Regulators' Roles?" *National Underwriter*, Vol. 78 (June 15, 1974), pp. 21–22.

The California experience has been a particular source of embarrassment to the "movement." The State of California did not, of course, simply hand over large blocs of the poor to be serviced by a commercial PHP; rather, it designated geographic areas to each group with permission to enroll a maximum amount. Under such contracting arrangements, one group might compete against another group, particularly when marketing areas overlapped. Salesmen marketing these programs were often paid on a commission basis, and were sometimes encouraged to employ misleading representations of service in order to make a "sale."

In one account, a salesman introduced himself by saying: "I'm from the Medi-Cal Center," thus creating the impression that he was a representative of the state explaining the obligations of the household resident to enroll in the program. Potential clients were often told they would enjoy a one-stop service center, taking care of all of their medical needs. While this reflected the ideal of the PHP program, it did not always reflect the realities. Most individuals probably did not fully appreciate that in signing up for the PHP program, they were denying themselves access to services from traditional sources, including care for their needs from a family physician and local druggist. The problems were compounded when it was realized, after the fact, that the service center might be located miles away, with no ready access to transportation facilities. Congressional committee analysis of the same problem has confirmed the "hard-sell" techniques, including the promise, in one case, of a free appliance as an inducement to subscription.[12] This unhappy experience has been given widespread publicity and has created a legitimate concern that group-practice plans may be pressed into vigorous hard-sell techniques to secure subscriptions.

There are obvious risks of unscrupulous selling programs to minority groups unfamiliar with what is being proposed. For example, in Los Angeles a "new" generation of HMOs was evaluated by a union-sponsored California Council for Health Plan Alternatives. Its study showed that 40 percent of one HMO's staff was made up of foreign medical-school graduates. Its small staff was supposed to provide care for more than 100,000 persons. Although most family subscribers had several children, the medical staff contained the full-time equivalent of only 2 pediatricians and had no obstetrician. Fewer specialists were available in internal medicine than in other major prepayment plans, and the organization provided about one-half the amount of hospital care used in other well-recognized group-practice prepayment plans. In an area where excellent hospitals abound, these relatively small HMOs provided less-than-ade-

[12] Robert Fairbanks, "Medi-Cal Reform: Favoritism and Shoddy Services," *The Los Angeles Times,* May 23, 1974.

quate care. In observing the evidence, the Dean of the School of Public Health at UCLA cautioned:

> The record of the "new" California HMO points up that in the search to make health care more equitable, more economical, and more available, it's also essential to avoid becoming entrapped in supporting enterprises that provide poor health care.[13]

Another physician fear is that, however rational the service plan, he will inevitably get caught up in a labyrinth of administrative controls and political encounters. Whatever the conceptual simplicity of the group plan, it does involve an overlay of rules and authority absent in solo practice. Proponents speak cheerfully about the internal review mechanism as a safeguard for individual physician performance, but the regular judgment of one's peers is fraught with tension and demand great objectivity and analytic ability.

Nor is there uniform evidence of a dramatic reduction in the hours of work for those serving in groups. It is agreed that a doctor is not likely to perform at his best when he is rushed and tired:

> The average self-employed physician, according to *Medical Economics*, works more than 60 hours a week, including all professional activities. The Permanente work weeks vary, but physicians interviewed reported working 50 to 60 hours a week, including a 40-hour office schedule, hospital rounds before and after office hours, rotation on night calls, staff and committee meetings, and educational activities.[14]

Related to this is the high-paced scheduling of visits with patients, often no longer than fifteen minutes. Although the Kaiser-Permanente plan provides for one hour a day for emergency calls, patients typically have to wait from four to six weeks for an appointment. Such a delay is as embarrassing to the physician as it is irritating to the patient. He may not begin his interview with his physician on cordial terms, particularly if there is an additional delay of an hour or so in the waiting room.

It is assumed that economies of equipment will afford the patient more effective technical services, but the physician may resent his small and spartan office facilities. David Mechanic found that the physician's greatest sources of discontent were the time available per patient, his income levels, his office facilities, and his community status.[15]

One may conjecture, too, that the federal government's enthusiasm

[13] Lester Breslow, M.D., "Health Care: Assuring Quality," *The American Federationist*, Vol. 80, no. 5 (May 1973), p. 8.

[14] Greer Williams, "Kaiser: What Is It? . . . ," *Modern Hospital*, February 1971, p. 84.

[15] David Mechanic, "Physician Satisfaction in Varying Settings," University of Wisconsin, mimeographed.

for prepaid group practice is alone sufficient reason for physician concern about such programs.[16] To the physician, the rapid increase in government funding of medical services is but one of the successive steps of a federal takeover, of a pending nationalizing process. The skeptics might retort that modest funding to encourage the establishment of HMOs reveals wavering support for this delivery mode. The $325 million budgeted to facilitate their growth is a modest investment compared with $32 billion now spent on Medicare and Medicaid. On the other hand, a cynic might charge that such underfunding is designed to ensure the failure of the movement and thus set the stage for more aggressive plans for intervention. In another version, other cynics might charge that both the funding of the HMO (with provisions for lay influence on its policy board) and the system of community ratings represent the formidable thin edge of government intrusion. In Act I of this plot, the physician anticipates legions of meddling bureaucrats in every doctor's office. In Act II, he sees dominance by the "slide-rule set" in Washington, looking over the shoulder of every physician as he labors in a government-prescribed group-practice setting. The physician may view the present opportunity in a *Catch 22* setting. If he participates in a group-practice plan, he surrenders vital freedoms to the group and sets the stage, through peer review, for national standards of both performance and pay. If he fails to participate, he is confronted with more ominous forms of federal intervention.

The issue of freedom is profoundly significant to the physician. He is immersed in a heavy workload and sees himself as a dedicated servant laboring tirelessly to serve his patients. If his 60-hour work week should yield an income over $100,000, that is only coincidental. There is some risk, in proposing alternative forms for the delivery of services, of neglecting the attractiveness of existing arrangements to the physician. As Reinhardt makes the point:

> . . . a society that places great value on individual freedom must surely give the American health-care system high marks for the freedom of choice it affords both the providers and the majority of the consumers of medical care. From the physician's point of view in particular, the American system is highly attractive, for it leaves entirely up to him the choice of a specialty, the choice of the mode and location of his practice, the determination of the length of his work week, of his patient load, of the level of his professional fees, and of the style and pace with which his practice is conducted. Finally, it is generally viewed as ap-

---

[16] *Health Care Crisis in America, 1971,* Hearings before the Subcommittee on Health of the Committee on Labor and Public Welfare, United States Senate, 92nd Congress, 1st session, on Examination of the Health Care Crisis in America, Part II (1971). The Hearings have reproduced a citizens' report, "Heal Yourself," largely critical of medical-care providers. George Besson, as a member of that citizen's group, offers a lucid rejoinder to those criticisms, p. 321.

propriate that, other things being equal, the financial rewards earned by health-care providers tend to vary positively with their own efforts. Indeed, some observers regard this relationship between effort and reward—as embodied in the fee-for-service system—as the *sine qua non* of high-quality care. . . .[17]

Capturing somewhat the same spirit of protest, C. Rufus Rorem reminds us that, however medical practice is organized,

. . . the throats will have to be swabbed by physicians with their instruments, not by slide rules. If the doctors like it, you're in, and if they don't like it, you're out. If they don't want it, can't see it, don't grasp it, if they don't understand that this is a way to organize their services more effectively so they can have more time to themselves, they will be indifferent. My observation has been that it isn't money particularly that physicians are concerned with. It's professional independence.[18]

George Besson is critical of the charges made about the fragmented system of medical care. He considers such fragmentation is essential to deal with the myriad needs of a highly scattered population:

The concept of disarray, in contrast to orderliness, is a semantic trap. One could hardly argue against rationality, responsiveness, or orderliness, yet what do we hope to achieve in providing personal health care if not, in the ideal, an intensively personal service responsive to the patient's needs? Disarray in one man's view may well represent ideal personal encounter in another man's view.[19]

In a similar vein, Russel B. Roth has testified:

I have yet to find a proponent of this charming idea who can tell me in any meaningful way what I and my associates in our urological group would be expected to do differently in a setting of contract or HMO practice. The talk invariably wanders to multiphasic screening, which is not half so much health maintenance as it is earlier discovery of disease, or it veers to immunizations and general health education against overeating, oversmoking, overdrugging, and the kind of thing which is far better done by individuals less highly skilled than those of us who were educated and trained to diagnose and treat the sick.[20]

There is one final aspect of the nonfinancial portion of physician services, which relates to the importance of personal care. Although the physician, regardless of the setting, has only a limited time to devote to an individual's problems, under solo practice he undoubtedly derives much

[17] Uwe E. Reinhardt, "Proposed Changes in the Organization of Health-Care Delivery," p. 174.
[18] Rorem, "Prescription for an HMO," p. 10.
[19] Dissenting Opinion, "Heal Yourself," *Health Care Crisis in America, 1971*, Part II, p. 320.
[20] Hearings, *Health Maintenance Organizations*, Part II, p. 339.

satisfaction from the respect, if not adulation, showered on him by loyal patients. The cult of personality characterizes solo practice, and the spirits of the physician are surely lifted by the regular praise or appreciation of patients. In a group setting, the opportunity to cultivate a coterie of loyal and appreciative patients is reduced. Although there is often provision for patients to select physicians, there is less opportunity for the physician to select patients. An unhappy match may prove discomforting on all sides. In solo practice, the patient is typically free to "vote with his feet" should he lose confidence in his physician. In a group-practice setting, awkward relationships may be more common, for neither the patient nor the physician has face-saving mechanisms for disengaging.

There is, in fact, only limited information about the complexities and subtleties of physician–patient relationships within group settings. We know that human relationships are critical to the patient's perception of the success of the production mechanism. Patients are sensitive to the promptness of care, the sincerity and thoroughness of the physician as he seeks the background for the illness, and displays of concern about the patient's welfare. He asks two questions: "Does the physician care?" and "Can the physician help me?" If the physician does not show that he cares, it is not illogical to conclude that disappointing treatment results reflect an indifferent or hurried diagnosis. Because of the inextricable connection between human relations and technical proficiency, the patient will judge the outcome of the treatment process by the quality of his physician contact. Can a congenial and responsive atmosphere be cultivated in the high-pressure clinical setting of group practice?

In a group setting, the so-called crock (a perennial patient) poses some unusual challenges to the physician. In a group practice, this sort of patient may resent being restricted to the physicians on his group's panel and because of that frustration be all the more demanding. In a thoughtful eighteen-month study of physician–patient relations in a group setting, Eliot Freidson reported the following caricature of the demanding patient:

> The seventeen physicians who generalized about the social character-
> istics of demanding patients yielded in sum a caricature of the demand-
> ing patient as a female schoolteacher, well educated enough to be
> capable of articulate and critical questioning and letter writing, of high
> enough social status to be sensitive to slight and to expect satisfaction,
> and experienced with bureaucratic procedures. In the physicians' eyes,
> they were also neurotically motivated to be "demanding."[21]

[21] Eliot Freidson, "Prepaid Group Practice and the New 'Demanding Patient,'" *Milbank Memorial Fund Quarterly* (Fall 1973), p. 484.

The physician is challenged (and strained) to pacify such patients by presenting complete explanations about the treatment process, along with candid discussion of its potential for success.

CONSUMER CONCERNS WITH GROUP PRACTICE

Our narrative of physician concerns inevitably brings to light issues of client concerns, for it is in the interaction that both parties define satisfactory treatment. As we noted above, the patient is highly sensitive to the quality of his interpersonal relationship with his doctor. At the time of serious illness, the patient's ability to seek out the best medical services is limited. Further, he may have only speculative information about his ailment. The patient seeks a congenial relationship as well as effective treatment, but the physician works within a tight schedule. By training, institutional pressure, and economic necessity, the physician moves swiftly. The emotional, social, and economic conditions that may interact with the biological problems cannot—except in unusual circumstances—command much attention. The physician cannot afford to spend much time assuring the patient that his problems are of major concern to him. How do patients participating in a PGP view the adequacy of attention received? More data are available on consumer than on physician satisfaction; so let us examine some of the results.

As the issue of the quality of health care becomes a political issue, client satisfactions with government-subsidized systems acquire fresh significance. There is less impulse to attribute shortcomings to imperfections of the medical market. Political sensitivities lead to issues of accountability and to the identification of persons with whom grievances can be filed. The customer emerges with a fresh degree of sovereignty. The same constraints operate on profitmaking group-practice plans. A disenchanted customer not only may withdraw from the group plan, but also may poison the attitudes of others about his group's services. Word-of-mouth attitudes determine public perceptions of group-health plans.

It might be reasoned that under solo practice, the consumer has equal influence in ensuring that he will receive high-quality health care. In a market that is highly fragmented, however, there is not the same facility for critical patients to jeopardize the revenue flow to the solo practitioner. As long as the consumer feels he has other options, as does the physician, there is less reason for individual grievances to fester. In medical markets characterized—as most are—by the shortage of physician services, the prospect of patient withdrawal from a treatment schedule is not a serious threat.

Equally significant is the charge that the consumer is not truly the best judge of what services are appropriate. Hence, medical policies would be distorted as the growth of the HMO movement gives more attention to the intuitions of the lay public and dilutes the influence of those technically proficient in medical care. No matter what the delivery mode, the case has been made that the benefits of "free choice" have been overemphasized. Esselstyn alleges that this freedom amounts to no more than "an obligation imposed on an unenlightened patient to choose from an unlabeled product."[22]

It is the fashion, in HMO literature, to emphasize the benefits that are achieved by "dual choice." But we should not neglect the competitive realities that serve to limit abuses in the private sector (the comments above notwithstanding). To the average citizen, his selection of a physician reflects his discretion. But not so when his selection is restricted to a closed panel. Further, in the consumer view, the solo physician has genuine economic incentives to deliver promised services.

> In the private-practice mode of organizing work, the physician makes a living by attracting patients and providing them with services paid for by a fee for each service. . . . He has no contractual relationship with patients. He must attract them by a variety of devices—accessibility, reputation, specialty, referral relations with colleagues—and maintain a sufficiently steady stream of new or returning patients to assure a stable if not lucrative practice. In theory, the patient is free to leave him for another physician, and relations with colleagues offering the same services are at least nominally competitive.[23]

The problems of launching a new HMO undoubtedly reflect the skepticism of both consumers and physicians about the potential for improving upon private or solo practice. It is difficult to determine whether that resistance reflects familiarity with unsatisfactory programs or simply ignorance. There is reason to believe that the latter may be the case. Merlin K. Duval, Assistant Secretary for Health and Scientific Affairs in HEW, has contended that a major barrier to the growth of HMOs is the unfamiliarity of both physicians and customers with their advantages and disadvantages. Just as the physician is cautious about the radical restructuring of services, so the patient may feel he has more to lose in an untested (or unfamiliar) innovation. It is probable, however, that consumer resistance does not reflect anxiety as much as ignorance.[24] As one writer explained:

[22] C. B. Esselstyn, "The Outlook for Group Practice Prepayment," Address before the Michigan State Medical Society, 1966, p. 10.

[23] Freidson, "Prepaid Group Practice and the New 'Demanding Patient,'" p. 476.

[24] "Development of HMOs: Concepts and Benefits," *Health Services Reports*, Vol. 87, no. 5 (May 1972), p. 407.

[The HMO] won't be an idea whose time has come unless those millions of housewives who make the decisions think it is. Consumers aren't demanding prepaid group practice now, because they don't know what it is.[25]

There is evidence, however, that the participant in prepaid group-practice plans is not uniformly pleased with the nature of services provided. According to most evidence, the deficiency is not perceived in terms of the quality of service or the technical skills of the attending physician. Discontent centers on the queuing problem—the delay involved in securing an appointment with a physician and the brief time allotted for each session. In the conventional view, there is a quality of impersonality, of haste (and sometimes delay) that tends to create a sense of unease about the system.[26]

Most participants in group-practice plans are satisfied with the technical competence of services provided. Surveys of consumer attitudes may be biased if those surveyed are not regular users of the system. Furthermore, measures of consumer satisfaction may not always reflect experience of actual services provided, but only the consumer's expectations. It is difficult to account fully for the influences of the latter. If the group payment plan has cultivated unrealistic expectations, it is only natural that the program be held fully accountable for its performance. But even so, perceptions of unsatisfactory service may reflect the nature of expectations rather than structural defects in the delivery system itself.

A further methodological problem is the absence of control groups in many studies. Measures of satisfaction must ultimately be relative. Those who participate in group plans may not have an experience of solo practice as a reference point, and many surveys neglect to consider the issue of relative performance. Also, because the service packages often vary from one plan to the other, consumer comparisons are not easily measured.

A study by Tessler and Mechanic of consumer satisfaction indicated high scores for both prepaid and Blue Cross plans. Blue Cross participants, however, indicated significantly higher levels of satisfaction on most items.[27] Satisfaction items included consumer satisfaction with his sense of privacy in the doctor's office, the amount of time the doctor spent with him, the doctor's warmth and concern about his health, the doctor's willingness to listen to a description of symptoms, and the friendliness of nurses and receptionists. In the question "Except in emergencies,

[25] Rorem, "Prescriptions for an HMO," p. 15.

[26] Paul Snider, "Health Maintenance Organizations: A Can of Worms?" *Personnel*, Vol. 51 (November 1974), p. 41.

[27] Richard Tessler and David Mechanic, "Consumer Satisfaction with Prepaid Group Practice: A Comparative Study," *Journal of Health and Social Behavior*, Vol. 16, no. 1 (March 1975), p. 98.

about how many days do you usually have to wait for an appointment?," the estimates of Blue Cross respondents averaged ten days.[28] Perceptions of accessibility were, as one might anticipate, a key element in measures of satisfaction. Although the prepaid-practice participants were very satisfied with the medical care they and their children had received, they expressed somewhat less satisfaction than their counterparts in Blue Cross plans. During the reenrollment period, approximately six percent of the prepaid-practice enrollees switched to the Blue Cross insurance option, while less than one percent of the Blue Cross participants changed to the prepaid-group coverage.[29] Although these results reflect a single sample of two study groups, Eliot Freidson's research underscores the conclusion that consumers perceive prepaid group practice as somewhat impersonal and unresponsive to individual needs and expectations.[30] The perceptions of impersonality may well reflect the consumer's more limited choice in selecting a physician. In a group plan, the physician may be under a more rigorous schedule, and the appearance of haste could convince consumers that the physician considers their problems trivial. Prepaid clients also resent, of course, any hint that they are equivalent to charity patients.

In a study of the Columbia Medical Plan, operated in Columbia, Maryland, by Johns Hopkins University, the Johns Hopkins Hospital and the Connecticut General Life Insurance Company, clients rated the program favorably. Only 1.3 percent defined their impressions as "poor." But when asked to indicate areas of needed improvement, 30 percent wanted improved appointment arrangements, 19 percent noted inadequate waiting-room arrangements, and 19.7 percent wanted improvement in after-hours treatment. Twenty-seven percent indicated an interest in periodic health-review examinations.[31]

In the Kaiser system, which also draws its share of criticism, the new patient is encouraged to choose his own doctor from the available internists, pediatricians, and obstetrician-gynecologists. Appointments are scheduled between nine and five, with new visits lasting thirty minutes and return visits fifteen minutes. Waiting times for appointments commonly run from three to six weeks. A physician may set aside one hour a day to see regular patients with acute illness or emergency needs. Such "squeeze-in" scheduling is intended to maintain order within the regular scheduling process. Making appointments through a central

[28] Ibid., p. 108.

[29] Ibid., p. 110.

[30] Eliot Freidson, "Client Control and Medical Practices," *American Journal of Sociology,* Vol. 65 (January 1960), pp. 374–82, and *Patients' Views of Medical Practice* (New York: Russell Sage Foundation, 1961).

[31] "Consumers Give Opinions on Columbia Medical Plan," *Modern Hospital,* Vol. 117, (August 1971), p. 43.

switchboard appears to be a problem. Between eight and twenty-four women sit around two circular tables. In the middle, a turntable is rotated to give each operator access to the appointment books for each doctor. Urgent calls are referred to another number, and in "true" emergencies an operator can dispatch an ambulance. Even with this arrangement, one patient complained of being "left hanging" for thirty minutes. Waiting time in the office may only be a few minutes. It is usually less than an hour, but may run as high as two hours, depending on patient loads and needs.[32]

Kaiser critics have been quick to point out how severely overloaded their system is. The San Francisco Medical Center receives an estimated 10,000 telephone calls per day, and occasionally the system breaks down under the weight of so many calls. A survey of Kaiser members who had been in the plan for more than 15 years uncovered some complaints about the telephone situation, but they generally felt that services had improved over the past several years. A Kaiser representative acknowledged that new members often have difficulty in "solving the system," whereas older members can usually get through to their doctor.[33]

Studies on consumer satisfaction typically indicate contentment with their health plan, regardless of its type. Also, most studies identify a hard core of dissatisfied customers, roughly 10 percent, who hold negative views on almost all aspects of their plan—again, regardless of its type. In a 1970 study of the Kaiser plan in the Los Angeles area, 87.4 percent of the members interviewed said they would renew with Kaiser, as compared with 94 percent in 1961. Eighty to 83 percent were satisfied with their doctors, 88 percent with the nurses, and 87 percent with the receptionists and other nonmedical employees. When asked how the plan might be improved, 25 percent pointed to the need to reduce the "long wait for appointments." Within the crowded schedule, physicians sometimes juggle the sequence in order to take the "sickest first." Because such disruptions cannot be fully explained to all patients, they are a ready source of resentment. One Kaiser physician explained the interruptions of scheduling as a source of discontent. He describes an emergency:

> The doctor may have to call for extra help, but what needs to be done must be done. Other patients may have to wait. . . . If it is necessary to pull half your internists, you will. You say to the patient, "It's nice talking about your ulcer, but let's talk about it next time; you can stew right now." Not quite that blunt, but that's the pattern.
>
> If I was a member and called up for a periodic health checkup, I would [have to] go to the end of the line. . . . The . . . [waiting time] would

[32] Williams, "Kaiser," p. 85.
[33] Tyler Marshall, "The Patients' View: What They Like and What They Don't Like," *Modern Hospital*, Vol. 116 (February 1971), p. 86.

be anywhere from two to three months, . . . which would leave you with a low satisfaction ratio if you had suddenly made up your mind—the wife was saying you were dragging around—why not get a physical examination? There is nothing worse than to say you are going to do something and your performance is poor. We have to live in a real world.[34]

This section has centered on attitudes, always a treacherous area of analysis. As we noted at the outset, perceptions may be ill-founded. Criticisms of the group-care operation may, in fact, be criticisms that can be generalized against all forms of medical practice. Certainly, for example, the solo practitioner has not solved the problem of waiting time or of the unanticipated interruptions of emergency surgery, and so on.

But the prepaid group practice does create difficulties that are peculiar to a "one-stop" service center. There is risk of bureaucracy, authority, impersonality, the chilling appearances of a factory. In a group-practice program, there is some risk that physicians may grow dissatisfied with obligations to treat the worried-well or others with trivial symptoms that are not of much interest to them. Despite this tendency, consumers who perceive a medical problem must be handled with diplomacy and care. If they are abruptly dismissed, they may leave feeling frustrated and dissatisfied. If a contract has promised care that has not been forthcoming, dissatisfaction can turn to angry resentment.

Sidney R. Garfield has advanced the concern that eliminating the price barrier can actually complicate the task of personal physician care. Within a group-practice plan, there is commonly

. . . an uncontrolled flood of well, worried-well, early-sick, and sick people into our point of entry—the doctor appointment—on a first-come, first-served basis that has little relation to priority of need. The impact of this demand overloads the system and, since the well and worried-well people are a considerable proportion of our entry mix, the usurping of available doctors' time by healthy people actually interferes with the care of the sick.[35]

He has proposed that a new entry regulator be designed, with health testing to separate the well from the sick and to establish priorities. Such an entry mechanism would also detect symptoms of early illness, provide a preliminary survey for the doctor, aid in diagnosis, and provide a basic health profile of the patient. All of this is intended to save time for both physician and patient.

This routing process is seen in Figure 15-1. One group of patients, the healthy, would be directed to a new form of health facility, where

[34] Williams, "Kaiser," p. 88.
[35] Sidney R. Garfield, "The Delivery of Medical Care," *Scientific American*, Vol. 222 (April 1970), pp. 19–20.

Figure 15-1 Flow model of medical-care delivery system

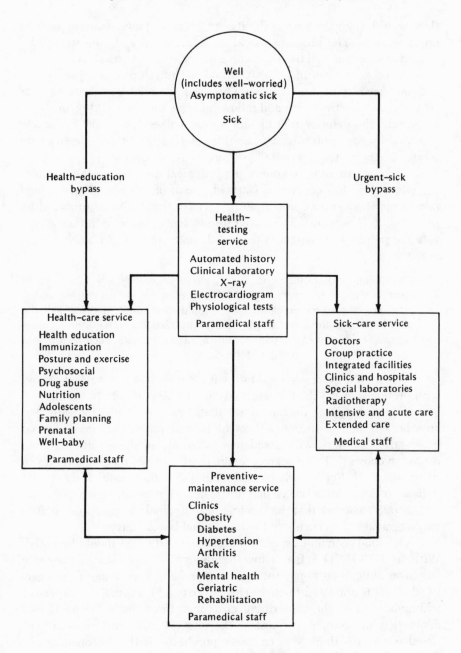

Adapted from "The Delivery of Medical Care," by S. Garfield.
© 1970 by Scientific American Inc. All rights reserved.

they would enjoy lectures, exhibits, audiovisual tapes, counseling, and other services. The program would be informative and educational, intended to keep the well from becoming either sick or worried-well.

A second stream of patients would be introduced to a preventive-maintenance service, providing support for high-incidence chronic illness requiring routine treatment and follow-up. This station would be intended to prevent the deterioration of illness, and its services could be largely provided by paraprofessionals. The third station would provide sick-care service whenever regular staff physicians are fully occupied.

Although there is no convincing statistical evidence of the "swamping effect" that has concerned Garfield, much of the physician's valued time is nonetheless used in diagnostic services that could be provided by paramedics. However, in the search for efficiency, we may further aggravate the patient's discontent with the adequacy of care. As Mechanic reminds us:

> A labeling and sorting process may make sense logically, but it might readily violate the psychological logic of effective doctor/patient understanding and communication. We should be careful in discarding the subtle skills of the sensitive physician, who recognizes that there is more to the problem than the patient will say, and who takes such factors into account in the management of the case.[36]

We should be concerned, too, with the mentally disturbed. Those with problems of psychiatric morbidity might be particularly hostile to a formal "gate-keeping" diagnostic mission. Some estimates indicate that anywhere from five to ten percent of patient populations have formal psychiatric disorders, with about one in twenty of these suffering from acute psychosis.[37] This suggests again there are no ready shortcuts in diagnostic work. For an early-classification system that would direct certain patients to alternative offices may ultimately require physician presence, and there is some risk that the labeling of individuals by paraprofessionals may aggravate concerns about the impersonal bureaucracy.

One final economic aspect of consumer satisfaction should be noted. With the 1973 HMO Act, a deliberate attempt is being made to eliminate employer obligations to pay for more comprehensive coverage than a certified HMO is obligated to offer. This, at first sight, shifts the prospect of additional cost to the subscribing customer. Furthermore, there is evidence that the competitive cost of the prepaid plan (and not differentiated service) is the key to customer purchases. If those economies are dissipated by further broad-coverage obligations, the consumer may be

[36] David Mechanic, "Human Problems and the Organization of Health Care," *The Annals of the American Academy of Political and Social Science*, Vol. 399 (January 1972), p. 10.
[37] Ibid., p. 9.

highly resistant to HMO participation. Specifically, he may not be attracted to various aspects of such broadened coverage. It is likely, for example, that many would resist paying for HMO coverage for problems of alcoholism and drug addiction.

ARE THERE ECONOMIES IN GROUP PRACTICE?

The HMO movement has drawn national attention because of evidence that it has reduced hospitalization by approximately 50 percent. The savings are substantial, but even more significant is the possibility for consumers to avoid the costs (and sometimes tragic penalties) of unnecessary surgery. There are few dollar estimates of these costs. It is hoped, too, that other economic benefits could be provided by the extensive use of paramedical personnel to reduce physician costs. There is little evidence this has happened. The integration of services within group-practice is more economical than the costs of private-practice services. Preventive care will sometimes minimize the heavy costs of curative treatment. The reduction in the physician–subscriber ratio to 100 to 100,000 (if uniformly available) would do much to "solve" the problem of the physician shortage. In 1973 there were about 325,000 professionally active physicians in the United States, or 155 per 100,000 population. If physician services could be provided through group services in major metropolitan areas at a 100 to 100,000 ratio, this would clearly leave a surplus to meet the need of the underserved areas of the country.[38]

But the critics are not persuaded that all these economies are, in fact, so substantial as they first appear. Let us enumerate some of the "costs" of the HMO movement, as represented by these economic considerations.

First, it is charged that we impute services to an HMO program that often do not become operational. This is most clearly seen in preventive and multiphasic screening. The principle of preventive care has obvious virtues, but there is considerable evidence that when such care is made available, even without charge, few individuals take advantage of it. The reasons for such indifference, as we have noted in an earlier chapter, are not clear. Nor, again, is there evidence that those who avail themselves of regular examinations have a better record of morbidity, mortality, or fatality.

A second, related criticism is that the HMO movement cultivates the illusion of health *maintenance*. There is persuasive evidence that a

[38] For data, *Basic Charts on Health Care*, Subcommittee on Health of the Committee on Ways and Means, U.S. House of Representatives, prepared for the Subcommittee on Health (Washington, D.C.: GPO, 1975), pp. 26–35.

person's abuse and neglect of his body does much more damage than can be repaired by any medical system. It is difficult for any "outside" health service to *maintain* health when we as the custodians of our bodies knowingly pursue lifestyles that are so destructive of health. In addition, there is that segment of society that may have incentives for body care but are prevented by environmental and income constraints. John R. Kernodle of the AMA has emphasized that a distinction must be drawn between a medical and an educational approach to health.

> You probably know as well as we do that our major killers—accidents, heart disease, and cancer—relate to lifestyle and environment as much as they do to the availability of medical care. I reaffirm this position simply to underscore the importance of health education.
>
> . . . But can HMOs discover a magic so far unrevealed to the rest of us? A magic that will somehow motivate people to drive more carefully, exercise more frequently, eat more sensibly, smoke less and worry less? Can the HMOs discover an educational magic, so far unavailable to the Public Health Service, which will reduce the incidence of the single most common communicable disease—gonorrhea—or the fourth most common—syphilis?[39]

A third economic criticism of HMOs is that there is not uniform evidence that the medical teams have made wider use of paraprofessionals. The pressures to preserve the occupational "turf" appear as well cemented inside as outside the HMO system.

Bailey has found no evidence that group practice increases physician productivity through the substitution of paramedical time for physician time. The rate at which internists treat patients is independent of group size.[40] Bailey contends that the earnings for group-practice physicians tend to be higher than for those in solo practice, and examines whether economies of scale permit those superior earnings. But his field studies show that the higher earnings do not, in fact, reflect greater physician productivity, in the sense that each physician sees a larger number of patients than in solo practice. The larger income can be largely explained by group practitioners obtaining income from ancillary services performed within the group. In solo practice, such services are obtained by sending the patient "out" for x-rays, tests, and so on. As another example, he found that pediatricians in solo practice were delegating more patient-care tasks and actually seeing more patients than pediatricians in large multispecialty group practices, holding the number of ancillary workers

[39] "Heal Yourself," *Health Care Crisis in America*, Part II (1971), p. 320.

[40] Richard M. Bailey, "A Comparison of Internists in Solo and Fee-for-service Group Practice in the San Francisco Bay Area," *Bulletin of the New York Academy of Medicine*, Vol. 44 (November 1968), pp. 1293–1303; "Economies of Scale in Medical Practice." In Herbert Klarman (ed.), *Empirical Studies in Health Economics* (Baltimore: Johns Hopkins Press, 1970).

constant. Yankauer and associates also found the number of physician visits per unit of time to be virtually constant with the increase in the size of the group practice.[41] The delegation of tasks by physicians tended to be confined to administrative, technical, and clerical functions, but not in patient-care functions. Delegation of patient-care functions appeared to reflect local shortages of pediatricians rather than a conscious redesign of job activities made possible by expanding the scale of group service. When allied health personnel perform some of the medical services, the patient usually receives additional services rather than a reduction in physician services. When there is an appearance of allied health personnel for physician services, these usually involve additional services for the patient, rather than reductions in the use of physician services. In one authority's review of the statistical evidence, the "economies of scale [in medical practice] have not yet been demonstrated empirically."[42]

This criticism can be countered by noting that there are many variables that account for the system's efficiency and productivity. Consider the number of physician visits. It would be naive to assume that all visits are uniformly productive and that a one-to-one relationship holds as the volume of such activity increases. In one sense, the flow of such service is paced by the system. By the analogy of industry, the productivity ratio is machine-controlled rather than worker-controlled. For example, Kaiser is experimenting with "mini, walk-in visits" designed for performing checkups and dispersing drugs; an estimated twenty such visits can be handled in an hour. It would be unreasonable to conclude that the system was thereby more efficient by a factor of five, since only four regular visits are handled each hour.

A fourth economic argument against the HMO structure is the larger issue of physician hours of service. The HMO is "sold" to physicians by the argument that hours are regularized and reasonable; the physician is not "on call" around the clock. Critics contend that benefits accruing to the physician must be set against costs to society. The reduction in hours of service per physician can be translated directly into larger needs for this expensive and scarce resource. More directly, the physician's gain is society's loss.

A fifth issue is the question of incentives. The Rand economist Joseph P. Newhouse contends that the larger the group practice, the more certain the physician's loss of interest in keeping his costs down and his

[41] Alfred Yankauer, John P. Connelly, and Jacob J. Feldman, "Physician Productivity in the Delivery of Ambulatory Care," *Medical Care,* Vol. 8 (January/February 1970), pp. 35–46.
[42] Herbert E. Klarman, "Analysis of the HMO Proposal: Its Assumptions, Implications, and Prospects." In *Health Maintenance Organizations: A Reconfiguration of the Health Services System* (Chicago: University of Chicago Center for Health Administration Studies), p. 31.

work effort high. The larger the group, the less likely the discernible consequence of a lagging effort and the smaller the reward from any additional work effort. The inference is then drawn that the larger the group, the higher the costs and the lower the productivity. Newhouse also predicts that as the group became larger, the "hours worked would fall as the individual physician's share of marginal revenue falls."[43]

A sixth economic criticism is that it cannot afford to give all segments of society the kinds of medical services promised in federal pronouncements. Subscriptions to group-practice plans usually exclude the very poor and the very wealthy. Membership is dominated by large segments of unionized workers and government employees. The government has insisted that "certified" HMOs have an open enrollment period during which the system would have to accept all applicants. Senator Kennedy has remarked that

> . . . the practice wherein low-risk persons are sold health insurance at preferential rates has been extraordinarily damaging to the entire health industry and to the . . . availability of services. This practice of "skimming the cream," of leaving those people most in need of health services to pay the highest bill, often without the assistance of adequate insurance, cannot and should not be encouraged by any program utilizing federal funds.[44]

The government has also insisted on "community ratings" in establishing the subscription fee. In brief, everyone would pay the same tariff. However, most experts in the health-care field contend that this arrangement simply will not work. Robert M. Yeyssel has noted:

> The HMO, if it is required to have an open-enrollment period, is very likely to enroll a population over time which is actuarially unsound and quite different from its competition. . . .
>
> On the other side of the coin, the problems of enrolling a representative sample of a metropolitan area . . . are enormous. One would need a fairly narrow corridor, running from the inner city out some place in the suburbs in order to do this.[45]

Under such arrangements, the sick are attracted to the plan. As the fee structure is raised to cover treatment costs for the seriously ill, the program becomes less competitive. To be "certified" under the 1973 Act,

> each HMO must have at least one open-enrollment period of at least 30 days once a year when it must accept (to its capacity) everyone in the community who applies, unless too many high-risk applicants threaten

---

[43] Joseph P. Newhouse, "The Economics of Group Practice," *The Journal of Human Resources,* Vol. 8, no. 1, pp. 37–38.
[44] Hearings, *Health Maintenance Organizations,* p. 119.
[45] Ibid., pp. 915–16.

to jeopardize its economic viability. There are provisions in the law for waivers of this requirement, but open enrollment remains one of the factors making the Federal HMO an expensive benefit package. In addition, the law provides that no person can be refused reenrollment or be expelled for any reason concerning health condition or need for service.[46]

There is evidence that the consumer is highly price-conscious when given a choice between alternative medical plans. If HMO coverage costs workers as much as eight to twelve dollars a month more than they are now paying, they will likely resist or reject the plan. Related to this problem is the fate of present insurance plans with fragmented participation of employees in two or more plans: "No one yet knows what will happen if, say, forty percent of the employees in an insured plan choose HMO coverage. There could be cancellations [of other plans] in smaller companies."[47]

The HMO will prove expensive—indeed far more expensive—than traditional insurance because of the absence of exclusions, deductibles, and coinsurance factors. The early experience of Blue Cross with the community-ratings structure is illuminating. Blue Cross used community ratings in setting premiums until employers with better records of good health sought out insurers willing to reduce premiums through an experience rating. The insurance principle—that the healthy help pay for the insurance protection of the less healthy—had become warped: the healthy abandoned the community-rated plans for those providing preferential treatment leaving the former plans with only the high-risk and high-expense clients. However, under the 1973 Act, with its mandatory open-enrollment period, the insurance principle has been restored. Paul Ellwood, Jr., President of InterStudy, has testified: "The HMO suicide pact is the requirement that all HMOs be community rated with everyone paying the same price. I feel that the open enrollment plus community rating are the scariest part of the bill for HMO insurers."[48]

Finally, critics of the HMO movement have questioned the circumstances surrounding the more modest use of hospital services. There are complex circumstances that account for the demand of such services. The solo physician may be seeking the "best" care possible, anxious to avoid any charge of neglect in a malpractice suit, eager to share responsibility of diagnosis with the backup facilities of the hospital, and so on. And of course the insured patient may see this as a costless exercise. The allegation that we have excessive hospitalization and surgery is challenged, simply because we do not have output measures that precisely establish

[46] Snider, "Health Maintenance Organizations: A Can of Worms?" p. 39.
[47] Ibid., p. 42.
[48] Paul Ellwood, Jr., "Risk Managers Take a Look at HMOs," *The National Underwriter*, October 18, 1974, p. 52.

just what is necessary. Russel B. Roth, Speaker for the House of Delegates of the AMA, explained that the entire issue of too little or too much reliance upon health-care procedures was offensive to the professional integrity of physicians. In this view, any alleged excess does not reflect an effort to increase income. As Roth explained:

> Of one thing we are quite certain: competent, conscientious, well-motivated physicians clearly practice good medicine in any setting, ranging from practice in the Armed Forces and the Veterans' Administration to fee-for-service partnerships and solo practice. If physicians for some reason are not competent, conscientious, or well-motivated, we doubt sincerely that a change in practice patterns will make them that way. We believe that the emphasis on the system is misplaced.[49]

CONFLICTS OF INTEREST

An additional set of criticisms concern the conflicts of interest created by the HMO arrangement. First, there is concern that a hospital-based HMO will be reluctant to reduce hospitalization. Depending on the management of the HMO, there will be varying pressures on the staff to make use of available facilities. If a hospital-based HMO has excess bed capacities, the board may be caught in a dilemma: unit costs of limited hospitalization will soar in order to absorb the large overhead. A new HMO designing its own hospital facilities would be sensitive to appropriate bed ratios and avoid this trap, but the conflict could be meaningful in coalitions of physicians with existing hospital operations.[50]

A second conflict of interest is the traditional struggle for control. As noted above, there is much skepticism about the effectiveness of lay control, both inside and outside the medical-care industry. It is not easy to achieve consumer sovereignty.

A third issue pertains to the treatment strategy itself. To what extent can a group practice afford generous and extended treatment of those who are chronically ill? In most situations, of course, the unhappy choice might be bypassed by the simple expedient of not admitting high-risk individuals into the system, even though the tactic of "skimming" runs counter to the regulations provided in the 1973 HMO Act. Nevertheless, the physician and the plan have a financial interest in a profitable HMO.

[49] Hearings, *Health Maintenance Organizations*, II, p. 340.
[50] "The Secretary of HEW, among others, has said that the administration's encouragement of health-maintenance organizations is aimed at emptying hospital beds; and the secretary and others have noted the extraordinary fact that hospital people have been among the leaders in a movement that will have the result of emptying the beds the hospitals have to keep full, in order to earn the revenues they have to have to do all the things they are expected to do." "Prescriptions for an HMO," p. 5.

Thus, the dilemma of what to do when an HMO appears headed for bankruptcy remains.

A fourth conflict of interest is the unsettling influence of requiring many options for workers when collective-bargaining contracts come up for renewal. If a certified plan exists, employers are legally obligated to give their employees a chance to vote for it. Many well-established plans now reflect the carefully cultivated relationships between major unions, corporations, and private insurers. Thriving and prosperous brokerage arrangements exist with a vested interest in ongoing arrangements. The issue is not whether it is appropriate to challenge vested interests in existing arrangements, but to appreciate that such a challenge will create resistance among many of the parties that have grown comfortable with them. The government's publications on the feasibility of HMOs notes that the presence of brokers serves as a major challenge to the introduction of a new HMO option.

A further challenge is the unsettling influence on collective bargaining of the legal obligation to consider the HMO option if a certified plan exists. Peter G. Nash, general counsel of the National Labor Relations Board, has contended that offering the HMO option "is inconsistent with the law and policy of the National Labor Relations Act." In his view, it undermines basic concepts of good-faith bargaining by giving employers a predetermined position at the bargaining table. Nash also pointed out the legal precedents for the union to make decisions on fringe benefits during collective bargaining. Other employers confessed that they would not welcome the inevitable charges of union busting that might arise should they be forced to the HMO option in defiance of union wishes.[51]

Fifth is the reality that physician interest in the HMO is likely to be strongest in an area having young physicians without established private practices, where there may be some surplus of such skill. "The paradox is that the HMO structure gains more physician support when there is already adequate existing service to the area's population by established physicians."[52]

SUMMARY

In this chapter, we have filtered the viewpoints of one stream of opinion, to identify some major concerns. Although the issues identified here are not exhaustive (nor their treatment complete) the concerns, for the most part, are sobering. They lend credence to the view that PGP is not a panacea. Perhaps we have expected too much from these systems and are, under present federal regulations, requiring too much of such

[51] See "The HMO Movement Stalls Once More," *Business Week*, April 21, 1975.
[52] Testimony to authors.

group-practice plans. There must be some reasonable opportunity for the mechanism to behave the way society expects it to behave. Harry Becker, professor of community health at the Albert Einstein College of Medicine, captured some elements of the excessive expectations placed on the HMO movement:

> New community structures will grow as the issues of full public accountability and patient relevance emerge in the struggle to make the HMO concept a reality. As now conceived, the HMO cannot act on behalf of the total community. The HMO cannot be an agency for outreach nor can it coordinate or develop a total community-wide system for care.

> The paradox of health care in the 1970s is that the HMO idea has set America toward the goal of an all-inclusive public and national health service. Before this becomes a reality, today's nonsensical, costly, and regressive mixture of manipulative financing arrangements will have to be replaced.[53]

If the HMOs offer such obvious improvements of service, with more generous rewards to the physician, one would wonder why they did not spawn earlier and why they have not thrived. The critics are quick to point out that the Kaiser-Permanente example is unusual: few such plans have the unique support of a major industrial enterprise. If these plans provide such a natural combination of advantages to both suppliers and subscribers, these would emerge as natural coalitions of interest groups, without encouragement and "seed money" from public sources.

The government is wary of liabilities inherent in the "takeover" of the health industry. In reality, the HMO movement gives the government an excuse for doing almost nothing when it doesn't know quite what to do. Pressed to do all things for all Americans (at the same time that it faces a taxpayer revolt), the federal government seems to have abandoned its support of the HMO concept. In this view, the fault is not that we are searching for improved forms of delivery, but rather that we expect too much from them.

Whether the pragmatism of group practice will satisfy the aroused public clamor for "more" remains to be seen. In the health-care field, rhetoric has whetted appetites. It has, in some cases, cultivated an illusion that we have escaped the constraints of scarcity. If we are, in fact, on the edge of abundance—a concept that most economists consider an obscene illusion—the abundance of quality health-care service will require a rapidly growing HMO movement. But it will probably require much more. The cornucopia of care is not yet here. We have, meanwhile, overloaded the fragile vehicle of HMO delivery with excessive expectations and responsibilities.

---

[53] "Development of HMOs: Concepts and Benefits," p. 408.

SUGGESTED READINGS

GLASGOW, JOHN M., "Prepaid Group Practice as a National Health Policy: Problems and Perspectives," *Inquiry*, Vol. 9 (March 1972), pp. 3–15. Glasgow is doubtful of the prospects for HMOs in our health-care system.

HAVIGHURST, CLARK C., "Health Maintenance Organizations and the Market for Health Services," *Law and Contemporary Problems*, Vol. 24, no. 4 (Autumn 1970). Provides a pro and con on the HMO issue, with special emphasis on legal cases challenging the HMO structure.

ROEMER, MILTON I. and W. SHONICK, "HMO Performance: The Recent Evidence," *Milbank Memorial Fund Quarterly*, Summer 1973, pp. 271–315. A survey of HMO performance.

SCHNEIDER, ANDREAS G. and JOANNE B. STERN, "Health Maintenance Organizations and the Poor: Problems and Prospects," *Northwestern University Law Review*, Vol. 70, no. 2, pp. 90–138. A legal treatment of HMO obligations to serve the poor.

SCHWARTZ, HARRY, *The Case for American Medicine: A Realistic Look at Our Health Care System* (New York: McKay, 1973). Most proponents of HMOs begin with criticisms of the current health-care system, whereas Schwartz's defense of health care today leads to the opposite conclusion about the desirability of HMOs.

SEWARD, E. W., "The Relevance of Prepaid Group Practice to the Effective Delivery of Health Services," *Proceedings*, 18th Annual Group Health Institute, Saulte Saint Marie, Ontario, Canada, June 17–18, 1968, GHAA, Inc., Washington, D.C. A conservative presentation of HMO planning.

WEIL, PETER A., "Comparative Costs to the Medicare Program of Seven Prepaid Group Practices and Controls," *Milbank Memorial Fund Quarterly*, Summer 1976, pp. 339–65. Examines treatment levels for Medicare patients in prepaid group plans.

16

WHAT MAKES DOCTORS SICK:
THE MALPRACTICE CRISIS

A California bumper sticker reads: "Feeling sick? Call Your Lawyer." A *New Yorker* cartoon pictures a doctor tapping the knee of his patient, whose head pops off: "Damn! I suppose this means another malpractice suit!" Another cartoon pictures a stiff-legged, stitched monster standing at the desk of the Acme Insurance Company. The insurance agent is on the phone: "Dr. Frankenstein: Your monster is suing you for malpractice." In yet another cartoon, the physician and patient eye each other suspiciously. The patient is picturing a bundle of his dollars flying away for the physician's fee. The physician is picturing a bundle of his dollars that will go to pay for the malpractice suit. At a Washington conference on malpractice, an attorney described his visit to a physician. As the doctor began his examination, he noted a nurse waving a sign behind him: "He's a lawyer!"

The malpractice issue is front-page news. In the past two years we have witnessed physicians on strike, marching with pickets, and jeering state governors. We have seen physicians' wives photographed at a "sleep in" in a governor's office. We have seen the unusual spectacle of two of our most prestigious professions attacking each other in a highly unprofessional manner, with the lawyers occasionally alluding to the "butchers" whose misdeeds have been covered by self-serving medical associations, while physicians charge lawyers with parasitic behavior, trafficking in the human tragedy of illness and practicing a form of extortion. Each week we are confronted with the details of tragic medical "maloccurrences," with lawyers skillfully playing on jury sympathies on behalf of comatose patients. Jury awards have gone "out of sight" and, with them, insurance premiums for physicians. We are told that malpractice premiums now exceed $1 billion annually, that fees paid to attorneys exceed $2 billion annually, that defensive medicine—extensive testing and consultation—add another $5 to $10 billion to medical costs. Meanwhile, we are told that the hapless patient cannot expect—even when winning an award—to recover more than 17 cents on each premium dollar spent for such protection. And we have evidence that the majority of physicians avoid any involvement in highway accidents. Some are refusing to treat "new" patients. Some refuse to administer tests, having considered the risks of toxicity. Many have threatened to retire early. Some already have. Some are stripping themselves of all assets except a 20-year-old Volkswagen and "going bare" or abandoning insurance coverage. Most tragically, at a time when all agree that we must humanize the physician–patient relationship, it is now represented as an adversary relationship. For the medical sector, it is clear that times are out of joint. The consuming public is confronted each week with evidences of excessive surgery and with the high costs of overmedication and unnecessary mortality. He is given weekly counsel on "How to Pick a Physician," replete with such aphorisms as "The Life You Save May Be Your Own." Physicians, for their part, are bewildered about how best to protect their patients, their professional integrity, and their incomes. An advanced treatment regimen may become a legal risk should it prove, after the fact, to have failed. But the failure to use an advanced technique may itself set in motion litigation if what is perceived as "traditional" treatment proves ineffective. Paradoxically, one suspects that it is the very best physician who is most vulnerable to litigation because of his courage in undertaking the most difficult surgical assignments.

In all of this, it is difficult to determine winners and losers. It is probable that attorneys have enjoyed substantial fees and that newspapers are enjoying subscriber appreciation for the grisly accounts of medical "accidents." It is not clear that the insurance companies emerge the winners. But it is clear that the losers are the patients, the mass of Americans paying health-insurance premiums, the taxpayers, and physicians.

In this chapter we shall focus on the costs of malpractice insurance, of necessity drawing on current periodicals rather than technical journals and government monographs because of the fast-breaking nature of this crisis. We shall review the dimensions of the problem in terms of the frequency of physician–patient contact, and the quality of that personal relationship.

Let us begin by summarizing the published accounts of some of the more dramatic medical and insurance episodes. These will set the stage for the discussion of the causes of the physician's concern with premiums and the customer's concern for receiving quality care.

Driving alone on Christmas Eve in 1972, Leonard Tolley, then a 55-year-old dentist practicing in Lake Worth, Fla., had an auto accident that left him paralyzed in all four limbs. During the next few weeks, Tolley regained partial movement on both sides of his body, but his neurosurgeon recommended spinal surgery as the best hope for full recovery. On Jan. 12, 1973, the surgeon performed a decompression laminectomy . . . to relieve pressure on the spinal cord. The operation failed to help. After surgery, Tolley, who had been earning $100,000 annually, was again totally paralyzed, unable even to control his bowel and bladder functions. Last summer Tolley and his wife filed a malpractice suit against the doctor. . . . After a nine-day trial this spring, with testimony from 28 witnesses—including eight neurosurgeons—the jury awarded Tolley and his wife $1,685,000. The neurosurgeon's malpractice coverage will pay $1.1 million; he must raise the rest himself (Newsweek, June 9, 1975, p. 64).

Gail Kalmowitz was born prematurely in 1953, and doctors at New York's Brookdale Hospital used a procedure that was common medical practice at the time: they kept the $2\frac{1}{2}$-pound infant in an atmosphere of highly concentrated oxygen. Two months later an ophthalmologist discovered that Gail had a form of progressive, incurable blindness called retrolental fibroplasia. Much later, Gail's family learned that exposing premature babies to too much oxygen had been suggested as a cause of subsequent blindness as early as 1952—though it is not clear just how widely disseminated this knowledge was when Gail was born. In 1972, the Kalmowitzes filed a $2-million malpractice suit against Brookdale Hospital and the pediatricians who had attended Gail. . . . Just as the Brooklyn Supreme Court jury was about to hand down its verdict, Gail—now a 21-year-old psychology major at Brooklyn College and almost totally blind—lost her nerve and decided to accept an offer of a $165,000 settlement from her doctor's insurance company. Only a few minutes later, she found out that the jury had been about to award her $900,000 in damages—more than five times the amount she had accepted (Ibid., p. 65).

Mrs. June Walker, 52, now lies in a coma in a San Gabriel, California, nursing home, as a result of a series of improper medical procedures that occurred in a UCLA clinic. Faced with charges that ranged from unnecessary surgery, falsification of records, and failure to monitor the patient, University of California regents have agreed to pay Mrs. Walker's daily medical expenses—currently about $350 and going up all the time—for as long as she lives. Though Mrs. Walker may never come out of her coma, doctors estimate that she still might live for 23.5 years. If she survives that long and inflation does too, the settlement could cost California taxpayers more than $4.5 million (Time, December 30, 1974, p. 50).

After 40 years of medical practice in Aurora, a northern Illinois town with a population of 79,000, Dr. Eugene Balthazar, at age 70, decided to retire. Instead of taking up golfing, he opened a store-front clinic. In the first two years, Balthazar and his wife (who has since died of cancer) spent $30,000 of their own money to keep the clinic going. On a typical day, Balthazar may see as many as 100 patients. Aided only by a nurse, a receptionist, and 25 part-time volunteers, he treats almost every conceivable illness—heart disturbances, abscessed ears, broken bones, malnutrition, and once even a case of leprosy. He accepts no money. He estimates his treatment costs at about $1 per patient. He refuses Medicare or Medicaid payments, because it costs more than $1 to process a claim. He serves a stream of Aurora's poor—Mexicans, Appalachian whites, Indians, and blacks.

For Dr. Bal (as patients call him) the most satisfying tribute is from his own patients, who eagerly do anything they can to please him—from scrubbing floors, washing windows, even baking casseroles for his lunch. In fact, when a woman patient recently sued him for malpractice (because of a scar left by the successful treatment of facial malignancy), other patients were incensed. "Around here," said one, "suing Dr. Bal is like suing God." Balthazar, who refused to carry malpractice insurance, easily won his case (*Time*, January 26, 1976, p. 70).

Except for the last case cited, this selection of malpractice cases illuminates the sources of public interest and anxiety: there are indeed astonishing episodes of serious patient neglect with tragic consequences for the patient. We see, in addition, remarkably generous awards issued in jury trials. Many juries are obviously overwhelmed with the sense of grief that befalls the paraplegic, who may also suffer blindness and deafness. It is clear, too, that many juries believe that physicians, hospitals, and major insurance carriers have adequate resources to recompense the afflicted. Settlements are not designed to substitute for the interruption of the afflicted patient's income. They are clearly intended as punishment for what is considered an avoidable tragedy. Impersonal commercial-insurance carriers have generous reserves to "make good" the irreversible injuries inflicted by health providers whom they insure.

THE COSTS AND FREQUENCY OF MALPRACTICE CLAIMS

The costs of medical care continue to soar, accelerated by increases reflecting the "add-ons" of malpractice insurance. Such costs are estimated to be as much as $10 per patient day in hospitals and as much as $2 per visit to a physician. Total premium costs for professional-liability insurance for providers was $60 million in 1960. This increased to $300 million by 1970, and (as noted above) is currently estimated to be well over $1 billion annually. The increase of premiums was dramatic from 1950 to 1960. In that 10-year period dentist malpractice-insurance premiums rose 115 percent, hospital premium costs 262 percent, physician premium costs (other than surgeons) 541 percent. For surgeons, the 10-year increase was 950 percent. It is difficult to get firm estimates of rate increases in the 1970s, but in many reports, these appear to be doubling annually. A 1975 report noted that doctors were then anticipating that new annual premiums would be as much as three times higher than their current rates, with some costs running to $22,704 for high-risk specialties, such as neurosurgery and anesthesiology. In 1975, Los Angeles doctors participated in a 1-day walkout to protest the prospect of a 100-percent increase in insurance premiums.[1] In 1975 New York physicians in low-risk specialties, such as psychiatry, paid an average of $776 annually. But annual premiums increased to $14,329 for such high-risk fields as plastic and orthopedic surgery, and anesthesiology.

> In Cleveland, the average premium rose from $2,300 in 1972 to $4,000 in 1974—with specialists paying as much as $30,000 a year. One Miami obstetrician paid $3,500 for insurance when he opened his office a year ago; this year, his insurance will cost $11,000. "If my training had taken one year longer," says the 34-year-old physician, "I could not have gone into business."[2]

In January 1975, the Argonaut Insurance Company announced that it would raise its premiums in May for Bay Area physicians in northern California by 200 to 300 percent. The area's anesthesiologists found their premiums rising from $5,377 to as high as $22,704. By May of that year, some 307 northern California anesthesiologists had refused both to renew their insurance policies and to practice without coverage. They walked off their jobs.

By 1976, the Travelers Insurance Company, which covers 70 percent of the Bay Area's doctors, hiked premiums by an average of 400 percent, with some specialty rates reaching $40,000.

> Dr. Paul Muchnic, a Los Angeles orthopedist, found that his premiums had suddenly risen from $6,500 to $36,000 a year. He angrily announced that he was quitting his $65,000-a-year practice. Others have pulled up stakes and moved to other states where there are fewer malpractice suits, smaller judgments, and thus more reasonable insurance rates.[3]

During each year since 1970 the press has carried regular accounts of these premium rate increases. In one account, Dr. Julius Jacobson, a vascular surgeon at New York's Mount Sinai Hospital, explained: "Suits are driving good men out of practice. It's an absolute disaster."[4] Dr. Rosamond Kane, who runs the Children's Foot Clinic at New York's Columbia Presbyterian Medical Center, maintains a small orthopedic practice in Rye, New York. She informed her private patients that she would no

[1] Jean Seligmann, "The Doctors' Revolt," Newsweek, May 12, 1975, p. 71.
[2] "Malpractice: M.D.'s Revolt," Newsweek, June 9, 1975, p. 60.
[3] Time, January 19, 1976, p. 42.
[4] "Malpractice: The High Cost," Newsweek, December 23, 1974, p. 50.

longer be able to treat them. To cover the increase in malpractice-insurance premiums would require her to add $54 to each of her bills.[5] The Medical Society of New York State conducted a poll of physicians and found that unless relief from malpractice premiums were found, one-third intended to move out of the state. Forty-two percent said they would retire early. Others have been seeking a sanctuary in military service:[6]

> After twenty years of private practice, Dr. Berly E. Bridges, Jr., a Los Angeles anesthesiologist, was earning $130,000 a year. . . . Soon he will be practicing at March Air Force Base near Riverside, California, at an annual salary of $46,900. Bridges is one of scores of physicians who are giving up civilian practice, often at a financial sacrifice, for the security of new careers in military medicine.[7]

But there is a rapid increase of malpractice suits in military service, too.

As we noted above, the pressure of premium increases is also influencing hospital costs. The Michael Reese Medical Center in Chicago planned a daily rate increase of $12 a bed. In New York, where 23 hospitals were faced with a 600-percent increase in malpractice costs, officials estimated an increase of $50 in the average patient's bill.

There is a temptation to infer from all of this that the insurance companies have overreached themselves in exploiting demand pressures in the rapidly expanding health-care field. Some medical providers have intimated that with the decline of the stock market in the early 1970s, the increase of premiums appeared an all-too-tempting expedient. The insurance companies, however, have been befuddled by large awards and by the long delay in the adjudication process. As we will note shortly, the statute of limitations, typically two years, does not apply from the time of the alleged negligence, but from the time of its discovery. Further, upon reaching the age of 21, a youth can sue on his own behalf for incidents of malpractice that occurred in the delivery room. Generous court decisions, the rapid increase of activity in this area, and the sharp increases of medical-care costs have created bewildering actuarial problems for commercial insurers. Companies find that their current premium income is not covering current expenditures; as a consequence, they are abandoning service to this area. The Argonaut Insurance Company of Menlo Park, California, decided to pull out of the state of New York when doctors there refused to agree to a 200-percent rate hike. It has also announced that it will not attempt coverage of hospitals in at least 14 states. In 1975, the Pacific Indemnity Company of Los Angeles and the Star Insurance Company of Milwaukee dropped coverage for 2,000 Los Angeles physicians.

[5] "The Doctor's New Dilemma," *Newsweek*, February 10, 1975, p. 41.
[6] "Malpractice: The State Steps in," *Time*, May 5, 1975, p. 82.
[7] "Doctors at Arms," *Newsweek*, March 10, 1975, p. 56.

One of the main problems that malpractice insurance poses for the companies is the fact that most policies are written on a so-called occurrence basis. This means that the company is liable for any malpractice episode that occurs in a given year, even if the claim isn't filed until a subsequent year. Thus, the total amount of premiums received by companies reporting data to the American Insurance Association in 1966 was $13.6 million. But by 1974, those companies had paid out a total of $18.2 million in losses on the 1966 policies. This "long tail" of claims, say the insurers, makes it hard to reach actuarial estimates on which to base premiums from year to year. "It's as if a car manufacturer tried to set a fair price today for a car he would not deliver until 1980."[8]

Tort, or malpractice, claims in medicine have been rather uncommon until recently. Now, though, the number of malpractice claims filed is increasing at about 8 to 9 percent annually. In 1966, 1.7 physicians per 100 were being sued.[9] But with the present growth rate, according to one estimate, one physician in three can expect to be sued sometime during his career.[10] Others indicate that it is much likelier that the specter of a malpractice suit will haunt every physician at least once. As further evidence of the enormous growth compression of this phenomenon, David S. Rubsamen notes that ninety percent of all malpractice suits ever filed have been brought since 1964.[11]

The basic reference work in the malpractice field is the Secretary's Report on Medical Malpractice, commissioned with a $2 million grant by the Secretary of HEW in 1970.[12] This two-volume study is in two parts. The first summarizes some of the findings of its technical appendix and offers a series of recommendations in a breezy and informal style. In essence, the report fails to anticipate the serious dimensions of the growing problems and provides a series of gentle admonitions, which seem to say little more than "Physician, heal thyself." Perhaps its tone reflects the fact that a majority of the expert review panel were trained in law rather than medicine. The major part of the report is its appendix, dubbed the "telephone book." It represents technical studies commissioned by the expert panel and is a veritable gold mine of statistics and insights for the serious student. The chairman of the commission staff complained of the obligation to prepare its conclusions and recommendations before all of

[8] "Malpractice: M.D.'s Revolt," p. 63.

[9] *An Overview of Medical Malpractice,* Prepared by the Staff for the Use of the Committee on Interstate and Foreign Commerce, U.S. House of Representatives, March 17, 1975, 94th Congress, 1st Session, Committee Print No. 4 (Washington, D.C.: GPO, 1975).

[10] *Medical Economics,* October 29, 1973, p. 93.

[11] *Medical World News,* January 1975, p. 66.

[12] *Report of the Secretary's Commission on Medical Malpractice,* Department of Health, Education, and Welfare, January 16, 1973, DHEW Publication no. OS 73-88, GPO. Hereinafter, this important study will be referred to as *Malpractice Commission Report.*

its technical studies were in hand. When Eli P. Bernzweig was accused of preparing a report that came close to identifying the advantages of benign neglect of this issue by the federal government, he angrily retorted that the issue had exploded to its present crisis stage because of a deliberate government policy to ignore the panel's many recommendations. Although the statistical time frame for much of the analysis is 1970, it remains an authoritative contribution.

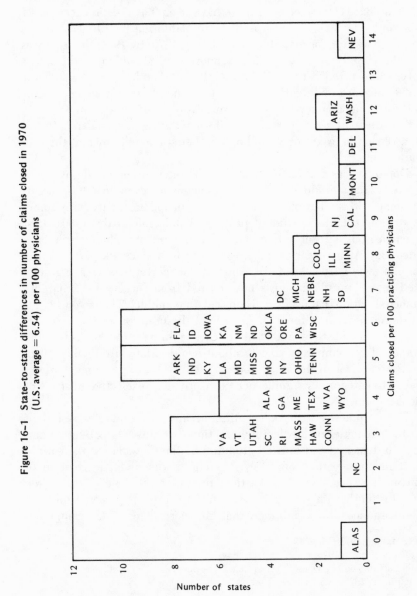

Figure 16-1 State-to-state differences in number of claims closed in 1970 (U.S. average = 6.54) per 100 physicians

Source: Commission study of claims closed in 1970; distribution of physicians in the United States, 1970, American Medical Association.

The Secretary's Report on Medical Malpractice emphasized the surprisingly moderate levels of settlements for cases closed in 1970. About 50 percent of these were under $2,000; 79 percent were under $10,000. Only three percent of the awards were over $100,000, and less than one out of every 1,000 claims was for $1 million or more. However, as we have emphasized, the size of claims has increased sharply since 1970.

For example, as of 1976, 20 awards for medical malpractice exceeded $1 million.[13] Until 1974, Chicago had never seen a malpractice judgment larger than $250,000. Since then there have been 3 awards in excess of $1 million, one of which was $2.5 million. In California by 1970, there had been only 5 awards for more than $300,000 in 1970; by 1974, the total was 36. Of the 19 settlements or awards of more than $1 million in the state's history, 13 occurred between 1973 and 1975.[14] Another report noted the national "blizzard of litigation," involving some 20,000 claims each year, with the average amount awarded in successful suits rising from $5,000 to $8,000 in the past four years. In California during the final months of 1974, a verdict in excess of $1 million was being handed down at the rate of one a month.[15]

Doctor strikes that have threatened the interruption of all but necessary services have produced substantial revenue losses to hospitals, threatening some with bankruptcy. The picketing of medical activists is somewhat reminiscent of the student protests that began in the 1960s. Lest the comparisons appear unfair, consider the picture photograph of a bearded Bay Area physician playing a flute in a sidewalk performance, garbed in white frock coat. In front of the performers is a carefully printed sign: "Anesthesiologists now barred from surgery by a liability insurance situation that needs revision. Take a pamphlet. Thank you."[16]

Many converging forces help explain the eruption of the malpractice problem at this time, and many of these represent the innocence and ignorance of contemporary society about health. Many are themes given separate treatment in the study. Let us identify these pressures, without reference to category or significance, as a prelude to selective analysis of particular themes.

The malpractice issue reflects the unrealistic consumer expectations about the capacities of medical intervention; it represents patient resentment with detached and hurried attention by the physician to their problems; it involves patient anxieties inherent in the divided attention of various health specialists to the patient problems, the generally mistaken public illusion that physicians have acquired enormous personal fortunes through practice, the assumption that commercial insurance companies

[13] *Time*, January 19, 1976, p. 42.
[14] *Newsweek*, June 9, 1975, p. 59.
[15] "Malpractice: The High Cost," *Newsweek*, December 23, 1974, p. 50.
[16] *Time*, June 2, 1975, p. 63.

have unlimited capacities to reimburse persons for negligent service, the substantial publicity given to cases involving generous awards, the neglect of evidence for the proportion of cases that involve modest settlements, the increase in the number of patient contacts with health-care providers, the increasing risks of heavy reliance on the so-called miracle drugs, the complexities of contemporary medical technologies, the cultivation of specialized skills by attorneys in eliciting favorable awards in court cases (including appeals to jury support by traumatic displays of crippled clients), gradual changes in legal philosophy in the courts that have tended to shift, in part, the burden of proof to the defense, the incapacity and/or unwillingness of physicians to police themselves through threatened loss of license and hospital staff privileges, the complexity of identifying causality of negligence in situations where illness or some physical malfunction is already present, the problems of identifying precedent for definitions of equity in the adjudication process, the ubiquitous presence of the so-called conspiracy of silence by practitioners themselves, the difficulties of identifying persistent patterns of malpractice (as contrasted with the single episode that might represent human frailty) in order to discipline medical negligence, the increasing publicity given to unnecessary surgery and to unnecessary deaths resulting from the same, the continuing shortage of physicians willing to serve the general needs of the public (necessitating hurried attention to individual needs), the growth of the consumerism movement, and the discernible erosion of public respect for the physician (for whatever reason). All of this has been represented cogently by *Newsweek:* the crisis is caused by "growing consumerism, the phenomenon of so-called runaway juries, the disappearance of the old family-doctor relationship, inflation and—to some degree—hungry lawyers and incompetent doctors."[17] Let us identify a few of these themes for elaboration.

THE PROBABILITY OF SUITS

In an era of proclaimed "rights" to medical services, not everyone is exercising that option. Even in prepaid group-practice plans, a substantial proportion of the insured never make contact in any one year with these standby services. However, there is a remarkable volume of daily contact with health-care providers, and one must orient the statistics on alleged negligence, with benchmark statistics on services in which we can presume reasonably adequate services are provided. In this context, the medical providers do remarkably well. The striking conclusion is not that we have so many suits, but that we have so few.

17 "Malpractice: M.D.'s Revolt," p. 58.

In 1970, some 206 million Americans were provided medical care by 279,000 doctors, 96,000 dentists, 694,000 nurses and 2,000,000 other allied health personnel. In 1970, the average physician treated 3,396 patients, and if we include patients seen in a hospital, the figure increases to 6,360. In 1970, the average patient visited a physician 4.6 times a year. The average dentist treated 3,219 patients in 1970, with an average of 1.5 visits per patient. In 1970, 1 out of every 6.5 persons was hospitalized. These statistics create an activity base against which to determine the extent of malpractice activity.

The Malpractice Commission's study of 14,500 "claims-producing incidents" in 1970 indicated that there was less than one chance in 100,000 of an incident occurring that would give rise to a medical malpractice suit each time a physician or dentist treats a patient.[18] But the occurrence of these claims is far from random: it falls with peculiar unevenness by geographic area and by physician specialty. The Commission noted that about 18,000 claims were opened in 1970. In that same year, 12,000 cases were closed. The 12,000 represents the number of "incidents," or patients. These cases involved 22,000 defendants, including doctors, hospitals, nurses, drug companies, and equipment manufacturers. Claims closed in 1970 could cover medical episodes dating back to 1960. Claims opened in 1970 were much more likely, of course, to cover recent incidents. But because of the time required to settle these issues, it might well be 1980 before the claims filed in 1970 are finally settled.[19]

In 1970, there were approximately 14,500 reported "incidents," prompting the opening of some 18,000 claim files. In 1970 there were 382,000 doctors, dentists, and hospitals at risk. Dividing 382,000 by 18,000 claims indicates that 1 out of every 21 health-care providers was the object of a malpractice claim. But some hospitals (just as professionals) appear more threatened by claims. Some 74 percent of all alleged malpractice incidents occur in hospitals, leading to the conclusion that the average hospital might be a party to a claim 1.9 times a year. If claims against hospitals were distributed randomly rather than uniformly, one would expect that 33 percent of the nation's 7,000 hospitals would have no claims filed against them during a year. In fact, however, 68 percent of all hospitals had no claims, and 15 percent of the hospitals accounted for more than half of the claims. Clearly, if the causes of such difficulties could be uncovered and corrected for this portion of hospitals, insurance costs—and patient difficulties—could be substantially reduced.

In launching the National Conference on Medical Malpractice in 1975, Robert W. Jamplis, president of the American Group Practice Association, took another slice at probability analysis:

[18] *Malpractice Commission Report,* p. 6.
[19] Ibid., p. 7.

We have roughly 300,000 doctors involved in patient care in this country. . . . [E]ach one of them sees approximately 138 patients per week. With simple arithmetic, this is approximately two billion doctor–patient encounters a year, or, to be very conservative, five million such encounters occur each day. I understand that there are approximately (and this again is on the high side) some 20,000 malpractice claims that are filed each year. These are claims, not suits that are won or lost. . . . [Thus,] there is only one claim for every 100,000 patient–doctor encounters.[20]

If we use the Commission's calculation that only 3 percent of the claims produce a settlement over $100,000, we have the probability of a payoff at this level of 0.0000003 per visit. In other words, 3 such awards are made for every 10 million visits. With odds so low, should we then encourage the conclusion that physicians (and hospitals) have become paranoid, that patients are remarkably inclined to give physicians or hospitals the benefit of the doubt when receiving disappointing treatment, and that physicians and hospitals perform to remarkably high-quality control standards? In truth, all elements are probably present. But what undoubtedly concerns the physician is that the older standards of avoiding the risk of suits are inoperative in the future, as a new culture relishes the prospect of "taking on" the physician.

There is considerable controversy and anxiety about the "tip of the iceberg" hypothesis. With such a small amount of litigation, it is not surprising that speculation has developed that patients are unusually passive in the face of negligence. As we shall review in our section on the criticisms of attorneys for "ambulance chasing," the defense is made that an insignificant proportion of episodes that justify consumer protection ever become cases. Undoubtedly the commercial-insurance companies realize that shifting the occurrence of litigation from .00001 to .0001 percent of patient contacts would increase litigation activity by a factor of ten. Attorneys clearly state that they are unwilling to represent patient grievances that would likely produce modest settlements, suggesting that a considerable number of grievances do not become cases. There is a strong presumption, too, that many American citizens still display a great respect for medical authority and are willing to believe that they have received excellent care, no matter what the setting for such services. Nevertheless, there has been some chipping away at the American impulse for patience, understanding, and even acquiescence when medical intervention has

[20] National Conference on Medical Malpractice, Subcommittee Print for the Use of the Subcommittee on Health and the Environment of the Committee on Interstate and Foreign Commerce, U.S. House of Representatives, June 1975, 94th Congress, 1st Session (Washington, D.C.: GPO, 1975), p. 3. Jamplis puts the ratio of charges at 0.00001 per patient contact. The ratio of a settlement involving a payoff to the patient at 60 percent of such proceedings is 0.0000006 per patient visit.

failed. The ingredient of respect, so critical to the operation of the health-care system, has not collapsed; yet there is evidence of wavering confidence. Not surprisingly, commercial insurers should be alarmed about the deluge, should the system fail to buttress public confidence.

IATROGENIC ACCIDENTS VERSUS NEGLIGENCE

One of the most important segments of the National Commission report was a study of the case records of 23,750 patients discharged from two hospitals. The study identified 517 patients who had received, during treatment, medical injuries caused by the negligence of health-care providers. But only 31 malpractice claims have been filed in that same period. If these statistics are at all representative, only 6 percent of those cases involving negligence led to a claim. This study concluded:

> On the basis of a review of a random sample of medical records drawn from medical, surgical, and gynecological services at two general hospitals, it has been found that 7.5 percent of the records show evidence of iatrogenic injury. *Several factors indicate that this number significantly underestimates the true rate.*[21]

Of that proportion of 7.5 percent, negligence was established in about 29 percent of the situations. But for this total of 29 percent, claims are filed in only 6 percent of the cases, an overall incidence of one-tenth of 1 percent. The potential for legitimate claims is 2.2 percent. For every case that is litigated, there are 17 that, in the view of the study, involved grounds on which litigation could be based. It is this factor that hovers over any actuarial analysis.

If this ratio of injuries in which negligence is established could be generalized to the national economy, we would have ominous statistics. We have over 30 million hospital admissions per year. Let us assume we have almost as many discharges. With the ratio of negligent injuries at 2.2 percent for all exits, we have a base of 660,000 episodes. This compares with the 12,600 claims asserted in 1970, or only 1 for every 52 claims in which negligence could be charged.

The consumer's impulse to consider the legal options in perceived cases of negligence reflects his familiarity with the malpractice issue. The growing publicity can only increase public awareness of the problem and hence the consumer reflex to call a lawyer. For example, *Newsweek* reports:

[21] Leon S. Pocincki, Stuart J. Dogger, and Barbara P. Schwartz, "The Incidence of Iatrogenic Injuries," Report of the Secretary's Commission on Medical Malpractice, *Appendix*, p. 63. Italics in original.

At least 154 million Americans were treated by a doctor last year, and Derbyshire's estimate means that 7.5 million of them may be in peril when they see a physician. The results can be costly—and deadly. Robert E. McGarrah, Jr., attorney for Ralph Nader's Public Citizen's Health Research Group, recently claimed that $21.5 billion of the $80 billion Americans spent on medical care is wasted on unnecessary hospital stays, unnecessary surgery, and unnecessary drugs and x-rays. Although an accurate count has never been made, such surgery takes thousands of lives each year, and thousands more die from reactions to drugs that have been improperly administered.[22]

If more technical sources are required to authenticate public concern, the *Georgetown Law Journal* notes that there is approximately 1 operation per year for every 13 people in the United States, involving between 12 and 15 million patients. This compares with the rate in England and Wales of only 1 out of every 26 persons. The journal points out that surgery is both dangerous and costly. The mortality rate for surgery generally varies from 0.5 percent to 3 or 4 percent. The mortality rate is higher if surgery is risky or if a patient is in poor condition. To this must be added the risk of the anaesthetic procedure, for which the mortality rate ranges from 0.05 to 0.1 percent. The journal observes that "unnecessary surgery, not a recent development, remains a serious problem today primarily because the medical profession, while recognizing the problem, has failed to initiate effective self-regulation. Williams has estimated that some 2 million operations are performed without justification each year, resulting in at least 10,000 unnecessary deaths!" He asks: "Who are these 10,000 that die unnecessarily? They are not the old and sick who would die soon anyway. Tragically they often include the young and healthy."[23]

If this account does not set the consuming public on edge, statistics cited in a five-part documentary on medical care written for *The New York Times* should. This exposé of malpractice has created an uproar and has been widely reproduced through the syndication of *The New York Times News Service*. Part I of the study explains:

> American surgeons, a Cornell University study indicates, are performing an estimated total of nearly 2,400,000 unnecessary operations each year in which 11,900 patients die as the result of complications.

> An estimated total of 10,000 Americans die or suffer potentially fatal reactions following the administration of antibiotics that are not needed, according to studies at the University of Florida and Ohio State University medical schools.

[22] *Newsweek*, December 23, 1974.

[23] L. Williams, quoted in "Unnecessary Surgery: Doctor and Hospital Liability," *Georgetown Law Journal*, Vol. 61 (1973), p. 807. Also see Bunker, "Surgical Manpower: A Comparison of Operations and Surgeons in the United States and in England and Wales," *The New England Journal of Medicine*, Vol. 282 (1970), p. 135.

As a result of errors in judgment, it is estimated that 260,000 women undergo needless hysterectomies each year and some 500,000 children are subjected to unwarranted surgical removal of their tonsils and adenoids, studies done in several medical schools suggest.

Each year, according to a drug industry marketing survey, doctors write about 161,000 prescriptions for chloramphenicol, one of the most dangerous antibiotics, for patients whose diseases are known to be unaffected by antibiotics or who could have been treated with safer alternatives.

About 2,200 hospitals, nearly one-third of the total in the United States, fail to meet the minimum standards of safety and adequacy of patient care required by the medical profession's Joint Commission on Hospital Accreditation. Despite this, there is no legal restriction on the medical and surgical procedures these hospitals may attempt.[24]

THE CONSUMER'S "PUSH-BUTTON" MENTALITY

We have noted previously that technical advances in medicine have provided prevention, cures, and remedies for many illnesses considered fatal a few years ago. These sweeping triumphs of both science and technology have created unrealistic expectations about what medical intervention can, in fact, produce. We have tended to forget the long way we have yet to go to ameliorate or cure cancer and heart disease or to deal effectively with stroke victims. In effect, the widely heralded triumphs have tended to obscure the new risks involved with new drugs, new techniques, new machinery, new operations. There is a tendency to neglect the delicate and fragile structure of the human system. We no longer accept illness as a usual or expected event in our lives. Today, most citizens lack an appreciation for both the complexities and the risks of contemporary medical practice. Increasing affluence has further served to increase "life" expectations: consumer-rights movements are insisting on quality care, and insisting, too, on the right for product evaluation. And they are increasingly insisting on recompense for negligence. The Malpractice Commission noted:

. . . the press and broadcasting media fostered greater public interest in medicine and particularly in its "miracles," leading the public to develop many unrealistic expectations about medicine's capabilities. Many Americans regard good health as though it were a commodity, something that the doctor can dispense at will. But good health is not a purchasable commodity. It is a matter, first, of heredity and, above all,

[24] Boyce Rensberger, "The Problem of the Incompetent Physician," *The New York Times News Service,* reproduced in *The St. Louis Post Dispatch,* February 15, 1976.

a matter of personal responsibility, choice, and self-governance. Unfortunately, the failure to achieve ideal health has caused great disappointment, with the results of treatment [for] some patients, and they turned with greater and greater frequency to the lawsuit as a means of resolving their disappointment.[25]

In a report to the national malpractice conference, Robert Maplis emphasized that "it is almost universally true that any drug (or indeed any operation), however beneficial, is almost always dangerous in proportion to its potential efficacy."[26]

It is paradoxical that the faith of the patient in the unusual skills of a physician may be warranted, not because the physician can achieve success, but because he offers at least a *chance* to avoid death. Often it is the most skilled physician who is invited to perform the most delicate operations in a desperate bid to ensure the survival of patients otherwise unlikely to survive. Furthermore, cultivating illusions of the possible, without acknowledging the high risk of the probable, may be as much a physician's as a patient's shortcoming. The experience of Dr. Thomas G. Baffes, chairman of the department of surgery at Chicago's Mount Sinai Hospital Medical Center and a pioneer in heart surgery, is instructive:

> Dr. Thomas Baffes once repaired a heart valve in a 69-year-old patient, whose condition was complicated by high blood pressure and diabetes. The operation saved the man's life, but when he had a stroke nine month's later, he blamed it on Baffes and sued for $1.2 million. The surgeon was exonerated, but only after a four-year court battle, and he was so shaken by the experience that he made up his mind to go to school at night. "I decided it was important to learn what lawyers were trying to do."
>
> The legal training has helped Baffes a great deal in his practice. Today he's much more cautious about trying to accomplish too much in the operating room. He makes sure his department keeps adequate records and that his colleagues establish close rapport with their patients. "We can't play God any more," says Baffes. "We have to tell our patients straight away what the risks are and ask if they want to take them."[27]

THE HUMAN ASPECT OF THE TREATMENT PROCESS AS A SOURCE OF ANTAGONISM

The Secretary's Commission on Medical Malpractice acknowledged the simple truth that suits often represent the tangible proof of the final

[25] *Malpractice Commission Report*, p. 3.
[26] *National Conference on Medical Malpractice*, Arlington, Va., March 20, 1975, p. 3.
[27] *Newsweek*, June 9, 1975, p. 63.

breakdown of the relationship between patient and doctor. If there is a collapse or failure of the treatment prospect, along with the breach of personal confidence in the physician himself, the chances for a lawsuit are much greater.[28] Individuals usually have the capacity to absorb the disappointments of unsuccessful therapeutic activities. They have much less capacity to absorb an inaccurate diagnosis by professions whom they consider both inept and indifferent. Physicians, both those who have been sued and those who have not, identify the most significant cause of malpractice suits as poor communication between physician and patient. The respondents to the Malpractice Commission also identified "declining public regard for doctors" as the third most significant cause of legal encounters.[29]

Because about seventy-five percent of patient challenges involve a hospital setting, it is probable that his anxiety and distrust may be sharpened by the nature of hospital treatment. It may be difficult to untangle resentments against the physician from resentments against treatment by hospital personnel. Hospitals often provide unhappy experiences. As one government study explains:

> Even under the best of circumstances, the hospitalization process tends to reduce the patient's sense of individuality and responsible self-assertion. The hospitalized patient is shifted from an active competitive world where he is aggressive and important, to a simplified world where even the smallest details of living—eating, eliminating, and physical position—are dictated by strangers. The deprivation of his sense of personal identity, coupled with his loss of privacy and control over his actions, places the hospitalized patient in a position of inferiority which tends to foster an unusual amount of frustration and resentment. The enforced passivity in the hospital, combined with the deindividualizing factors just mentioned, intensifies the patient's reaction to any dissatisfaction in the treatment process, whether real or fancied, which he is then likely to direct against the hospital or physician in a greatly exaggerated manner.[30]

Again, the impersonality and the indignity of such care may reduce frustration tolerance, particularly when such treatment is associated with disappointing outcomes. The remedy to this situation requires some redesign, if not rethinking, of the hospital regimen in order to improve the dignity and respect afforded patients. Efforts must be made to reduce the patient's anxiety and uncertainty over the treatment process, rather than to leave him with the feeling of being a trivial "input" to the mechanistic, disciplined, and efficient process. There must be occasions for privacy, for

---

[28] *Malpractice Commission Report*, p. 67.
[29] Ibid., p. 68.
[30] Eli P. Bernzweig, *Legal Aspects of PHS Medical Care*, U.S. Department of Health, *Education, and Welfare*, PHS Publication No. 1468 (Washinngton, D.C.: GPO, 1966), p. 43.

courtesies, for explanations, and for expression of interest. As the Commission noted, in pressing for the distribution of statements of patients' rights in the hospital setting, "to ignore the rights of the patient is both to betray simple humanity and to invite dissatisfaction that may lead to malpractice suits." Such care is warranted by consideration of both pragmatism and humanism.[31]

Profiles have been constructed of both the patient and physician likely to be a party to a suit. Such a patient is highly emotional, with unconscious fears of both his illness and the prospect of death. He has underlying suspicions about the technical skills of attending physicians, but he may compensate for such anxiety by displaying a childlike faith in the efficiency of the medical industry. He has, concurrently, a sense of inferiority but is sensitive to any treatment regimen that appears to be unimportant. The individual may also prove to be an uncooperative patient, declining to describe symptoms accurately or failing to follow a prescribed therapy while pretending to do so.[32]

The Malpractice Commission summarized a 1957 study of the human-relations aspects of malpractice litigation:

> The suit-prone patient was found to be a person who goes into a medical situation with a variety of unrealistic attitudes, including unreasonable beliefs about money ("The doctor should be paid only when he produces quick results"), about physicians ("I don't trust them; they can't really help me"), and about medicine ("Everything should be curable"). In addition he tends to be dogmatic and quick to blame others when things go wrong.[33]

The day-to-day interplay between the doctor's and the patient's personality is a key to malpractice prevention. "Ordinarily, too little attention is given to the interpersonal and emotional aspects of patient care, with a resultant failure to recognize the need of many patients for psychological as well as physical comfort.[34]

Some further insight into physician perspectives of patients likely to bring suit is provided by Nathan Hershey. Hershey undertook a study

---

[31] *Malpractice Commission Report*, p. 71.

[32] Bernzweig, *Legal Aspects of PHS Medical Care*, pp. 40–41.

[33] *Malpractice Commission Report*, p. 68, drawing on R. H. Blum, *The Psychology of Malpractice Suits* (San Francisco: California Medical Association, 1957). See also R. H. Blum, *The Management of the Doctor-Patient Relationship* (New York: McGraw-Hill, 1960), p. 253. Blum points out that at least half of all malpractice suits are preventable even after some malpractice has occurred, provided that the physician gives appropriate consideration to the danger signals of the hostile patient. Also see C. A. Levinson, "Beware the Malpractice Plaintiff," *Journal of American Dental Association*, Vol. 62 (March 1961) and "Breakdown in Doctor–Patient Relationships Is Shown by Malpractice Suits," *Bulletin of the American College of Surgeons*, Vol. 44 (May/June 1959).

[34] Bernzweig, *Legal Aspects of PHS Medical Care*, pp. 39–40.

of seventeen physicians in the Pittsburgh area. The study was a gentle probe of the physicians' practice of defensive medicine, in the course of which perceptions of patient personalities surfaced. The analysis was largely subjective, with an informal, open-ended conversation with friends about the reality of defensive medicine. The study, though in no way allowing generalizations to all physicians, illustrates some interesting aspects of the physician–patient relationship. The study noted that "defensive practice depends more on the patient's personality than on any other factor." What are those personality traits?[35]

High-risk patients are variously described as paranoid and hysterical and as exhibiting other psychoneurotic tendencies; they often have a low socioeconomic background and a demanding or belligerent attitude. "Sometimes you can almost smell trouble in certain people." Further symptoms include the "doctor shoppers," patients who go from physician to physician without ever being satisfied. Frequently these persons have unrealistic expectations, demanding immediate or complete disappearance of their symptoms. Another type are those who apparently need more emotional support than medical intervention. They are seeking a father-figure, a friend, or a confidant, and they grow hostile or impatient if such emotional support is not forthcoming. The paranoid patient is persuaded that physicians (or everyone else around him) is trying to hurt him. The "hysterical" patient is represented as likely to be a female with a preoccupation with her body or bodily symptoms. These types often elevate the physician to unrealistic roles or godlike figures. Another concern is with the patient who confronts the physician: "I've been coming here a lot and spending a lot of money, and I'm not getting any better."

Yet another group of patients who create concern are those who have good friends who are attorneys and who may be expecting VIP treatment, with sensitivity to physician responsibility at every stage of the treatment process. Yet another group that some physicians indicated they would wish to avoid are personal friends. Such friendships typically create unrealistic expectations for cures, and disappointing results could lead to both a loss of friendship and a lawsuit.

One physician explained the positive consequences of this new era of consumerism, in which physicians must make a fresh effort to communicate with each patient fully about his illness:

> It makes doctors talk to the patient, which they never really did before. Now you sit down and explain to them what you're going to do and what the possible consequences are. Everybody has become more aware of the patient's right to know what's going on. And this is why you do it, not because there's a lawyer breathing down your neck.[36]

[35] Nathan Hershey, "The Defensive Practice of Medicine: Myth or Reality?" *Milbank Memorial Quarterly*, Vol. 50, no. 1, Part I (January 1972), p. 294.
[36] Ibid., p. 298.

Interestingly, most of these 17 physicians do not regularly practice defensive medicine. Each explained, in one way or another, "I practice good medicine, and that's it." Four of the 17 had faced malpractice suits. A scale was developed to define whether the patient relationship was one represented by suspicion or an adversary posture (counted as 1), or by congeniality (with a score of 10). The responding physicians rated themselves between 9 and 10. The physicians who had malpractice claims made against them rated their patient relationships between 9.5 and 10. The group typified all other physician–patient relationships, however, as ranging around a value of 6.

There may, in addition, be physicians who are more likely to be party to a suit. He has an antipathy or indifference to the emotional needs of his patients. Even when sensing emotional anxieties, he maintains a posture of aloofness. He treats his patient as a mature, understanding adult. There is no time or reason to deal with emotional displays of anxieties. Instead of finding out how to make the patient feel less angry, less afraid, less depressed he may be more preoccupied with his own image; he may bolster his faltering ego by disclaiming any responsibilities for the "trivial" emotional aspect of a patient's behavior. Such a physician "is virtually begging for a lawsuit. Indifference to the patient's disappointment only adds fuel to growing feelings of resentment and may be indicative of the physician's own psychological deficiencies." Dr. Sidney Wolfe, director of the Public Citizens' Health Research Group (a Ralph Nader organization) has further confirmed the beleaguered doctor–patient relationship as follows:

> Aside from the more apparent attributes of modern medicine, such as increased specialization, the use of penning a prescription to avoid having to talk any more to the patient, and more machines, all of which are very understandably depersonalizing to the patient, there is an increased patient perception of the low regard many doctors have for their human rights.

The issue is most conspicuous in the areas of informed consent; for here, Wolfe charges, there are hundreds of thousands of women who have had hysterectomies and tubal ligations "without the most primitive semblance of informed consent." In his view "the absence of allowing patients an informed choice is a major contributing factor to the steady flow of unnecessary surgery, misprescribed drugs, and other unchecked therapeutic and diagnostic excess of American doctors and hospitals."[37]

Much of the criticism of hurried or impersonal attention to patients must ultimately reflect imbalances of physician supply and demand. Since the medical associations have done much to influence or regulate the flow of physician supply, we cannot always exonerate the individual

[37] *Malpractice Commission Report*, p. 63.

physician for pressures placed on his time. Indeed, to realize the unlimited public clamor for attention serves to lift the physician's self-esteem and to secure the conviction that he has "unique" qualifications to advance society's welfare. It is hardly persuasive for physicians to seek sympathy (or understanding) for the time pressures imposed on them when they have collectively (however unconsciously) done much to "rig" that scarcity. The matter is not, however, an issue simply of aggregate balances between supply and demand, but of the distribution of skills.

We entitled this section "What Makes Doctors Sick." The experience of malpractice activity is traumatic for physicians in this country, for it is alien to a value structure steeped in traditions of self-sacrifice and service. An AMA spokesman, John Coury, explained the emotional impact of the issue:

> Physicians are not, by and large, insensitive or callous. They are trained carefully to make decisions which are hard and are trained not to show their emotions. It has not been recognized generally that being sued by a patient, for whom the physician has developed an attachment and for whom he has done his best, is a devastating occurrence. All of us have seen what it does to our colleagues. Even when they win the trial, they are no longer the incisive, effective, optimistic surgeons which they were before. A court of law may be the workroom for the attorney, but is the torture chamber for the doctor. Frivolous suits initiated by attorneys are a disaster.[38]

One physician member of the malpractice panel felt so moved by his reactions to the entire issue that he wrote an essay to his colleagues serving on the panel. In his statement, George Northrup acknowledged: "Medicine is a proud profession—on occasion, perhaps, too proud." He added that "a medical degree does not confer an intelligent knowledge of government, law, insurance, and consumer action. Medical-legal problems, complexities of the insurance industry, governmental function, and consumerism are subjective areas of intellectual destitution for many physicians. And ignorance breeds fear."[39] He explained that the cost of malpractice activity was more psychological than economic:

> Community reputation is a socioeconomic asset for a physician. The malpractice problem, he believes, tends to destroy this. His self-interest, if you want to call it that, and his reputation and credibility, are of far greater personal concern to the physician than the availability of professional-liability insurance and its cost. The portrait of a doctor—seemingly portrayed by some as an overpaid, callous, inhuman individual—disturbs his ego.[40]

38 Ibid., p. 24.
39 Ibid., p. 106.
40 Ibid., p. 107.

He further explained:

> As a physician, I live in an aura of fear—fear of suit. Fear contributes to hostility and rarely contributes to constructive action. Medicine has some bad doctors and some bad health-care institutions. We are not proud of them, nor do we defend them, and we are concerned with the correction or elimination of that element.
>
> The House of Medicine feels belabored. Medical organizations are trying their best to overcome their deficiencies, but in my opinion, malpractice litigation is not the best incentive to improvement. It places medicine in an adversary position, and hostilities too often result. . . .
>
> It may be hard to believe, but we are a frightened profession. The doctor feels put upon. . . . He often tries to cover himself with pride, and even occasionally arrogance, only to find himself being castrated. He really doesn't want to believe the hostility he feels. . . . The faith of the patient is important to the patient and to his physician. Faith is a power, and the physician continually feels it eroded by sometimes-justified (but frequently unjustified) attacks.[41]

The Commission also noted an episode in which an internist establishing the treatment required by a seriously ill patient. He and a colleague had pondered the question at length, for the literature reported only two instances of treatment through which other patients had lived:

> The doctors pulled their patient through, though he suffered a double leg amputation. The patient sued, and through legal proceedings which the doctor-witness believed to have been most unfair, won a judgment. The event had a considerable effect upon both his professional practice and his outlook on life. Asked what a doctor should do, he replied: "Practice the best medicine possible. . . . Retire earlier and seek medical employment which involves less patient contact, which I have done. Practice defensive medicine. And above all, and this to me is the most important thing, despise what could and should be honored, jurisprudence."[42]

SUGGESTED READINGS

ANDERSON, JOHN T., "The Physician Testimony—Hearsay Evidence or Expert Opinion: A Question of Professional Competence," *The Texas Law Review,* Vol. 53, no. 2 (January 1975), pp. 296–322. Considers the ethical issue of physician testimony.

AUGER, RICHARD C. and VICTOR P. GOLDBERG, "Prepaid Health Plans and Moral Hazard," *Public Policy,* Vol. 22, no. 3 (1974), pp. 353–93. A re-

---

[41] Statement provided by George Northrup, ibid., p. 20.
[42] Ibid.

view of the issue of the moral hazard of inundating the system with either prepaid plans or private insurance.

HARRIS, ROY J., "Nevada Doctors Beat Insurance Rate Rises by Dropping Policies," *The Wall Street Journal*, January 27, 1976. An example of how one state's physicians handled the malpractice problem by discontinuing their insurance coverage.

HAVIGHURST, CLARK C. and LAURENCE R. TANCREDI, "Medical Adversity Insurance: A No-Fault Approach to Medical Malpractice and Quality Assurance," *Milbank Memorial Fund Quarterly*, Vol. 51, no. 2 (Spring 1973), pp. 125–68. An examination of no-fault insurance, including a proposal to develop a reimbursement schedule.

HEINTZ, DUANE H., "Arbitration of Malpractice Claims: A Hospital-Based Pilot Project," *Inquiry*, Vol. 13, no. 2 (June 1976), pp. 177–86. A discussion of arbitration as an alternative method of conflict resolution.

NARAGHI, WENDELL J., "Res Ipsa Loquitur in California Medical Malpractice Law: *Quintal v. Laurel Grove Hospital.*" A commentary on the obligation of providers to establish their innocence.

O'CONNELL, JEFFREY, "Extending the 'No-fault' Idea," *Public Interest*, no. 36 (Summer 1974), pp. 112–19. A favorable approach to the idea of no-fault insurance.

PECK, CORNELIUS J., "Compensation for Pain: A Reappraisal in the Light of New Medical Evidence," *Michigan Law Review*, Vol. 72, no. 7 (June 1974), pp. 1355–96. An exploration of an unusual subject: should patients be compensated for the pain they experience during medical treatment?

ROYSTER, VERMONT, "The Malpractice Problem," *The Wall Street Journal*, March 24, 1976. A recent view of the malpractice problem.

RUBSAMEN, DAVID S., "Medical Malpractice," *Scientific American*, Vol. 235, no. 2 (August 1976), pp. 18–23. Overview of the malpractice issue.

SHENKIN, BUDD N. and DAVID C. WARNER, "Giving the Patient His Medical Record: A Proposal to Improve the System," *The New England Journal of Medicine*, Vol. 289, no. 13 (September 27, 1973), pp. 688–92. Examines the complexities of sharing with patients their medical records.

SPRINGER, ERIC W., "Law and Medicine: Reflections of a Metaphysical Misalliance," *Milbank Memorial Fund Quarterly*, Part I, Vol. 50, no. 3. A survey of the interrelationship between the legal and medical professions as these relate to key problems in the medical field.

PART FOUR

Prospects
for the Future

17

NATIONAL HEALTH
INSURANCE: ISSUES AND
IMPLICATIONS

All of the previous chapters in this book have primarily surveyed existing trends, characteristics, deficiencies, and benefits of the American health-care system. Accurate description and analysis of a system so complex is difficult enough; projection of its probable future is more difficult still. These last two chapters seek to provide some limited perspectives on the system's future.

At the time of this writing, analyzing the issue of national health insurance is troublesome. As we show below, there are substantial pressures supporting the rapid establishment of NHI, but there are many authors who predicted in 1970 that it would exist within five years. We cautiously assert that it still seems probable we will have some form of national health insurance by 1980, although national politics and the economy will clearly be determining factors in its establishment.

Today no one can be sure what form our NHI will take. Congress is considering a number of plans, all of which have advantages, disadvantages, and powerful proponents and enemies. The following are the important aspects of national health insurance which can currently be understood: the conditions of the health-care system encouraging its establishment; what NHI is and isn't, and the basic characteristics (e.g., who is covered and for what services, etc.) that form the essence of alternative NHI formats; and the broad policy issues and processes that have been and will continue to be influential in this critical national question.

THE CURRENT SYSTEM AND PRESSURES FOR NATIONAL HEALTH INSURANCE

Although it is impossible to measure accurately the influence of the various pressures for changing the system, the enormous and growing costs of our national health-care system is the primary consideration of most supporters of NHI. Health-care expenditures were 4.6 percent of the gross national product in 1950, but are closer to 10 percent of the GNP in 1976.[1] Unless reform occurs, a projected health-care expenditure of $165 billion by 1980, which seemed unrealistically high when released in 1972, now seems unrealistically modest.[2]

No society, however wealthy, can afford everything it might like to have. Resources are limited; so priorities must be established, some things financed, and others forgotten or deferred. In this context, our growing health-care expenditures provide arguments for both the proponents and opponents of national health insurance. Opponents argue that the establishment of NHI will drastically increase these expenditures. Early in 1976, President Ford repeatedly opposed a comprehensive health-insurance plan, arguing the country could not afford it "under existing economic conditions."[3] This argument is particularly well received when the economy is depressed, unemployment is high, and taxes seem burdensome. Related to the issue of cost is the fear that it would also be wasteful. David Matthews, Secretary of Health, Education, and Welfare, has illustrated this position:

> If a national health-insurance system is not carefully designed, we could spend 20 or 30 billion dollars more than we are already spending for health care and not provide one more tongue depressor or put one more doctor into practice. . . . Another important consideration is timing. I think the President is right in saying that right now the economy could not sustain a program of national health insurance that both addresses the problems I mentioned [maldistribution of doctors and nurses, rising costs, etc.] and also assures every American the financial capacity to purchase the care he needs.[4]

Even those supporting NHI recognize that it will require large expenditures. Karen Davis estimates that federal expenditure for NHI, including any remaining aspects of Medicare and Medicaid, will range between $38 billion and $95 billion, depending on how the plan is finally constructed.[5] But she believes that large reductions in current expenditures can also result from NHI. This would occur principally because, unlike current private health insurance, NHI could be used to discourage

[1] Wesley W. Posvar, "The Doctor and Health Care." Delivered at Hershey Medical Center Commencement, The Pennsylvania State University, May 24, 1975. Reported in *Vital Speeches of the Day*, Vol. 41 (August 15, 1975), pp. 666–68.

[2] "Nation's Health Ills?" *American Druggist* (August 1972), p. 29.

[3] "National Health Insurance," *Congressional Quarterly*, Weekly Report, Vol. 34, no. 6 (February 7, 1976), p. 278.

[4] Interview with David Matthews, "Outlook for Health Insurance . . . ," *U.S. News and World Report*, Vol. 80 (April 12, 1976), pp. 41–44.

[5] Karen Davis, *National Health Insurance: Benefits, Costs, and Consequences* (Washington, D.C.: The Brookings Institute, 1975), pp. 132ff.

inpatient care and encourage the provision of many medical services on a less expensive outpatient basis. It seems certain that NHI can indeed replace some current health-care expenditures and not simply result in additional costs to society. There is little doubt that private health-insurance policies covering inpatient care force many patients to make expensive short-term hospital visits in order to make their policies effective. In addition, we should remember that private health-insurance expenditures have grown from $1 billion in 1950 to over $35 billion in 1975, thereby comprising a significant proportion of our national health expenditures. This might be reduced under NHI. According to a strong proponent of a national plan:

> In fiscal year 1975, American expenditures for health care reached $118.5 billion, a figure that is 8.3 percent of the gross national product. Remember, this astronomical sum is what we pay now, without national health insurance. Opponents of the plan say that national health insurance inevitably will mean higher health-care costs for the individual citizen. But why should that be? Dollars paid in premiums to a national-health-insurance program will cancel out the dollars we now pay in medical bills and in private and semiprivate health-insurance premiums. And for our money, we should have better-distributed and more-inclusive health-care services. For all of us.[6]

The proponents of NHI further argue that private health-insurance plans encourage financial and medical extravagance and have few if any cost controls. We have already noted that most private policies cover the more expensive inpatient care and have limited outpatient and extended-care benefits. Private health-insurance policies are also ineffective in controlling the prices and charges of physicians and hospitals. Hospitals predict the revenues they will receive from insurance payments and then expand their facilities to include the more elaborate services and expensive equipment that this guaranteed revenue enables them to afford. Few hospitals want to have a large surplus of funds; therefore the inclination is to increase expenditures to match anticipated income, a cycle that encourages higher hospital costs.

Another argument in favor of NHI as a cost-reduction factor pertains to the appropriateness of the medical services covered. Private health policies tend to provide comprehensive coverage for services during hospital stays. Thus, neither the patient nor the physician has any financial reasons for limiting the services delivered. "If the insurance will pay for it, why not do it" seems to be the response. We must note, however, that most supporters of NHI want to increase the coverage of outpatient services.

The health expenditures of individuals and families are also influ-

[6] Robert Massie, "The Politicians vs. Our Health," *Newsweek,* March 29, 1976, p. 13.

ential considerations in the debate over NHI. About eighty percent of our population under sixty-five has some form of hospital and surgical insurance. Almost all of the elderly and permanently disabled have coverage under Medicare. In the past, therefore, the growth in hospital and related physician charges were not directly felt by the insured consumer. But there is now evidence of dramatically increasing commercial health-insurance premiums. These increases are producing demands for change from labor unions and from large employers paying part or all of their employees' health-insurance costs.[7]

The financial burden of a major or catastrophic illness and limitations on the coverage of major medical expenses by commercial health insurance are the source of additional support for NHI. Only about half of the American people are covered by some form of major medical insurance. The rest of those who have private health insurance have policies that limit the amount they will pay for a major illness. In addition, since chronic illness often means a lifetime of outpatient visits to a physician, the limited coverage of these visits by private insurers is a major weakness.

It is with regard to major medical expenses that humanistic values in support of NHI become quite appealing. Even noncatastrophic illness is expensive, and "with the rapid rise in medical care costs, the ability to afford adequate medical care is no longer a problem only for the poor."[8] But the problem of excessive medical expenses is particularly severe with a chronic or terminal illness. It is tragic that some persons are seriously ill but are denied sufficient care because they cannot afford it. It is even more tragic that families and patients involved with terminal illness must suffer the burden of debilitating expenses as well as the trauma of impending death.

The current patchwork of private and public health insurance also fails to provide coverage for an enormous number of American citizens. Although Medicaid covers millions of our impoverished citizens, over 5 million poor do not benefit from the program at all. Even Medicare has severe limits on its benefits. The average yearly medical expense for someone over 65 is over $1,200, with Medicare paying about $460 of that total. In the decade or more of its existence, Medicare has paid an ever-smaller share of its recipients' medical expenses. As one report notes:

> Neither part [Parts A and B—two basic parts of the program, as outlined in chapter 8] covers long-term illnesses or preventive-health services. In 1974, Medicare paid only 62 percent of older people's hospital bills and only 52 percent of covered doctor bills. It paid nothing for their out-of-hospital prescription drugs and medical appliances (eyeglasses,

[7] John K. Inglehart, "$119 a Car, $1,700 an Employee," *National Journal,* May 1, 1976, p. 598.

[8] Davis, *National Health Insurance,* p. 3.

hearing aids, dentures, and so forth) and next to nothing (3.3 percent) for nursing-home expenses.[9]

Furthermore, about eighty percent of all private health insurance is offered through employers, but not all employers offer adequate benefits. Many Americans from the low-income working class are without coverage. Temporary employees are often excluded from coverage, and persons working for very small employers may have no health benefits, or their policy premiums may be based on individual rather than group rates. Private health-insurance companies offer lower "group rates" for employers with large numbers of employees, and persons working for small employers often find the "individual premium rates" too high to purchase the coverage. In addition, less than one-third of those who lose or leave their jobs retain their private health-insurance policy. Thus, those who become unemployed can lose their income and their health insurance at the same time. The self-employed often have difficulty getting group rates, and, if covered at all, they pay the higher individual premiums. In addition, about one million Americans are considered by private insurers as too ill to warrant health coverage. For example, hypertension or other serious existing illnesses are often grounds for denial of coverage. Finally, the benefits offered by "group-rate" policies are usually the result of agreements between employers and the insurance companies, and are often deficient, in coverage, especially in major medical benefits.

As we noted in chapter 8, Medicare and Medicaid were our first major attempt at publicly funded medical services for large segments of our population. The benefits, deficiencies, and experiences of those two programs provide support for the establishment of national health insurance. The principle of assisting the elderly and disabled with their medical expenses is now well established, and few of our nation's leaders oppose it. The important services and sizable expenses not covered under Medicare lead to arguments for "filling the gaps" with NHI. The disclosures of millions of dollars lost through "rip-offs" and fraud by medical providers involved in these two programs have been used to illustrate the need for stronger controls on medical providers, which NHI might provide.

It seems likely that the major deficiencies in our current health-care system used commonly as arguments for national health insurance will

[9] "Health Insurance for Older People: Filling the Gaps in Medicare," *Consumer Reports,* Vol. 41 (January 1976), pp. 27–34. The 3.3 percent figure of Medicare support tends to underestimate the extent of government support for nursing-home care. In FY 1975, for example, total expenditures for such support were $9 billion. Public-assistance payments from both federal and state governments met $4.8 billion of those costs, with Medicare expenditures providing only $257 million. See *National Health Insurance Resource Book,* prepared by the Staff of the Committee on Ways and Means, U.S. House of Representatives, August 30, 1976 (Washington, D.C.: GPO, 1976), p. 109.

worsen in the immediate future. The total federal expenditure for health care will probably continue to grow in staggering proportions, as will health-insurance premiums. Although there are limited attempts to shift some illness treatment from inpatient to outpatient care, the results are as limited as the attempts. We find little evidence in the direction of the national economy or in the proposals for partial reform of Medicare/ Medicaid to suggest that the approximately fifty million Americans without health insurance will soon be covered.

In the long run, the major pressure for change may well result from the fact that our current mixture of private and public health-insurance coverage is based on the illness patterns of the first half of the twentieth century, rather than on those patterns as they exist today and will most likely exist into the foreseeable future. Coverage today essentially assumes acute, short-term illness; treatment during a short-term hospital stay, as a result of which the patient either gets better or dies; and expenses that are high during the duration of the illness, but that do not continue to grow for months or years. Currently, both our private and public insurance programs emphasize short-term inpatient care, limit outpatient coverage, seldom assist in extended care, and offer few preventive services and little home health care. But cancer, diabetes, stroke, and heart disease tend to last a lifetime. Even if the original medical episode is fatal, elaborate medical technology has made it overwhelmingly expensive for all but our upper-income citizens. If patients survive the early stages of these illnesses, continued treatment and mounting costs are required. Finally, since more and more of us live long enough to experience the various, largely incurable illnesses of aging, our health-insurance programs again prove outdated.

WHAT IS NATIONAL HEALTH INSURANCE?

One's ideas about the characteristics of a national health insurance program and what consequences and benefits it should have are clearly influenced by how one sees the strengths and weaknesses of the current health-care system.

We shall begin . . . by postulating that there are two archetypical and opposing views about the nature of our problem, and [about] the contribution of health insurance to its solution. On the one hand are those who believe that our medical-care system is essentially sound; that it is in a process of healthy growth and evolution; and that the major role of health insurance is to provide protection against the unpredictable costs of illness. On the other hand are those who believe that our medical-care system has failed to produce health services efficiently or to distribute them equitably; and who regard a national health insurance scheme not only as a means to achieve protection against the costs of illness, but also as a powerful force that should be used to reshape the medical-care system itself. Obviously, our assessment of any given proposal will be deeply influenced by which of these viewpoints, and their associated objectives, we accept.[10]

The authors of this textbook essentially accept the more critical viewpoint.

Broadly defined and viewed in the context of the United States, national health insurance will be a program in which the federal government will finance and guarantee a broad range of medical services to all (or virtually all) of our citizens.

Current discussions of national health insurance are based, first, on a commitment that medical care should be available to everybody and, second, on a belief that the costs of medical care should be met through group payment. The commitment to availability reflects a basic social policy stemming from widespread belief that no one in modern society should suffer because medical care is not available when and where it is needed. The consensus favoring group payment, or cost sharing, derives from the fact that the costs of medical care are not readily manageable on an individual or family basis because of the uncertain and variable nature and the potential size of the costs for any particular family in relation to its private resources.[11]

National health insurance is considered to have several basic objectives. Perhaps the most commonly stated objective is ensuring and improving access to health services. In fact, all forms of health insurance seek to improve access to health services through minimzing the out-of-pocket expenses consumers must pay for the medical services that are covered. But the problem here, of course, is the absence of a guarantee that everyone will receive coverage.

The impact of NHI on access to medical care is complicated and not entirely predictable. We do believe that the medical services covered by NHI will be used more than they currently are, especially by those millions who now have no health insurance. But some observers believe that services not covered by NHI might also be increasingly used. They feel that consumers will be willing to spend their "savings" from services that are covered for those desired services that are not covered. Most supporters of NHI disagree.

[10] Avedis Donabedian, M.D., "Issues in National Health Insurance," *American Journal of Public Health*, Vol. 66, no. 4 (April 1976), p. 345.
[11] I. S. Falk, "National Health Insurance: A Review of Policies and Proposals," *Journal of Law and Contemporary Problems*, Duke University School of Law, Vol. 35 (Autumn 1970), "Health Care," Part II, p. 669.

In analyzing this issue, we must remember that we seek or avoid medical care for numerous reasons. People who do not obtain medical services when they ought to may not want to hear what they fear. Others may avoid needed medical care out of ignorance or a fatalism about their health. National health insurance will not be directly concerned with removing these psychological barriers to receiving care. It will, however, remove the cost of health services, which is perhaps a higher barrier. Thus, under NHI, not everyone will obtain medical services when needed, but the cost of those services will not be the barrier it is today.

A second objective commonly attributed to national health insurance is the reduction of financial hardship that can result from medical bills. The "national" in NHI means that the entire society will finance the medical costs for each individual and family. No one will be forced to pay enormous medical expenses because of major illness. In theory, we will all pay something, through taxation or insurance premiums, but no one will pay the larger medical expenses out of his pocket. Even the most modest NHI proposals provide coverage for major medical expenses.

A third objective of NHI is to reduce or limit the total cost of health care or at least to limit its cost increases.[12] This objective is one of the most controversial. Opponents of NHI believe it will actually increase our health expenditures, whereas supporters say that NHI can shift emphasis away from expensive medical services, such as those provided on an inpatient basis. Opponents counter that this will lead to administrative red tape, will deny needed services, and produce bureaucratic costs.

Other benefits are also frequently ascribed to NHI. A major argument is that the current fragmentation of the health-care system, with its waste and inefficiency, will be alleviated by the nationalization of the system. In this vein, both proponents and opponents of national health insurance see current government efforts at rationalizing the health system, such as by encouraging the growth of health-maintenance organizations, as preparing the way for the creation of NHI. By implication, the government's involvement in the system, through improving the efficiency of delivery and planning the allocation of resources, has provided us with a growing recognition of current deficiencies and with the experience and knowledge necessary to establish a national system. Thus, despite the increasing involvement of the federal government in improving the health-care system, "many deficiencies in the health-care system remain, and it is widely maintained that the case for a unified, coordinated national health-care policy is becoming steadily stronger."[13]

It is at this level of "rationalizing" the current "nonsystem" of American health-care delivery and of reorganizing the delivery of medical serv-

[12] Davis, *National Health Insurance,* chapter 1.
[13] Davis, *National Health Insurance,* p. vii.

ices that objectives for national health insurance seem at best wishful thinking, rather than certain and predictable benefits. Currently, both the desirability and the possibility of using NHI as a mechanism for major system reform in the delivery and quality of care are being questioned.

> There is some agreement among health planners that national health insurance should be strategically organized to create incentives to affect the behavior of medical-care delivery systems. In order to avoid substantial escalations of health-care costs under . . . national health insurance, runs the argument, government will almost certainly need to use the financing tool as a lever to promote desirable utilization, production, and distribution of personal health services.

> Other health planners do not concur with the assessment that national health insurance should be used to induce change in delivery systems. . . . Thus, the national health insurance debate involves multiple objectives in the absence of precise knowledge about probable effects of different policies on health-care systems.[14]

It seems clear that the system is in need of major reform and reorganization. But it may be unrealistic to hope that national health insurance will lead directly to improvements in such widespread difficulties as the unequal distribution of physicians and the uneven quality of care. At least as currently conceived, national health insurance is a plan for changing the structure of financing health services. We can only make educated guesses about its major consequences for the rest of the health-care system.

We should not underestimate the capacity of the current health-care system for avoiding change or minimizing its extent. Attempting to discourage the use of more expensive and often unneeded medical services through NHI may or may not work, depending on whether consumers decide to pay for these services out-of-pocket. Seeking to reorganize health-service delivery into (for example) HMOs may or may not work, depending on the power of governmental incentives and on innumerable decisions by physicians, potential HMO enrollees, and local community leaders. Many NHI proposals encourage the continued establishment of HMOs, but the resistance to these organizations will remain strong. National health insurance can certainly improve access to care and can minimize the medical costs paid by individuals and families. Whether it can reduce our national health expenditures is less certain; and its ability to "rationalize" the health system seems even more uncertain. We are tempted to conclude that NHI may be less than its proponents want and less a threat to the status quo than its opponents fear.

[14] Stuart H. Altman and Joseph L. Falkson, "National Health Insurance and the Health Care Delivery System, Social Security—Issues and Trends," Industrial Relations Research Association, 25th Annual Proceedings, 1972, p. 231.

SOME BASIC ISSUES AND DECISIONS

Policy makers must face a number of basic issues and decisions in establishing public policy on national health insurance. First is the question of who should be covered and how that coverage would be established. The most modest advocates propose that only the poor and those facing catastrophic medical expenses should be insured by NHI. On the other extreme are those who propose that coverage be universal. The issue is partly one of cost: the more people covered, the more expensive the program. But the issue also has philosophical aspects. Is health care an absolute right or not? Should the benefits be available only to those employed full-time, only to those poor who qualify for welfare, or to everyone? The weight of current opinion seems to favor a nearly universal coverage. "Universal coverage without regard to family composition, employability, or social-security contribution history seems to provide the most equitable solution."[15]

A related issue is how to establish the coverage. What methods and systems do we use to bring people into the national health insurance program? Some have recommended the Social Security Administration, which already has related experience through its involvement with Medicare. But this would exclude many of the poor who do not participate in social security. Others recommend using the place of employment as the site and means for enrollment. But the unemployed, again, would be excluded, as would the self-employed.

An additional consideration is whether national health insurance coverage should be voluntary or compulsory. Although making it compulsory will anger some citizens, making NHI voluntary has even greater problems. Certainly the very wealthy might choose not to participate, but so would many of the very poor.

> Voluntarism will never produce universal coverage, for there will always be those who opt out due to ignorance, undue optimism, or neglect. A national health insurance program which does not provide universal coverage will unquestionably perpetuate the two-class system of patient care it is designed to eliminate, as afflicted individuals without health-insurance protection will have to be treated on a charity basis.[16]

Perhaps the most difficult decision is choosing what services should be covered. The question of who should be covered is partly economic, partly philosophical, and clearly political. The decision about what serv-

---

[15] Davis, *National Health Insurance*, p. 57.
[16] "National Health Insurance," editorial, *Journal of Medical Education*, Vol. 49, no. 7 (1974), p. 708.

ices should be covered is all of these and medical as well. Again, we find a range of proposals from the more modest ones, which would insure only the most frequently used services of general physicians, specialists, and hospitalization in medical emergencies, to those seeking to insure almost all medical care. The following is illustrative of the second approach:

> A national health insurance plan should finance the most comprehensive package of health-care benefits within the resources available. As a general rule, all necessary health-care expenditures should be covered without quantity limits. Exclusion from coverage should be well defined and well reasoned. All exclusions should be periodically reviewed and reevaluated in light of new federal initiatives and new developments in health-care management and delivery.[17]

This view illustrates the difficulty of deciding what medical services should be covered, for it asks more questions than it answers. What is meant by the "resources available"? Are these "resources" medical—the ability of the health-care delivery system to provide medical care—or are they financial—the monies available to the federal government to pay for these services? Should "resources available" include monies made available through additional taxation of the citizenry? Who will decide which health-care expenditures are "necessary" and which are not?

This thorny problem of choosing what services should be covered under NHI is indicative of the fact that the objectives can be contradictory. If we opt for more comprehensive coverage, then we minimize our ability to reform the system. Including services under NHI coverage should encourage their use; excluding them should discourage frequent or unnecessary use. Davis provides an apparently reasonable set of criteria for NHI coverage. She would give high priority to the following:

1. those services that reduce mortality or disability—prenatal care, immunizations, well-baby care are examples
2. medical services that are so expensive that they add substantially to the financial burden of individuals and families—cancer and expensive chronic illnesses are examples
3. medical services that will be sought regardless of their cost
4. medical services constituting lower-cost alternatives to important medical care—examples are minisurgery in lieu of inpatient surgery and the use of extended-care facilities[18]

There are many proposals for what services to include under NHI coverage. Most would insure physician services and needed hospitalization, but there is less agreement from there on. Prescription drugs are often included, whereas mental-health services are sometimes excluded,

[17] Ibid.
[18] Davis, *National Health Insurance*, p. 58.

partly because of a lack of faith in their curative ability. Cosmetic surgery is almost always excluded from NHI plans, while dental services are sometimes included and sometimes not. Laboratory and x-ray charges are often included in the benefits, and maternity and at least some pediatric services are almost always listed for coverage.

The financing of national health insurance raises additional problems and serious considerations. A basic and unresolved question is what the country can and will spend for NHI. Behind this question is the apparent difficulty of estimating how much the various proposals for NHI would actually cost. There are often major differences between two or more estimates of the costs of any one plan. In 1971, for example, a plan proposed by Senator Edward Kennedy was estimated to cost between $44 and $77 billion a year; the AMA estimated that its own plan would cost about $8 billion, whereas the Social Security Administration estimated that the tab for the AMA's plan would be twice that amount.[19]

There are various options available for raising revenues to pay for national health insurance. One method is through the payment of premiums by employers, employees, and individual citizens. A payroll-deduction method could be used, but this again would exclude all those who do not receive salaries or wages. If we have a fairly uniform premium charge for everyone, that cost will be disproportionately heavy for those with lower incomes. Many favor financing NHI through general revenues accruing to government largely through the various income taxes. This would mean a progressive financing of the system: those with larger incomes would pay more.

Another issue is the question of whether consumers should be required to share the cost of certain services. The arguments favoring such co-payments, as established by government policy, seem compelling. There are often many ways in which an illness may be treated, and patients paying some share of the medical expenses will want the less expensive method. This could assist the NHI in meeting the objective of reducing the total national health expenditure.

The involvement of various agencies and population groups in the stucturing of NHI provides a fascinating challenge. There is great controversy over the potential role of private health-insurance companies. Some favor a major role for private insurance companies, which would include selling the NHI plan, underwriting coverage and paying medical expenses, and making a profit from NHI. Others argue that private health insurance should have little or no involvement with NHI. They note that Blue Cross and Blue Shield have demonstrated inefficiency and an inability to control physician and hospital costs during their administration of Medicaid and Medicare. They also argue that private insurance compa-

19 "Health Care for Everybody," *U.S. News and World Report*, Vol. 70 (January/March, 1971).

nies would be an unneeded bureaucratic layer between consumers, providers, and NHI administrators. Some take an intermediate position by suggesting that the plan be monitored and financed by the federal and state governments, with private health-insurance companies involved in administration and claim review. At this point the debate over the involvement of private health insurers seems largely emotional and political.

More-complicated questions exist in discussions about the role of state and national governments. Many argue that we have retained our system of federalism, with power for public programs distributed among the various layers of government. They continue by saying that since state governments are involved in licensure, certification, insurance regulation, and Medicaid, a nationally controlled NHI managed by Washington would be wasteful and inefficient and would alienate state officials.

It is probably desirable to have the involvement of both national and state agencies in national health insurance. Different sections of the country, different states, even different regions within the states have their own health delivery systems and attitudes. The federal government should set the broad guidelines for NHI policy but leave much of the program's administration to state and local governments.

> The major roles that have been proposed for state governments in national health insurance are to regulate the private insurance industry, establish standards for participation and payment methods and levels for medical-care providers, and administer and subsidize coverage for low-income families.[20]

Perhaps the central questions pertain to the potential impact of NHI on providers, consumers, and on their interactions. The fundamental reality is that NHI must have the reasonable support and participation by physicians, hospitals, and consumers. Doctors choosing en masse to fight NHI can severely hamper it. This is not to say that we must fear giving in to any potential political blackmail. But we must have enough provider participation to make the system work.

A major question for physicians is how NHI will affect their income. They are the highest-paid professional group in the country, and a rapid and dramatic change in that status will not favor their happy participation in such a plan. National health insurance could continue the status quo by paying physicians a fee for service. In this case, many related questions must be answered. What fee level should be used? Most argue for paying physicians the usual and customary fees, but this fluctuates over time and is less precise than often assumed. Different physicians in the same location or physicians in adjacent areas may have different fees for the same services. Still, some use of usual and customary fees may well be the best short-term answer for physician compensation.

[20] Davis, *National Health Insurance*, p. 75.

Some proponents of national health insurance recommend the capitation method for paying physicians. Although many medical providers consider capitation payments a frightening prospect, some find it increasingly attractive. The method permits physicians and other medical providers to predict income quite accurately. It can also result in an income "windfall" for physicians who are able to reduce their costs for providing care by hiring lower-paid associates and making use of auxiliary medical personnel.

Physicians seem most strongly opposed to being paid predetermined salaries for their services under NHI. To many this seems somehow less than "professional," and it clearly creates the possibility of limiting their income. A salary is essentially a fixed sum, and physicians would be less able to increase income through extra work. Again, the potential conflict between NHI objectives becomes apparent. We need enough physician participation in NHI to provide the services, and this goal would seem to depend largely upon how much money they could make. But we also want to cut health-care expenditures, and minimizing physician income is one way to do that.

Some have argued that we should find a compromise between physician demands for maintaining their income and the social objectives of limiting health-care expenditures. One method would be to reimburse physicians for services provided under NHI, while not prohibiting them from making additional charges to patients for those same services. This may make physicians happy, but it would probably be inflationary. In addition, it would again be burdensome to lower-income patients. The system of co-payments mentioned above seems more equitable.

The participation of physicians in NHI is as much a sociological and political problem as it is economic. We have for many decades believed that doctors epitomized free enterprise: the harder they worked and the more efficient they were, the higher their income; the delivery of their services was based on skills and knowledge, and government should leave them alone. Yet we see that the current health-care system has enormous deficiencies. The literature on national health insurance illustrates this conflict. Proponents of NHI support its establishment and yet are deeply troubled by proposals for limiting physician compensation.

This same conflict exists in considering how to ensure high-quality care under a national health insurance program. We have for many years believed that the individual physician delivering care to "his" patient knows best what should be done. Yet we are troubled by the revelations that thousands of people die from unnecessary surgery, that most hysterectomies are ill advised, and that at least some doctors and hospitals are willing to indulge in questionable billings to Medicaid and Medicare. If we are to put billions of dollars into NHI, we must have assurances that we get what is paid for. But fears of bureaucratic control and destruction of the "doctor–patient relationship" remain and will not easily be overcome.

Nor does the adequate participation of consumers in NHI seem any easier to plan. We clearly must establish methods by which consumers can register complaints against policies and practices of the government and medical providers. What is perhaps most critical is that this complaint system not be so complicated and time-consuming that consumers decide it is not worth using. Administrators of many hospitals and HMOs use their complaint system as a way of getting rid of the troublesome patient rather than as a useful method for righting wrongs and improving services.

The presence of consumers on various NHI policy boards at federal, state, and local levels is also usually proposed. On the face of it, it seems as though they have as much right as government officials and medical providers to be involved in policy formulation. But numerous complications exist. Aren't we all medical consumers? Even doctors go to doctors. Being a medical consumer is usually defined as not being a medical provider, a loose definition at best. In addition, since policy-board members are usually chosen by administrators or existing board members, there is a strong tendency to choose highly active citizens, members of the local community elite, and cooperative rather than contentious persons. This is not to say that consumer participation in NHI policy formulation is not important. Nevertheless, it remains a participation that needs clarification and significance beyond the current practice in the planning of health care.

A FINAL LOOK

National health insurance in America will have major problems. It will be opposed by many physicians as "socialized medicine," by many hospital administrators as unduly bureaucratic, and by many citizens as an additional tax burden. It will at least occasionally suffer from conflicts between state and federal officials, much in the same way as Medicaid. Its opponents will consider it a disaster; its proponents will consider it a panacea for the deficiencies in our health-care system. It will probably be neither.

Perhaps the most important consideration is that it must be understandable and manageable. If it is to work, millions of citizens must know what services are and are not covered. If it becomes a program so complex and vague as to require constant interpretation for provider and consumer alike, its costs could be astronomical and its benefits limited. National health insurance could be a method for making health care a right rather than a privilege. It could also be a costly contribution to confusion, chaos, and political warfare.

SUGGESTED READINGS

ARROW, KENNETH J., "Problems of Resource Allocation in United States Medical Care." In Robert M. Kunz and Hans Fehr, eds., *The Challenge of Life: Biomedical Progress and Human Values* (New York: International Publishers Co., Inc., 1972), pp. 392–408. Studies problems of resource allocations as viewed by economists.

BLOOM, BERNARD S. and SAMUEL P. MARTIN, "The Role of the Federal Government in Financing Health and Medical Services," *Journal of Medical Education,* Vol. 51, no. 3 (March 1976), pp. 161–69. A survey article identifying some of the data on the proportion of income spent on health care.

CAREY, WILLIAM, "Policy Making in a Negotiating Society," *Journal of Medical Education,* Vol. 51 (January 1976), pp. 14–18. A commentary on the politics surrounding the issue of national health insurance.

COOPER, JOHN A. D., "Institutional Response to Expectations for Health Care," *Journal of Medical Education,* Vol. 44, no. 1 (January 1969), pp. 31–35. A commentary on public clamor for improvement in the health-care delivery system.

CULYER, A. J., "The Nature of the Commodity 'Health Care' and Its Efficient Allocation," *Oxford Economic Papers,* Vol. 23, no. 2 (July 1971), pp. 189–211. The perspectives of a British economist on national health insurance.

FEIN, RASHI, "On Achieving Access and Equity in Health Care." In Spyros Andreopoulos, ed., *Medical Cure and Medical Care* (New York: Prodist, 1973), pp. 157–89. A discussion of the issue of federal intervention in the health-care system.

INGLEHART, JOHN K., "Health Report: State, County Governments Win Key Roles in New Program," *National Journal Reports,* Vol. 7, no. 45 (November 8, 1975), pp. 1533–39. The consideration of state and local governments' influence on national health insurance.

INGLEHART, JOHN K., "Kidney Treatment Problem Readies HEW for National Health Insurance," *National Journal,* June 26, 1976, pp. 895–900. A discussion of how the crippling financial aspects of chronic illness have paved the way for national health insurance.

KOHLMEIER, LOUIS M., "Overseeing the Health Care Industry," *National Journal Reports,* Vol. 7, no. 16 (April 19, 1975), p. 591. A progress report on the development of support for national health insurance.

MASSIE, ROBERT K., "The Politicians versus our Health," *Newsweek,* March 29, 1976, p. 13. A commentary on the political pressures that influence the fate of national health insurance.

MITCHELL, BRIDGER M. and WILLIAM B. SCHWARTZ, "Strategies for Financing

National Health Insurance: Who Wins and Who Loses," *The New England Journal of Medicine*, Vol. 295, no. 16 (October 14, 1976), pp. 866–71. Examines proposals for financing national health insurance.

NEWHOUSE, JOSEPH P., CHARLES E. PHELPS, and WILLIAM SCHWARTZ, "Policy Options and the Impact of National Health Insurance," *The New England Journal of Medicine*, Vol. 290, no. 24 (June 13, 1974), pp. 1345–59. A survey containing ninety-one additional references to sources dealing with the impact of a national insurance plan.

ROOS, NORALOU, P., "Influencing the Health Care System: Policy Alternatives," *Public Policy*, Vol. 22, no. 2 (Spring 1974). A description of the health-care system's policy options and alternative strategies for change.

WERLIN, STANLEY J., ALEXANDRA WALCOTT, and MICHAEL JOROFF, "Implementing Formative Health Planning Under PL 93–641," *The New England Journal of Medicine*, Vol. 295, no. 13 (September 23, 1976). An approach to implementing national health insurance.

18

ETHICAL ISSUES: GENETIC CONTROL, SELECTIVE BREEDING, AND THE HUMAN PROSPECT

Throughout this book, we have noted how the triumphs of medical biology and technology have transformed the nature of the curative process. We have described how these have compelled radical alterations in the delivery of care and how these have radically altered the patient–physician relationship and the morbidity patterns of society.

In this chapter, we will turn to the genetic explorations that now pose unprecedented challenges to society. The history of medicine is a narrative documenting our success in extending life. We have also developed the "technology" for the control of birth. But we are now on the threshold of one of the most remarkable innovations of all: within our lifetimes, we shall be able to control the sex of our offspring and to participate in genetic manipulation not only to control disease, but also to shape the very form and character of the human being itself. With cloning we shall be able to produce carbon copies of ourselves, literally a duplicating process. In brief, we are moving from an era of organ transplants to an era in which we are quite literally designing the human being. Such intervention sets a course that will have implications for generations to come.

Increasingly, the medical field is confronted with questions that are more ethical than medical. Should we legalize abortions? Who controls the life of the fetus? Should society allow a woman autonomy in the "uses" of her body? Should society intervene in the reproduction process when its certain consequence is a malformed baby, with the prospect of serious costs to society? Should women have access to artificial insemination, so that the father of her child might be some distinguished figure? Should a mother wanting to avoid the discomfort of carrying her baby have the option of having the baby carried by a "rented mother"? Should the mother and father encourage *in vitro* growth of their eggs to the blastocyst stage to circumvent infertility? If so, should they make use of the sperm of a Henry Kissinger, or a Paul Newman, or from a catalogue of men with remarkable physical and mental prowess? Should they seek to fertilize a female egg from a similar catalogue of distinguished females? What is the laboratory meaning of parenthood if neither "parent" contributes to this asexual union of sperm and egg and if they have the baby carried to term by a borrowed "mother"? What appears as the science fiction of the future is rapidly becoming the science of today. In our lifetime, these questions, while appearing fanciful, will require answering.

At one end of the age spectrum, we have the problems created by the use of artificial-support systems to sustain life. In traditional medical terminology, a person was dead when his heart stopped beating. But today we can sustain the heartbeat indefinitely. How are we, then, to define death? It is clear that the definition must involve the human being in the life-or-death decision-making process.

Behind this moral question is the larger issue of whether persons should not have the right to opt for a short life—if possibly a merrier one— or should society intervene to insist on the prolongation of life? Kenneth Boulding, in drawing analogies of the human to the machine, notes that the scrap value of the machine includes consideration of amortizing future production potential against future maintenance costs. But the human has more than instrumental values. By our value structure, each person has a positive value until the moment of his death, simply because society has identified life as something inherently valuable. However, with the intervention of life-prolonging techniques, death is no longer an "act of God" but increasingly an issue of excruciating public choice.

Society has a strong appreciation for the view that each person must decide for himself just when life has lost hope—particularly for those who, in the judgment of medical science, are terminally ill and are confronted with a downward projectory to painful death. Should this decision be modified? The respect we have for the autonomy of individual choice is modified, of course, for those who are mentally ill and for children. But at what point does the judgment of those in failing health remain operative? Should the decision, in such situations, be left with guilt-ridden or distraught relatives, the family physician (if such exists), a lawyer, a judge? We see, then, that technological developments have transformed death from an unavoidable, natural event to one that demands the active participation of decision makers.

The American Hospital Association issued its Bill of Rights for Patients in November 1972, and again in January 1973, to its seven thousand member hospitals. Its twelve-point protocol includes, as point four: "The patient has the right to refuse treatment to the extent permitted by law and to be informed of the medical consequences of his action." But what guidelines do such statutes provide? Amitai Etzioni asks the hard questions:

> If the patients themselves have the right to insist . . . that life-extending machines be turned off, they must be conscious when they so choose, but their action would be tantamount to suicide. On the other hand, if the patient has to be unconscious beyond recall before the machines can be turned off, the right to refuse service is not his. Who, then, exercises the right—one doctor? . . . two? . . . three? . . . with or without consultation of the next of kin? . . . under what medical conditions?[1]

The intervention of the federal government in providing dialysis support for those afflicted with kidney ailments will reach an estimated $1 billion annually within a few years. Is this the "best" allocation of our medical resources?

The problem of defining death assumes significance, not simply because we can maintain artificial life, but also because effective organs that are to resume their life in a new host must be provided by a donor with a sustained heartbeat who is close to the hospital where the organ transfer will take place. We have the obligation to define the mutuality of interests. Can society properly "speak" for the comatose patient, with no prospects for recovery, in the surrender of his organs to another living person?

Defining appropriate measures of postponing death is as critical to our society as its renewed hope that, through intervention in the processes of conception, we can limit the spread of genetic defects. Between these twin issues, we are confronted with ethical issues about the appropriate forms of experimentation with human beings. How do we secure informed consent from the mentally retarded, children, prisoners, and even college students? For such groups, there is always the risk of coercive influences and the risk that the advantages secured from the experimentation may be for society alone, with no therapeutic benefit for the subject.

Also, as we noted at the outset, the ability of genetic control to influence the physical and mental characteristics of the human race are now before us. What are the implications of our search for a "more perfect" human specimen? Should we have the arrogance to presume that contemporary definitions of the "best" should influence future civilization in perpetuity? What are the implications of cultural differences in the definition of the "best"? Is there the risk of a "genetic gap" as one nation undertakes to produce its crop of supermen, with the prospect of world dominance by the super race? What would remain of the family structure and of the values implicit in that structure if we synthesize the human species, in or out of the laboratory? Let us touch briefly on a few of these issues.

[1] Amitai Etzioni, "The Genetic Fix," *Society*, Vol. 10, no. 6 (September 1973), p. 38.

DEFINING VALUES: THE ETHICAL DILEMMA

Before we view specific issues in terms of the "correct" response of society, we must emphasize the proliferation of values within contemporary society. In the absence of a single ethical structure, there is no single "good" answer to the questions we face. This is not to say we must be cultural relativists in dealing with ethical issues, but only to emphasize that we have conflicting value systems producing contradictory responses.

Let us briefly sketch two major value systems that reflect differences of methodology and philosophy about the meaning of life itself. As we noted earlier, primitive cultures viewed illness and all other aspects of fate as the workings of gods, often working through nature. Hippocrates, in about 500 B.C., was among the first to challenge the proposition that all ills could be attributed to the supernatural. At the time, epilepsy was considered a sacred disease because victims appeared to be overcome by the gods or demons.

> Hippocrates wrote: "It seems to me that the disease of epilepsy is no more divine than any other. It has natural causes just as other diseases have." Then he added, "Men think it is divine only because they do not understand it." Here we find one of the first statements rejecting supernaturalism and miracle thinking, and it is from this perceptive man that we derive our Hippocratic Oath.[2]

By the Renaissance, three distinguished professions had emerged—theology, medicine, and law. Of necessity, medicine became particularly concerned with the practical issue of whether affliction had natural or supernatural origins. If it were the latter, how would one reconcile the affliction of disease with God's purpose? And as we defined different gods, we had varying interpretations of the causes of disease and varying notions about man's obligations to assist the afflicted. On the issue of personal obligation, many religions emerged with a version of the Golden Rule.

With the emergence of rationalism, empiricism, and critical thinking, even the doctrine of the Golden Rule came under attack. As George Bernard Shaw reminded us, we should *not* do unto others as we would have them do unto us, for they may have a different value orientation. The utilitarian "radicals" charged that depending on altruism alone meant the blind leading the blind to the abyss. And the physician might charge

---

[2] This section owes much to Richard Thomas Barton, "Sources of Medical Morals," *Journal of the American Medical Association*, Vol. 193, no. 2 (July 12, 1965). The quotation above is drawn from pp. 127–28.

another defect: all too often we do not know what we wish to have done unto us.

In dealing with the mystery of life and the intriguing question of moral purpose, we can distinguish two major trends of thought. First, we have the natural-law theory of morality, drawing inspiration from Catholicism, but by no means limited to Christianity. It emphasizes that man, by his reasoning, can synthesize a code of conduct or moral directives from nature. The answers, in brief, can be found in the study of history, the analysis of man, and the realization of ethical imperatives that survive time and transcend man. In this context, our problems today reflect a corruption and moral bankruptcy, for we have given up our search for, and even appreciation of, these eternal verities. We must, in this view, return to a moral universe through an unending search for those universal laws applicable to all men. The discovery of natural law is not simply the product of civilization; it is written in the hearts of men. Man has God-given capacities for identifying these essential values. It is charged that such a viewpoint is conservative, antiscientific, and absolutist, for it emphasizes certainty, with eternal rights applicable to all men in all circumstances at all times.

A second strand of philosophic perspective finds its roots in empiricism, with a school of philosophers that includes Bacon, Locke, Berkeley, Hume, and John Stuart Mill. Although drawing on elements of natural law, empiricists believe that moral directives should be derived from experience rather than from revelation or simple idealism. This viewpoint set the stage for scientific inquiry, rationalism, and pragmatism. In the context of pragmatism, man acquired a position on center stage, with the tenet "Will it work for mankind?" Pragmatists are more concerned about the quality of life in this world than with preparing for another world. They hold that attitudes about right and wrong are acquired through human experience, through trial and error. All existing judgments must be challenged to identify the potential for improvement. Pragmatists are pluralistic, are tolerant of the diversity of viewpoints, and carry on a constant search for an improved understanding and morality. One has written of the "mountain-range effect": we climb one mountain range only to look across the range to another. Science will show us no certainty about moral imperatives.[3]

A related branch of philosophy—existentialism—contends that man must accept responsibility for his existence, his freedom, and his actions. We cannot place the blame for events or mistakes upon God, the environment, race, caste inheritance, childhood traumas, or misdirected education. Man is condemned to freedom, to making his own decisions. He alone is responsible and must cultivate a self-awareness of the awesome

[3] Ibid., p. 137.

influence that his own actions might have upon the change of civilization.

It seems clear that the mere act of genetic engineernig involves profound philosophical issues. To the "natural law" group, such tinkering with the design of nature may well prove the undoing of mankind, for truly the scientist, in "making" man, is assuming functions ordained by and for nature. The existentialist may have similar concerns, reflecting again the arrogance of the scientist's convictions that his values—advanced through genetic engineering—are appropriate in perpetuity.

Typically, the scientist is not a student of either ethics or philosophy, but of the scientific method. For the most part, he is inclined to the view: "If it can be done, it will be done." A new generation of philosopher-geneticists is emerging that appears to be succumbing to the view: "If it can be done, it should be done." Moral sanctions are now being extended to genetic explorations, with the prospect that mankind can finally lift itself, by its genetic bootstraps, to higher levels of consciousness and civilization.

HEREDITARY DISEASES: THE CASE FOR
GENETIC INTERVENTION

The genetic lottery has produced some unhappy losses to society. These are all the more tragic because they strike young children and mean anguish for parents and burdens to society. It seems reasonable to try to decipher the code that accounts for some two thousand identifiable genetic ailments. Today, these diseases afflict twelve million Americans, or about one in eighteen. They account for a third of the admissions to pediatric wards and for forty percent of all infant deaths.[4] Every person is a carrier of some genetic flaw, and it is probable that not all problems can be eliminated by any program—no matter how ambitious or authoritarian—to reduce the transfer of these traits from one generation to the next. Some flaws (such as early baldness or color blindness) may be relatively minor, but others have lethal consequences. There is a genetic "predisposition" to some of our more common ailments, including heart disease, schizophrenia, manic depression, ulcers, and diabetes. There is also a racial or ethnic disposition to some afflictions. The most widely recognized is Tay-Sachs disease, afflicting Jews with forebearers from Eastern or Central Europe, and sickle-cell anemia, afflicting blacks. Cystic fibrosis is largely confined to Caucasian children, afflicting between 20,000 and 25,000 children and young adults. Another major genetic affliction produces Mongoloid children. Some 50,000 such children in the United

[4] Gene Bylinsky, "What Science Can Do About Hereditary Diseases," *Fortune*, September 1974, p. 148.

States today require an estimated annual support cost to both family and society of $250 million. There are now some 70 genetic abnormalities that can be diagnosed during pregnancy. These problems can be "treated" by aborting the fetus, but another 40 diseases can be treated and alleviated by diet and drugs.[5]

Ethical questions have been raised about the appropriateness of requiring tests during the early stages of pregnancy to detect abnormalities, the problem of who should pay for such tests, the uncertainties of risk to the fetus, and the stigma attached to both parent and infant with "probablistic" estimates of deformity or affliction. Also, what is the appropriate response to evidence of a malformed fetus? If parents are unwilling—because of economic circumstance or even emotional impulse—to provide support and care for a Mongoloid child, does society have a moral right to determine whether such a child should be born?

Prenatal examination of the delicately balanced biochemical machinery to detect possible chromosomal abnormality involves a process known as amniocentesis, in which a needle is inserted through the abdomen into a pregnant woman's uterus to draw out a small amount of the amniotic fluid surrounding and protecting the fetus. Through examination of cells shed by the developing fetus, one can identify the genetic makeup of the child and determine whether the baby will be "normal." For reasons that are not understood, the risk of bearing a Mongoloid child increases with age. About half of the five thousand Mongoloid born annually in this country are the offspring of mothers past thirty-five years of age.[6]

Only about 3,000 amniocentesis tests have been performed in the United States in the past 2 or 3 years, or less than 1 test per thousand pregnancies. The tests require skilled practitioners and a well-equipped laboratory to evaluate the results. Amniocentesis is usually performed around the fifteenth week of pregnancy. Most chromosomal defects are voided through spontaneous abortion, but Mongoloid children slip through nature's genetic screen at the rate of about 1 in each 600 births. Although half of all Mongoloid children die before they reach 5 years of age, some live, with the help of modern medicine, to 50 years of age.

In dealing with society's obligation, we should realize that not all parents suffer an overwhelming sense of grief with Mongoloid children. Charles Lowe of the NIH has testified:

> As a pediatrician, I have cared for families who didn't want to get rid of a child with Down's syndrome [Mongolism]. These children have a sunny disposition, they are very responsive, and their demands are not excessive. It would be wrong to say that all families with a defective

[5] Ibid.
[6] Ibid., p. 152.

child want to get rid of it, or that if they had it to do again, wouldn't have the child. It's not that black and white. Sometimes a defective child plays an important part in keeping a family together. The big problem is, who will look after the child after the parents are gone?[7]

With limited screening now a reality, and with improvements in support systems to sustain life for the crippled, the social and economic costs for such children will increase substantially. Health-systems analyst Terrance E. Swanson observed that "if we allow our genetic problems to get out of hand by not acting promptly to ameliorate the situation, we as a society run the risk of overcommitting ourselves to the care and maintenance of a large population of mentally deficient patients at the expense of other urgent social problems."[8]

No one is proposing the forced abortion of Mongoloids or other defective fetuses. But programs of testing, counseling and voluntary abortion could save society from $75 billion to $100 billion over the next 20 years. Amitai Etzioni explains:

> It's clear that a woman has the right to bear a defective child if she wants, but there is a question whether she has the right to give birth and then charge it to the state. Very often parents just dump children in an institution and never even visit them. People just don't worry about the social costs. I say, in our kind of society, individual needs should come first, second, and third; but in the fourth place there's room for social considerations.[9]

We also have a genetic-screening device for the detection and treatment of phenylketonuria, PKU. Although comparatively rare, this affliction produces severe mental retardation. Through a chemical imbalance in the fetus, the baby develops abnormal concentrations of phenylalinine in the blood and spinal fluid, a problem that can be either solved or sharply reduced through detection and appropriate diet. Testing is inexpensive, costing one dollar or less per infant. In some states testing for PKU is now mandatory.

Even more lethal is Tay-Sachs disease, again involving a biochemical abnormality. Tay-Sachs babies are often beautiful and display no outward signs of difficulty until about 6 months of age. They then suddenly begin to deteriorate physically and mentally. They go blind, become helpless, and soon die. Life can be sustained in a vegetative state until the child is about 5, with support costs of $45,000 annually.[10] It is estimated that the risk of both husband and wife carrying the defective gene is 1 in 900 couples. Blood tests can anticipate the presence of the diffi-

[7] As quoted by Bylinsky, ibid., p. 152.
[8] Ibid., p. 154.
[9] Ibid.
[10] Ibid., p. 156.

culty, but counseling young couples of its presence requires skill and diplomacy. High-risk couples can refrain from having children, adopt children, use artificial insemination, or undergo amniocentesis to allow the abortion of fetuses with the ailment. In a test of 10,000 persons (on a voluntary basis), 11 couples both had defective genes. Of these, 5 proceeded with pregnancies, with the screen of amniocentesis to detect abnormality.

Much more controversial are the widely publicized programs to control sickle-cell anemia. Black activists and others concerned about minority deprivation have launched educational and fund-raising campaigns to mount detection and remedial programs. This effort brings into sharp focus the problems created for society when tests are devised to identify the presence or the "trait" of sickle-cell anemia, without the full realization that no cures are in sight. The ethical issue of arousing concerns within even the very young of the black community about their impaired genetic structure can do lasting damage.

The faulty molecular structure of the red blood cells distorts these normally disc-shaped cells into the form of a crescent or sickle. Such disfigured cells have a life of only ten to twenty-five days instead of the normal life expectancy of four months. The result is anemia with misshapen cells, causing miniature logjams in small blood vessels, as well as pain and tissue damage. It is ironic that the defective gene, the sickle-cell trait, protected black Africans against malaria. This trait represented a biologic or genetic response to a killer disease. Blacks could thrive in malaria-infested areas in Africa known as the "white man's graveyard." With malaria control now a reality, the sickle-cell has lost this defensive function.

It is estimated that this trait afflicts 1 black of each 600 born, with about 8 percent of the black population, or 2 million persons, now possessing the trait. But presence of the trait is not always debilitating. The purpose of uncovering its presence is to counsel both husband and wife, when both possess the trait, about the possibility of producing an afflicted child. But distinctions have not been made between the "trait" and the crippling affliction. One consequence of the widespread testing campaign was the stigma attached to persons who were found to have the trait. Children were made to feel like freaks, and employers sometimes fired blacks because of their supposed high-risk status, and insurance companies increased rates. There were no uniform laws to protect the confidentiality of the test results. A *Fortune* study speaks of the "sickle-cell fiasco" and the "new ghetto hustle"—the exploitation of inner-city residents because of the unhappy consequences of diagnosis. As Dr. Ernest Beutler of the City of Hope Medical Center in Duarte, California, explained:

> The only good that could come would be predicated on the assumption that you could materially alter people's reproductive patterns by giving

them advice. This is dubious under the best of conditions—and the sickle-cell programs were carried out under the worst conditions.[11]

One group studying this kind of testing proposed guidelines in screening for all genetic diseases, emphasizing the importance of identifying goals of the program, the sharing of those goals with persons being screened, the opportunity for individuals to have an informed choice about risks of reproduction, and alleviating anxieties about the prospect of serious genetic disease. Because virtually everyone carries a small number of deleterious or lethal recessive genes, distinctions must be drawn between those afflicted with the trait only and those suffering from the disease. In some screening programs, there is admittedly no therapy immediately available for the uncovered pathologic condition. Thus, the case for such testing must rest with therapeutic benefits anticipated in the future. There must be informed consent and the protection of subjects from relatively untried testing procedures. Counseling should be nondirective, with an emphasis on informing the client and not making decisions for him.[12]

TECHNOLOGICAL TRANSFERS AND MEDICAL SERVICES

We are entering an era of "spare-parts" replacement. We are simulating human functions with prosthetic and other mechanisms: dialysis machines, iron lungs, ventricular bypass functions, artificial limbs that respond through fusion of nervous and electronic energy sources, and so on. For example, it is now estimated that as many as 40,000 of the 17 million Americans now afflicted with arthritis each year may be able to walk again with hips that have been replaced by artificial sections. The invention of a biochemical compound, methyl methacrylate, now has the capacity to bond these sections to the body's bone structures.[13] Dr. Christian Barnard, who performed the first heart-transplant operation, has devised a technique for implanting a second heart along with the old one. An artificial lung machine has also been devised.[14] Electrodes have been implanted in the inner ear in experimental projects to overcome deafness,[15] and brain pacemakers have been implanted to control not only epileptic seizures but also other forms of spasticity and tremors associated with

[11] Ibid., p. 158.
[12] For full discussion, see Marc Lappe, et al., "Ethical and Social Issues in Screening for Genetic Disease," *The New England Journal of Medicine*, Vol. 286, no. 21 (May 25, 1972), pp. 1129–32.
[13] *U.S. News and World Report*, March 18, 1974.
[14] "An Artificial Lung," *Newsweek*, August 4, 1975, p. 64.
[15] "The Electric Ear," *Newsweek*, April 1, 1974, p. 50.

cerebral palsy or the aftereffects of a stroke.[16] University of Western Ontario surgeons have placed electrodes within the visual centers of the brain of a patient in a search for an artificial system of vision.[17] Reid Hilton of Santa Ana, California, has been fitted with a $40,000 arm. Unlike other artificial arms, Hilton's is directly connected to the nerves in the stump of his severed arm and is equipped with a feedback device affording him a sense of touch.[18] A new artificial kidney machine (about the size of a cigar box), planned for production can be self-operated for a yearly cost of $1,000, compared with present costs of $25,000. The La-Barge corporation of St. Louis has marketed an air-bypass voice prosthesis for persons who have had their larynx removed because of cancer. The instrument permits effortless speech without training.[19] Equally significant are the manipulative effects upon the nervous system of chemotherapy and psychopharmacology. For example, studies report the chemical control and improvement of memory, although the very concepts of choice, chance, selfhood, and rationality—so central to our philosophic structure—are thereby subjected to influence, if not manipulation.[20]

Such technology appears to have a momentum of its own. It is clear, however, that the benefits have been unevenly applied in the medical field.[21] The innovations require a combination of biology, chemistry, psychology, engineering, physiology, and electronics, among many other specialties. Because changes have often been sweeping, they have been self-reinforcing.[22] The ethical implications of all of this are suggested by Joseph Fletcher. In his view, we have reached the end of the age of innocence—that is, of ignorance. And the end of ignorance means the end of our excuses. Should we undertake the possible?

Both the origin and consequences of technological change have long fascinated the academic community. The truly creative individual is often considered somewhat of an intellectual ragamuffin, a beachcomber on the edge of the sea of the unknown. He is sometimes as unfamiliar with elements of reality as he is unappreciative of his own contributions. He seeks to understand the unknown; yet because his creative efforts are so often a "leap into the dark," it is difficult to hold him accountable for the conse-

---

[16] "Pacemaker for the Brain," *Newsweek*, October 1, 1973, p. 72.

[17] "Light for the Blind," *Newsweek*, February 11, 1974, p. 48.

[18] "The $40,000 Arm," *Time*, December 1, 1975, p. 63.

[19] Stanley Taub and Lloyd H. Bergner, "Air Bypass Voice Prosthesis for Vocal Rehabilitation of Laryngectomies," *The American Journal of Surgery*, Vol. 125 (June 1973), pp. 748–56.

[20] Joseph Fletcher, "Technological Devices in Medical Care." In Kenneth Vaux (ed.), *Who Shall Live? Medicine, Technology, Ethics* (Philadelphia: Fortress Press, 1970), p. 122.

[21] Cf., Charles D. Scott, "Health Care Delivery and Advanced Technology," *Science*, Vol. 180 (June 29, 1973), pp. 1339–42.

[22] Fletcher, "Technological Devices in Medical Care," p. 118.

quences either before or after the fact. Should we expect these remarkably creative individuals to be philosopher-kings as well?

The traditional Catholic morality holds that we are only tenants of our bodies; and as such, rather than as proprietors, we are permitted no mutilation beyond efforts to preserve life. But this old morality of nature has, to some extent, given way to new values that could accept the notion of organ transplants. In its contemporary form, this is often known as "situation ethics," in which the axiom is advanced that the abuse of the thing by some does not bar its use. In this context, it is not against nature to place a pig's liver in a dying woman. We have witnessed the "demythologizing" of moral prohibitions, with accommodations to medical technology rationalized by a new situational ethic. Raymond Queneau boldly asserts: "The people who whine about naughty robots and inhuman machinery have never proved anything except their own lack of imagination and fear of liberty."[23]

Even so, there are difficult ethical issues, even with the freedom to treat each case on its own merits. One can respect Immanuel Jakobivits' assertion that "even a fraction of life is precious. Therefore, no one must hasten the death of a donor."[24] There is a risk, however, that affirmations of patients' rights may become pretentious posturing or moralizing, without the realization that almost every element of experimentation involves some risk. To deny experimentation is simply to deny innovation or the advance of our understanding. When the New York State Assembly introduced a bill restricting research in the medical care of children, several physicians testified that such a law, if it had existed in the early 1950s, would have meant that polio, measles, and rubella would still be widespread hazards. There is, in reality, a contest between the uncertain therapeutic benefits for individuals participating in the experiments and their potential benefits for society. Fletcher explains:

> Ethical plain speaking calls for a hardnosed formula: the welfare of the many comes before the welfare of the few, or, if you prefer, the individual may rightly be sacrificed to the social good. It is ethical infantilism to suppose that there is a comfortable harmony between the private and the social interest. It was never shown to be so by the laissez faire theory of Manchester economics and it cannot be shown in the realms of medicine and sanitation. . . . We have to . . . [calculate] our moral decisions, our choices between value alternatives. This is properly called "statistical morality." Ethics cannot escape calculative interests, playing the numbers game, nose or head counting. We have to make responsible choices in medicine, all the way from an almost one-to-one choice by selection committees trying to decide who shall live and who shall die when there is only a limited supply of kidney machines available for

[23] Ibid., p. 125.
[24] *Newsweek*, December 18, 1967, p. 87.

dialysis, up to such massive enterprises as the historic yellow fever studies in which thousands of ignorant people were inoculated with no hope of personally benefiting. (After all, juries and draft boards also decide who shall die and who shall live.)[25]

The new morality, then, includes an element of pragmatism and the realization that we cannot constrain every potential advance of medical science by realizations that not all individuals participating in the experiment will benefit from the discovery. Even in a prison setting, inmates condemned to death may conclude that such participation is a contribution to posterity. There is need for such opportunism, rationalized by the prospect of long-term general benefits for mankind. Bernard Bard and Joseph Fletcher charge that the "natural-order" moralists are hopelessly out of tune with contemporary reality:

> The belief that God is at work directly or indirectly in all natural phenomena is a form of animism or simple pantheism. If we took it really seriously, all science, including medicine, would die away because we would be afraid to "dissect God" or tamper with His activity. Such beliefs are a hopelessly primitive kind of God-thought and God-talk, but they hang on long after theologians generally have bid them good-bye.[26]

In this new era, it is not surprising that we should be seeking moral standards. Even if we recognize that the scientist may assume the airs of a demigod when he is only a petty magician, even when we recognize what Veblen called the "trained incapacity of the specialist," we have the obligation to define appropriate and inappropriate research and methodologies. It is acknowledged that machines transcend some of the limitations of their designers. Thus, we cannot resolve the moral choice before society by relegating all decision making to the scientist. The scientist may take the position that his research activities are morally neutral, but we have the obligation to determine whether the results of such experimentation will do good or evil. In terms of a situational ethic, how do we establish the moral guidelines that determine who shall live and who shall die, or (in contemporary jargon) who will have authority to "pull the plug"?

ETHICAL ASPECTS OF THE RIGHT TO DIE

Because of the growing ability of modern medicine to extend the limits of human life, the issue of determining the right to die—or its counterpart, the right to live—is creating a widening debate between physi-

[25] Fletcher, "Technological Devices in Medical Care," pp. 130–31.
[26] Bernard Bard and Joseph Fletcher, "The Right to Die," *The Atlantic*, Vol. 221, no. 4 (April 1968), p. 64.

cians, lawyers, theologians, economists, Congress and state legislators, sociologists, and philosophers.

The issue is even a reality for those who want to take their own life. A Humanist Manifesto was recently signed by 250 intellects asserting the absolute right of the individual to control his own bodily destiny in regard to reproduction, medical treatment or lack of it, and termination, including euthenasia and suicide.[27] An emerging attitude holds that individuals (not God, the physician, or the state), "own" their bodies. Increasingly, society is willing to acknowledge that terminally ill cancer patients have the right to take their own lives. The corollary is drawn that the right to live—so much more clearly supported by contemporary ethics—is the complement of the right to die. To exercise a "right," one must have discretion or choice. (By analogy, the right-to-work movement has reasoned that the constitutional warranties for freedom of assembly are not valid if the individual does not enjoy the right *not* to assemble. A union security contract that requires a worker to join a union as a condition of employment thus violates constitutional rights assuring the individual freedom to assemble.) By the same reasoning, can one have the "right" to live if he is denied the "right" to die?

A 1975 Gallup poll found that forty-one percent of Americans believe that a person has the moral right to end his life when suffering great pain and having no hope of improvement. Fifty-one percent said no, while eight percent had no opinion. Forty percent approved of the right to end life in the case of an incurable illness, while twenty percent approved of that right when a person is "an extremely heavy burden on his or her family."[28]

There is also a growing interest in "living wills" in which individuals declare themselves willing to die rather than be kept alive in an unconscious or semiconscious state. One such statement, prepared by the Euthenasia Education Council, states:

> If the situation should arise in which there is no reasonable expectation of my recovery from physical or mental disability, I request that I be allowed to die and not be kept alive by artificial means or "heroic measures." I do not fear death itself as much as the indignities of deterioration, dependence, and hopeless pain. I, therefore, ask that medication be mercifully administered to me to alleviate suffering even though this may hasten the moment of death.[29]

Such wills, however, are not legally binding.

In 1973 the Supreme Court held that no state could ban abortions

---

[27] "Now, a Right to Suicide?" *Newsweek,* October 29, 1973, p. 78.
[28] "Medical Ethics: Who Decides the Life-and-Death Issues," *U.S. News and World Report,* June 16, 1975, p. 63.
[29] Ibid., p. 63.

during the first six months of a pregnancy. But state sentiment runs high against abortions, and many states have also passed legislation restricting experimentation on the living fetus. Responding to the rising moral indignation over such experimentation, the National Commission for the Protection of Human Subjects of Biomedical and Behavioral Research was formed. The Commission urged, however, that research be permitted on a fetus during an abortion, even in cases in which there were no clear benefits to the mother or the child. Such "nontherapeutic research," it noted, had led to amniocentesis. The debate continues. In his dissenting vote on the Human Subjects Commission, David W. Louisell alluded to the too-recent violations of human integrity, presumably a reference to the atrocities committed by the medical profession—in the name of medical research—during the Nazi regime. But Willard Gaylin and Marc Lappe took the opposite view:

> At some point it becomes unethical *not* to do fetal experimentation. We believe that point has been reached when the research has as its objective the saving of the lives (or the reduction of defects) of other wanted fetuses.[30]

Each month, evidence is uncovered of controversial methodologies in medical research. There is the "infamous" study of syphilis control in the South, in which medication was withheld from a control group to see how it would fare. It did not fare well. Is there not, as Gaylin and Lappe emphasized, something immoral in the use of control groups being denied medication to establish the effectiveness of a new treatment regimen? If new medication is to prove itself economically feasible, certainly it must do so in a test against the best-known (and proven) techniques, not against no treatment at all. In an editorial in *The New England Journal of Medicine,* Daniel S. Greenberg explains:

> Hitting old ladies over the head and stealing their purses provides no substance for ethical meditation. Similarly, it is difficult to perceive any ethical quandary in the application of psychosurgery to prisoners who are advised that cooperation with prison authorities is a condition of parole.
>
> . . . But then comes the question of what should be required if a defective fetus is found. It is unthinkable, at least as far as current social values would have it, that abortion be required. Not infrequently, however, the unthinkable quietly turns up as social practice, if not formal policy, as witness the revelations of coerced sterilizations of welfare recipients. Park Avenue patients would, of course, remain uncoerced, though in virtually all instances it may be assumed they would opt for abortion. But what of the downtrodden folk who are enmeshed in well-

[30] *The Atlantic,* May 1975. The above discussion is drawn from commentary in the *U.S. News and World Report,* June 16, 1975, p. 64.

intentioned social-service bureaucracies? And what happens when the capacity for testing goes beyond mongolism to other characteristics, such as a purported tendency toward "antisocial" behavior, low, but not dismally low, IQ, or sexual deviation?[31]

GENETIC DETERIORATION OF THE SPECIES: A CASE FOR SELECTIVE BREEDING

Is it possible that the success in limiting infant mortality has interceded with the process of "natural" selection, leading to an unprecedented number of individuals with flawed genetic structures? In 1850, about twenty-five percent of all children born in the United States died before the age of five. But by 1959, the death rate was such that sixty-three years would have passed before this proportion of the population died. In effect, natural selection has been seriously modified by the intervention of medical care. What are the implications for medicine of this reduced opportunity for genetic selection by death? James F. Crow acknowledges that the proliferation of genetically flawed individuals is partially offset by an improved environment. As he describes the process:

> Despite the fact that many of the deaths in the past were accidental or caused by diseases that are not now relevant, some of them were genetically selective in eliminating mutants that otherwise would now be causing harm. To the extent that these deaths no longer occur or are reduced in number, the genetic makeup of the population is deteriorating. We may not be conscious of this, for the environment is improving too rapidly, but the damage is still there to be reckoned with by any society that is conscious of its genetic future. The question is: can we use birth selection in an effective and socially acceptable way to compensate for decreased death selection?[32]

Nevertheless, Crow is not impressed with the beneficence of nature's selective process:

> We must remember that natural selection has been cruel, blundering, inefficient, and lacking in foresight. It has no criterion of excellence except the capacity to leave descendants. It is indifferent to whether living is a rich and beautiful experience or one of total misery. Postreproductive ages are of no consequence except in so far as older parents and grandparents aid in the survival of the young.[33]

[31] Daniel S. Greenberg, "Ethics and Nonsense," *The New England Journal of Medicine*, Vol. 290, no. 17 (April 25, 1974), pp. 977–78.
[32] James F. Crow, "Mechanisms and Trends in Human Evolution," *Daedalus*, Vol. 90, no. 3 (Summer 1961), p. 428.
[33] Ibid., p. 430.

Because survival involves only this limited definition of the fittest, he sees every logical reason for trying to improve the stock. This would, at the very least mean counseling and the hope that society would ultimately revise its notions about therapeutic abortions and make wider use of artificial insemination whenever genetic diseases are present. Historically, in his view, society owes much to a small minority of gifted intellectual leaders. If we practiced artificial insemination by donors of outstanding intellectual or artistic achievement, the occasionally highly gifted children might greatly benefit society.[34]

The opportunity to reverse the trend toward the genetic deterioration of society through "selective" breeding (artificial insemination) has gained much attention since it was advanced by Nobel Prize winner Hermann J. Muller. In Muller's view, communities can no longer support a situation in which everyone is helped to live according to his need and to reproduce according to his greed or his lack of foresight. Through our efforts to save lives, we have suffered an increasing accumulation of detrimental genetic mutations, and our policy of genetic "laissez faire" can lead to serious genetic problems. Muller estimates that medical techniques can now save some nine-tenths of the otherwise genetically flawed twenty percent of the population. Although there are many offsetting influences that could affect this trend, it is not conceptually impossible that much of the energies of future societies could be absorbed in ministering to social infirmities. Are we confronted, then, with a genetic cul-de-sac?

What we require is a new morality in which the purpose of having children is not simply the glorification of the parents, but also the well-being of the children—and the welfare of subsequent generations. We seek children who are happy and healthy, and we want to avoid as much as possible the prospect of children who are crippled and possibly resentful of both parents and society for not having taken advantage of measures that might have given them a better heritage.

One major opportunity for improving this situation is selective breeding through artificial insemination. Thousands of children are born each year through this method, but with a process that is done furtively, almost as though everyone concerned were guilty.[35] Muller proposes a rational-selection process, with deep-frozen spermatozoa stored indefinitely without deterioration. A sperm bank would be available, made up of contributions from individuals with brilliant academic, artistic, and scientific achievement. The resulting children would have high endowments and the potential for making substantial contributions for the betterment of society. Muller also identifies the opportunity for selective con-

[34] Ibid., pp. 428–30.
[35] Hermann J. Muller, "Should We Weaken or Strengthen Our Genetic Heritage?" *Daedalus*, Vol. 90, no. 3 (Summer 1961), p. 440.

trol of the female, a technique that has now been accomplished. Methods have been developed for

> flushing out . . . [the] eggs from the female reproductive tract, to be fertilized *in vitro* with chosen sperm, and then implanted in selected female hosts at the appropriate stage of their reproductive cycle. This procedure would be parallel to artificial insemination. It would permit the multiple distribution of eggs of a highly selected female into diverse recipient females; yet when so desired, it would enable the child to be derived on its paternal side from the recipient's husband.[36]

How would we determine the traits most appropriate for procreation? Muller sees an excess of egotism, ethnocentrism, and selfishness in contemporary society. He hopes society could cultivate persons with cooperative dispositions, a depth and breadth of intellectual ability, moral courage and integrity, an appreciation of nature and art, and so on. We want to lessen the tendencies to quick anger, blinding fear, strong jealousy, and self-deceiving egotism. We want to avoid cultures in which men are mere cogs in their work and pawns in their play. Muller seeks a deeper and broader vision. As he explains:

> Our imaginations are woefully limited if we cannot see that genetically as well as culturally, we have by our recent turning of an evolutionary corner set our feet on a road that stretches far out before us into the hazy distance.[37]

It is not surprising that such a daring program, now available to us through the technique of artificial insemination, should evoke a sharp and spirited debate. Let us review those concerns.

CRITICISMS OF SELECTIVE BREEDING

It is charged that the attempts to shape the human species to be less egotistical is itself a form of egotism. By what logic should we presume to have the appropriate map for future generations? By what logic should we presume the capacity to improve on nature's selective process? To recall the aphorism, most hell on earth has been the consequence of man's effort to create heaven on earth. Isn't this more of the same?

Mankind's capacity for survival reflects his remarkable diversity, his ability for accommodation. As Huxley reminds us, man is the least specialized of all organisms, and it may well account for his survival. By se-

---

36 Ibid., p. 443.
37 Ibid., p. 448.

lective control of the gene pool, we may lose that resiliency or plasticity in the survival process.

There is also an interaction of the biological and environmental structure that accounts for "animal" behavior. For example, studies of male baboons in their natural state reveal an aversion to conflict and a relative tranquility within the basic organization of the group. But within the context of a "socially disorganized" group of strange adults in the London Zoo, males fight over the possession of females, sometimes literally pulling one another to pieces. Certain kinds of environments appear conducive to our goal of congeniality and tranquility, but we have little insight into how future environments might prove appropriate to a genetically controlled population.[38] Dobzhansky confirms the view that there is a genetic environment that appears congenial to biological structures:

> What is good in the Arctic is not necessarily good on the equator; what was good in man in the ice age is not necessarily good now; what is good in a democracy is not necessarily good under a dictatorship. This is really so elementary for a geneticist that it would seem a waste of time to talk about it, if it were not for the fact that it is so often forgotten in discussions of human evolution. . . .[39]

Another consideration is the assumption that we can predict the consequence of such a union, that we can simply fit together the genetic structure of idealized males and females to produce a composite that enjoys the best of both.[40]

Again Dobzhansky explains:

> It is too easy to let our imagination strive for something with a body as beautiful as a Greek god, healthy, resistant to cold and to heat, to alcohol and to infections, with the brain of an Einstein and the ethical sensitivity of a Schweitzer, the musical talents of an Oistrakh and the poetical talents of a Shakespeare. In the first place, it is quite possible that all of these qualities just cannot coexist in the same person, and that even several of them cannot, for genetic or physiological or psychological or educational reasons. I do not mean that a beautiful body is necessarily incompatible with a beautiful mind, but rather that a peak performance in each field may depend on a very special genotype. . . .[41]

There is also the issue of the family itself. Standards of performance will undoubtedly be influenced by the genetic structure of the child, cre-

[38] Cf. J. P. Scott, in "Comments on Genetic Evolution," *Daedalus*, Vol. 90, no. 3 (Summer 1961), pp. 456–57.

[39] Theodosius Dobzhansky, ibid., pp. 461–62.

[40] This issue is reminiscent of the invitation allegedly extended to George Bernard Shaw by a shapely female that Shaw father her child, with the prospect that the progeny would have his intelligence and her beauty. He responded: "What if the child has my looks and your intelligence?"

[41] Ibid., p. 472.

ating tensions and disappointments for both "parents" and the child if these expectations are not realized. These disappointments might aggravate the parents' guilt as they try to understand why their own best efforts to provide a congenial environment for their children's maturation have failed.

Another concern is the parents' attitudes toward children they themselves have not created. Would they feel any loss of pride for not having created their own children, particularly if their other children disappoint them? Also, will such parents be able to feel the same sense of responsibility for either the success or failure of their children? If disappointed, they may instead conclude that recessive genes have taken control, with the mischief created by the unanticipated signals of sperm secured from the local market. Related to this are the attitudes of the children themselves:

> The whole idea [of selective breeding] bristles with problems. . . . What psychic burdens would bear down on youths of distinguished genetic parentage and undistinguished achievements? What forms of sibling rivalries might develop? (My genetic father was a great athlete and yours was only a President.)[42]

Who will organize the frozen-sperm bank, and who will determine access to or allocations of its resources? Again Dobzhansky poses the right question:

> Are we to have, in place of Plato's philosopher-king, a geneticist-king? And who will be president of the National Sperm Bank and of the National DNA Bank? What checks and balances are to be imposed on the genetic legislature and the genetic executive powers? Who will guard the guardians?[43]

Finally, there are concerns that our own nationalism will dominate in public decisions on the directions and quality of future generations. Rather than cultivate strains characterized by compassion, it may be concluded that such sentimentality is a luxury we can ill afford when we are surrounded by hostile forces. Hermann Muller has expressed concern about the possibility of a "germinal race" somewhat similar to the present armaments race.[44] Roger Shinn adds:

> I have occasionally tried to imagine a secret meeting of the National Security Council at which the CIA reports that the Russians or Chinese have "cracked the genetic code" and are preparing to produce a race of

[42] Roger L. Shinn, "Perilous Progress in Genetics," *Social Research* (Spring 1974), pp. 91–92.

[43] Theodosius Dobzhansky, "Changing Man," *Science*, Vol. 155 (1967), p. 413.

[44] "What Genetic Course Will Man Steer?" In J. F. Crow and J. V. Neel (eds.), *Proceedings*, Third International Congress of Human Genetics (Baltimore: Johns Hopkins Press, 1967).

super warriors. My scenarios saw the launching of an Operation Gene-war, akin to the Manhattan Project that produced the atomic bomb. I assumed that my speculations were pure fantasy—until one day I read press reports that Russians were worried that the United States was applying genetics to warfare.[45]

THE PROBLEM OF ETHICAL CHOICE

In this chapter, we have selected only a few aspects of the many changes now confronting both the medical sector and society. We have identified the issue of genetic control to avoid crippling afflictions, simply because the techniques of such control are now in hand. The questions we have posed are being answered daily, if not through the consensus of the collective society, then in the decisions of individuals and the judgments of medical-care providers. And we have identified the prospects—and problems—of another process now in hand: selective breeding. We have not touched on a third category of influence: genetic engineering. Techniques now appear feasible for the cloning of man, as well as for controlling the signaling process of the chromosomes to determine the "mix" of traits in the offspring. By the year 2000, in conservative estimates, we should be able to produce duplicates of ourselves. Most of the billions of cells that make up each person contains within it the genetic code for the reproduction of its owner's entire body. It is now established that we can implant a new gene into the DNA ring that has been chemically split. The genetically altered DNA ring can then be reintroduced into another bacterium. "The fresh plasmids thus created can then be introduced into other bacteria, where the genes start to change the hereditary characteristics of their new host bacteria just as if they had been there all along."[46]

In all of this, we are confronted with speculations that we can so transform the human agent at the very source of its creation as to resolve many of our medical problems. By analogy, we are less concerned now with the "safety" or performance of existing automobiles. We have in mind the opportunity to "melt down" the existing stock and to start all over again with quality control of the product. This will minimize the importance of repair garages (hospitals) and our dependence on mechanics (physicians). The mischievous characteristics of existing products, obligating their recall for replacement parts, will become less and less a problem. The techniques that have served animal husbandry so well can now serve the human race.

[45] Shinn, "Perilous Progress in Genetics," pp. 99–100.
[46] Peter Gwynne, Stephen G. Michaud, and William J. Cook, "Politics and Genes," *Newsweek*, January 12, 1976, p. 50.

It is difficult to avoid admissions of exaggeration in the above analogy, for certainly we are confronted with evolutionary changes rather than with any "melting down" of our imperfect human stock. Surely, too, the consequences of quality control are themselves uncertain. But it *is* certain that we have in hand the techniques and opportunities for genetic manipulation. In his critical essay, Leon R. Kass explains that "the mysterious and intimate processes of generation are to be moved from the darkness of the womb to the bright (fluorescent) light of the laboratory, and beyond the shadow of a single doubt."[47]

We are reminded of Jean-Paul Sartre's observation that "man is condemned at every moment to invent man," which now has not only philosophic but also biologic force. As Garrett Hardin notes, the issue of whether man shall direct his own evolution is no longer in question. Hardin explains we have only the option of doing so consciously or unconsciously, of minimizing or maximizing the role of chance, of controlling individual actions on a directive basis or not, of setting up one system or many to influence outcomes.[48] In reflecting on the prospects for genetic change, Robert Sinsheimer has said:

> For the first time, . . . a living creature understands its origin and can undertake to design its future. Even in the ancient myths man was constrained by his essence. He could not rise above his nature to chart his destiny. Today we can envision that chance—and its dark companion of awesome choice and responsibility. . . . We can be the agent of transition to a wholly new path of evolution. This is a cosmic event.[49]

We can be certain that what can be done will be done. Perhaps only posterity can conclude whether what will be done should have been done.

SUGGESTED READINGS

BARBER, BERNARD, "The Ethics of Experimentation with Human Subjects," *Scientific American*, Vol. 234, no. 2 (February 1976), pp. 25–31. A recent article on the ethical implications of medical research with humans.

BERRY, CHARLES A., "Health as the Physician Views It, and the Use of Space Technology to Achieve and Maintain It." In Robert M. Kunz and Hans Fehr, eds., *The Challenge of Life: Biomedical Progress and Human Values* (New York: International Publishers Co., Inc., 1971), pp. 379–90. An analysis of the use of the systems approach to avoid the inundation of health-care facilities with the worried-well.

[47] Leon R. Kass, "Making Babies: The New Biology and the 'Old' Morality," *The Public Interest*, no. 26 (Winter 1972), pp. 22–23.
[48] Garrett Hardin, "Comments on Genetic Evolution," *Daedalus*, Vol. 90, no. 3 (Summer 1961), p. 453.
[49] As quoted by Kass, "Making Babies," p. 54.

Bok, Sissela, "The Ethics of Giving Placebos," *Scientific American*, Vol. 231, no. 5 (November 1974). A opinion on the effectiveness and ethical meaning of physicians deceiving their patients with harmless placebos.

Fletcher, Joseph, "Technological Devices in Medical Care," *Who Shall Live? Medicine, Technology and Ethics* (Philadelphia: Fortress, 1970), pp. 116–42. A forthright discussion of techniques to sustain human survival.

Freund, Paul A., "Introduction to the Issue 'Ethical Aspects of Experimentation with Human Subjects,'" *Daedalus*, Vol. 98, no. 2 (Spring 1969), pp. vii–xiv. A commentary on the ethical aspects of human experimentation.

Inglefinger, F. J., "Informed (but uneducated) Consent," *The New England Journal of Medicine*, Vol. 287, no. 13 (1972), pp. 465–66. Although physicians and researchers justify the use of human subjects because they have their informed consent, the subjects often fail to understand the true nature of the experiments.

Mann, Kenneth W., *Deadline For Survival: A Survey of Moral Issues in Science and Medicine* (New York: Seabury, 1970). An analysis centering on human experimentation and informed consent, organ transplants, sex reassignment, genetic and fetal engineering, birth control, and sterilization.

Michaelson, Michael G., "The Failure of American Medicine," *The American Scholar*, Vol. 39, no. 4 (Autumn 1970), pp. 694–706. An attack on some contemporary writers who treat the major health problems and their inadequate treatment with clinical detachment.

Muller, Hermann J., "Should We Weaken or Strengthen our Genetic Heritage?," *Daedalus*, Vol. 90, no. 3 (Summer 1961), pp. 432–50. A contribution to the symposium on genetic engineers.

Pappworth, Maurice H., *Human Guinea Pigs* (London: Routledge & Kegan Paul, 1967). A discussion of medical experiments that use human subjects.

Rosenfeld, Albert, *The Second Genesis* (Englewood Cliffs, N.J.: Prentice-Hall, 1969). Major sections on the "refabrication" of the individual, the exploration of prenativity, and the control of brain and behavior.

Watson, James D., "Moving Toward the Clonal Man: Is This What We Want?," *The Atlantic*, Vol. 227, no. 5 (May 1971), pp. 50–53. A review of the techniques of cloning.

Wertz, Richard W., ed., *Readings on Ethical and Social Issues in Biomedicine* (Englewood Cliffs, N.J.: Prentice-Hall, 1973). A gathering of articles concerned with experimentation on human subjects.

Will, George F., "Discretionary Killing," *Newsweek*, September 20, 1976, p. 96. A consideration of the problem that arises when there are only limited resources available and the physician must decide who shall and who shall not receive treatment.

Williams, Preston N., *Ethical Issues in Biology and Medicine* (Cambridge, Mass.: Schenkman, 1973). A commentary on the ethical problems surrounding medical research.

INDEX

Abel-Smith, Brian, 54*n*, 89, 90
Abkhasian people, 106–7
abortions, 393–94
absenteeism, work, 112
access to medical care:
  national health insurance and, 369–71
  by the poor, 105
  by prepaid group plan members, 303–5
  see also physicians, geographic distribution of
accidental deaths, 122, 147
accidental injuries, 122
activity analysis, 243
Aday, Lu Ann, 246*n*
administrators (managers):
  of educational institutions, 11
  health-care, 260–61
advertising by physicians, 315
age, appraised and compliance, 245
age categories:
  expenditures on health care by, 52–54
  major afflictions by, 121–25
aged, the:
  diseases of, 123–25
  expenditures for health care by or for, 53–54
  in Great Britain, 54
  under institutionalized care, 124
  see also extended-care facilities; Medicare; nursing homes; retirement
aging process, mental illness and, 184–85

alcoholism, 117, 150, 183
allied health professionals, 10–11
  see also paraprofessionals
Altenderfer, Marian E., 70*n*
ambivalence, sociological, 72–73
Altman, Stuart H., 208, 371*n*
American Association for Comprehensive Health Planning, 257–58
American Hospital Association, 46, 207, 381
American Indians, 148–50
American Journal of Psychiatry, 80
American Legion Magazine, 230
American Medical Association, 262, 281
American Nurses Association, 10
amniocentesis, 386
Anderson, Fred, 30*n*, 195–96
Anderson, Odin W., 303
Anderson, Ronald 246*n*
Andreano, Ralph L., 31, 32*n*
Andreopoulos, Spyros, 17*n*, 140*n*, 143*n*
anomie, 103
antitrust laws, 262
anxiety, neuroses and, 177–78
aphasia, 116, 117
Arehart-Treichel, Joan, 185*n*
Argonaut Insurance Company, 342, 343
arthritis, 120, 123, 389
artificial insemination, 396–97
asthma, 123
atomization of health-care industry, as planning option, 262–63
Avioli, Louis V., 133*n*